Instructor's Manual to Accompany

FUNDAMENTALS OF EMERGENCY CARE

Instructor's Manual to Accompany

FUNDAMENTALS OF EMERGENCY CARE

RICHARD W. O. BEEBE, MED, RN, NREMP-T
DEBORAH L. FUNK, MD, NREMT-P

DELMAR
™
THOMSON LEARNING   Australia Canada Mexico Singapore Spain United Kingdom United States

COPYRIGHT © 2001 Delmar, a division of Thomson Learning, Inc. Thomson Learning™ is a trademark used herein under license.

ISBN 0-7668-1494-7

Printed in Canada
 2 3 4 5 XXX 05 04 03 02

For more information, contact Delmar, 3 Columbia Circle, PO Box 15015, Albany, NY 121212-0515.

Or find us on the World Wide Web at http://www.delmar.com

For permission to use material from this text or product contact us by
Tel (800) 730-2214
Fax (800) 730-2215
www.thomsonrights.com

Library of Congress Catalog Card Number: 00-050889

Contents

Introduction

We, the students of today, attending schools of yesterday, being taught
by teachers of the past, with methods from the middle ages, to solve
the problems of the future!

—*Anonymous*

Every EMT instructor is troubled when a bright student, perhaps a "star" pupil, has difficulty in the field. When conscientious instructors inquire as to what the difficulty is, the responses often focus on the student's inability to get the big picture or troubles fitting in and working with others. In a phrase, these students are described as "book smart but not street smart."

Why do students have difficulties going beyond the facts? Why do these EMT students have difficulty connecting basic principles with essential applications? Why are these EMT students unable to grasp the special considerations that make every emergency scene unique?

Perhaps the problem stems from the method in which they were originally trained. Traditional instructional methods teach in such a way that the knowledge taught can be easily tested but may not transfer directly into practice. Yet, despite the fact that students must be successful with these written exams to succeed, most students do not take an EMT class to pass the tests. Students take EMT classes in order to learn how to do the work of an EMT. Passing the tests is just part of getting there.

Similarly, EMT instructors should not "teach to the test" even though the mark of a good instructor is, unfortunately, the number of students that pass certifying examinations. EMT instructors should be trying to graduate competent entry-level providers who can perform a service to the public.

Keeping these two key concepts in mind, how can an EMT instructor change the thought processes of students so that when they look at a situation in the field, they will look and act as other EMTs would in the same situation? How does an EMT instructor make a change in human disposition or capability and help the EMT learn how to think like an EMT?

PROBLEM-BASED LEARNING

The solution may be **problem-based learning (PBL)**. PBL is an adult-oriented, student-centered, problem-based small group learning experience based within a clinical context. While that defines PBL, what is PBL? PBL is a pedagogical strategy for teaching EMS. Its origins stem from the original dialectic method. The dialectic method of intellectual investigation utilized discussion as the main vehicle of inquiry. The most famous teacher to use this method was probably Socrates. Socrates would ask his students a question that posed a problem and that required the students to think deeply about the question and to formulate a satisfactory answer.

PBL is similar in that the students are given a problem that is similar to one they might encounter in the field. Then they are asked to analyze that problem and come up with a solution.

Problem-based learning theorizes that adult students will learn better if what they are learning can be applied directly to a real-life problem. In other words, the problem must be have a contextual setting for it to be interesting to the adult student. The ability of the student to take what has been learned and apply it directly to actual situations is a core concept in adult learning.

A student in the classroom learns how to manage a clinical situation while in the classroom by creating a mental "script" that is taken to the field and adapted to a current, similar situation while in the field, by generalizing the conditions from the first script and forming a new script.

Therefore, the goal of PBL is to teach the student more than mere fact acquisition, to be regurgitated at exam time. The goal of PBL is to educate the student on how to be an EMT. The students who have been educated with the PBL approach, will have a better working knowledge of EMS and should have an improved ability to problem-solve, using all available resources, while in the field. In short, they will have the necessary tools to be competent, entry-level EMTs.

WHY IS PBL A SUCCESSFUL EDUCATIONAL APPROACH?

Before answering this question, it may be helpful to understand the origins of PBL. PBL was advanced as a theory in medical education by the faculty of McMaster University of Canada in the 1960s. Since that time several prominent universities and colleges, such as Case-Western Reserve, the University of Delaware, and even Harvard Medical School, have adopted the PBL approach. In fact, over 80 percent of American medical schools utilize PBL for part or all of their medical students' education. Recently, schools of nursing and engineering, as well as K–12 education, have adopted PBL.

PBL has been so successful primarily because it has received widespread support from both teachers and students alike. PBL produces the results that these people were looking for—for the instructor, a competent entry-level provider, and for the students, an education that taught them how to be EMTs.

PBL is able to do this because it is firmly based on principles of adult learning. For one, PBL offers the student educational independence, or, in other words, student autonomy. Student autonomy is critical to adult learners.

PBL also focuses on building from the unique strengths of the different students. This draws on the students' own life experiences and education, as well as permitting students to appreciate others' life experiences. This diversity lends itself to discovery and invention, making the learning even more exciting.

The student learns to build, on previously laid foundations, new ideas and new applications of old ideas (constructivism). As the student learns, developing an analytical approach to each situation, she or he is creating the intellectual scaffolding for further learning.

Finally, the student learns that these problems are real and require the immediate application of new-found knowledge. This sense of immediacy generally improves the students' retention of the material.

THE ADVANTAGES OF PBL

With PBL, the student, not the instructor, directs the learning process. In some instances, artificial time constrictions have been removed to encourage the student to learn at his or her own pace and to attain the maximum learning from the potential.

The student then takes the problem, considers it thoughtfully, and starts to think about how to solve it. This self-discovery places emphasis on the meaning of the problem, and not just the facts. In other words, PBL tends to encourage authentic learning. As a rule, this self-discovery improves the student's motivation as well. Motivated, curious students are prime for an educational opportunity.

With the focus on teamwork, PBL also encourages the student to improve interpersonal skills and develop a sense of team that is often present in ambulance corps, rescue squads, and other close-knit groups.

Traditional "prescriptive" teaching assumes that the teacher knows best and that the student is simply an empty vessel into which knowledge may be poured, or pounded, into. This approach may be seen by adults as a kind of "educational communism." PBL, on the other hand, reaffirms the importance of the student as an individual, an adult, who is responsible for her or his own development and education.

Finally, PBL complements lab-based education. Skill training, coupled with real-life problems, allows the student to not only learn the psychomotor skills of an EMT but also how to integrate those skills into patient care. The student therefore practices skills within the context of the problem and learns by doing.

THE PROCESS OF TEACHING PROBLEM-BASED LEARNING

To start, the instructor typically divides the class into groups of five or more but no more than ten. (In EMS education a group of five or six is optimal as it represents a more natural crew configuration.)

The students are then presented with "the problem." The problem, which will be discussed in more detail shortly, should lead the students to ask more probing questions, and hence the learning opportunity is created.

Some instructors give the problems to the students one at a time and then give the students the class and/or the time between classes to discuss the problem. Internet "chat rooms" as well as e-mail may be used for discussion, if face-to-face discussions are impractical.

The questions usually cannot be answered by the students immediately. This "knowledge failure" requires the students to research the question and return with more information—another learning opportunity.

The students may research the questions using their textbook as a resource, or the Internet, or even "expert providers." Expert providers are seasoned EMTs who have a wealth of experience from which to draw on. As the expert carefully tells the tale of a similar experience, the EMT student first realizes the relevancy of the problem and then starts to see himself or herself in the role of the EMT. The EMT student should take away from the story the lesson that was learned as well as connectivity that the problem has to real life.

A word of caution is in order. As Paul Werfel, EMS educator, states: "war stories are like clipart, sometimes interesting but not always relevant." The instructor should carefully guide the student to the selection of experts for research, perhaps utilizing only selected faculty members.

The instructor may be used as a resource. However, the instructor's role is not to provide the solution, but to offer advice as to where the answer might be found. In other words, the instructor is a resource. A good instructor, who is monitoring the team's progress, offers advice periodically, even if it is not solicited.

Learning psychomotor skills is also a part of education. Certain problems, such as an unmanageable airway, lend themselves to the practice of certain skills, such as suctioning. The skills of an EMT should not be detached and taught as isolated exercises. Rather, skills should be taught as part of the resolution of the problem, and thereby integrated, often subconsciously, into the EMT's "routine" for a complicated airway, for example.

Finally, when the team is ready, they present the resolution to the problem. The resolution may be reported by demonstration within a patient scenario or by a verbal report. In either case, the instructor should take the opportunity to summarize the key points that the students have discovered, to compare them to the standard of care, and to generally bring closure to the problem before the team moves on.

Naturally, earlier problems should be simple and uncomplicated. Subsequent problems should build on the earlier successes of the team and develop a deeper understanding. Often the instructor ends up giving step-by-step instructions in the early cases, but as the team develops the instructor will eventually provide only general instructions to the team.

ROLES WITHIN PBL

One of the most remarkable differences between PBL and traditional instruction is the change in the role of the instructor. The instructor is no longer seen as the "sage on the stage" but like the "guide on the side."

A comparison can be made with an orchestra conductor. No longer playing the instruments, the conductor simply stands in front of a group of capable people and directs them to work together for a glorious result.

This paradigm shift can be confusing for some instructors, and may even be perceived as making the instructor obsolete. Nothing could be farther from the truth. The instructor has several prominent roles to fill.

First, the instructor must be an advisor to the student. The instructor must be constantly monitoring the teams, looking for progress, and more important, looking for blocking. Blocking represents a learning opportunity for the team. A few carefully chosen questions, asked by the instructor, can lead the team to the path of discovery. Enabling the team in this manner, the instructor acts as a facilitator for the team.

In his role as a facilitator, the instructor may occasionally encourage the group to outline their progress, to create a "concept map" of the ideas that they have generated. This often serves to focus the team and helps them discover errors or defects in their logic.

Finally, the instructor must serve as the evaluator. As students present their resolutions to the problems presented, the instructor must evaluate these answers with an unbiased eye. Often students will create original approaches to problems. However, in EMS there are certain basic principles, and the students' responses must be measured against the established standards of care.

Students often have the hardest time accepting problem-based learning. Conditioned to accept traditional instruction, students, especially younger students, are surprised when they are offered educational freedom.

But with every freedom comes responsibility. Students in a PBL class must take individual responsibility for their education. They should not expect to be "spoon-fed" the answers. Rather, hard study and even harder thinking are required.

Furthermore, PBL students also must learn about personal responsibility to the team. PBL is, by definition, a collaborative process, similar to many other work experiences. The PBL student must put input into the group to expect any output from the group. To get input from all of the team members requires dedication to the mission as well as individual integrity to the process.

THE PROBLEM EXAMINED

In order for PBL to work, the problem must, first, be compelling. It must be one that the EMT student could reasonably be expected to see in the field and would be required to resolve in the field, thereby making it inherently interesting to the student.

As an instructor develops problems, the problem sequence should be somewhat spiral in nature. Each subsequent problem should build on the experience the student has gained from the previous problem. When this is accomplished, each new problem becomes more significant to the student. These challenging problems are acutely interesting to the EMT student and therefore the most useful, from a PBL perspective.

The problem should be designed in such a way that the course objectives are being taught. First, all problems serve to facilitate the larger goal of training competent, entry-level EMTs. Moreover, each problem must incorporate within it subgoals, that is, objectives such as airway management, that every EMT student must master before becoming an EMT.

The last problem(s) should ultimately permit the student to care for a patient with a common chief complaint, such as chest pain, by incorporating all prior skills, such as AED use, and knowledge, such as cardiac disease, to permit indicated care for the patient.

These last problems serve to graduate the student from the classroom to the field. Under optimum conditions, the student continues education while in the field under the close scrutiny of a field preceptor.

ELEMENTS OF THE PROBLEM

Every problem should start with an introduction. This introduction should explain why the student needs to know this material and should work to gain an understanding. An example of this motivational material is illustrated at the beginning of each section of the national EMT curriculum. However, in most cases the EMT instructor can develop this introductory material using personal life experiences, knowledge of local EMS characteristics, and a personal passion for the subject.

Next, the problem is presented. The problem should involve a clinical situation that the EMT would be expected to encounter while in the field. The problem, being somewhat ill conceived, should raise more questions than it answers.

The students then discuss, in an open meeting, what is known and what is not known. Focusing on the unknown, the students develop a list of all the significant issues for investigation. Certain problems create fundamental questions. These fundamental questions need to be investigated by everyone in the group. Other less pressing, but nevertheless interesting questions should be investigated. These individual questions should be addressed by no less than two students in order to promote discussion later.

Having identified the questions, the students next identify the resources they will use to investigate the answers to the questions. Commonly, a section or chapter of the textbook will be assigned, by the student team, for review. But other sources of information exist as well.

The student may also elect to search the Internet. Resources such as Medline® and PubMed® are two examples of sources of Internet-accessible information. Or the student may elect to present the problem to a seasoned provider for his or her explanation.

The students can use the instructor as a "content-expert." However, instructors should be warned that the role of an instructor is not to provide "mini-lectures" during office hours. Students should be encouraged to refer to their textbook or other resources before requesting an audience with the instructor. Then when the student(s) approach the instructor he or she should ask more questions then provide answers.

In some cases the instructor can activate student learning by asking questions that are open-ended or that encourage students to make connections or that force them to explain their reasoning. In many cases, the hardest job of an instructor is to sit and listen!

Finally, the students meet at an information-sharing session. During this session the students discuss and put to rest any questions that arose previously. Often the result of the student inquiry will not only be answers to the previous questions but also more questions. It is at this point that the instructor must decide to intercede if necessary, before the group's progress is hampered by unimportant questions that exceed the course objectives.

In every instance the instructor should note the students' responses and compare them to the standard of care. While it is possible for students to develop novel approaches to a problem, the basic fundamental principles of emergency medicine are inflexible at this level.

Finally, the students should wrap up the session and proceed to the next problem. Again, the instructor must carefully monitor the students to ensure that they are actually ready to proceed. Remember, each successive problem is, in some aspect, based on a previous problem. A premature departure from the material at hand will surely result in confusion and frustration in later lessons.

Students should also expect and receive periodic assessments of their performance. In many instances the student's gradation is simple. As in life, the student's performance is either satisfactory or unsatisfactory. Elements of assessment typically include the student's skill at critical appraisal, group participation, attitude (affective), and willingness to direct personal learning.

The student's performance, on a topic or problem, may also be classified as either a strength or a weakness. This approach permits the student to honestly appraise his or her own knowledge of EMS. This can help the student to prepare for more traditional testing tools.

It is also in the student's best interest if she or he is occasionally tested using traditional testing tools. Since the objective for the student is attaining knowledge, some instructors elect to make these examinations open-book exams.

Finally, a demonstration of skills, again within the context of a problem, should be every student's expectation. Every student can anticipate and should be prepared for practical examination during the certification process. Again, to divorce the skill from the problem, that is, to make it stand alone and out of context, makes the skill meaningless. Without meaning the student quickly forgets how to perform the skill.

GOALS OF PROBLEM-BASED LEARNING

Outwardly, the goal of every EMT instructor is, in part, to develop a student who has a firmly established knowledge of EMS. The key difference between problem-based learning and traditional teaching strategies is the approach.

The problem-based learning approach strives to improve the student's attitude toward learning, to make the student motivated to learn more now and in the future. When a student learns, solving problems within a clinical context, he or she starts to believe that learning is valuable and important.

Next, problem-based learning encourages the student to learn how to attain that knowledge, to problem-solve. A student who can use reasoning to resolve problems in the future will continue to learn for a lifetime. In fact, the student will quickly see the unique opportunities that EMS offers as it brings novel situations/problems to the attention of the EMT each day. The adage "I learn something new every day" could not be truer for an EMT trained in problem-based learning.

Problem-based learning does all this within the context of a team. Learning teamwork may be one of the most valuable lessons in PBL. A student cannot, and should not, expect to be an expert on every topic. However, with the support of a team of fellow professionals, the EMT can have a reasonable expectation of success with every mission.

CLOSING COMMENTS

The intention of this introduction to problem-based learning is to introduce the EMT instructor to the topic, somewhat like a survey course in college introduces a topic. For further information about how to implement problem-based learning, the instructor is encouraged to use the resources listed below. Several textbooks have been listed as well as several on-line PBL sites for your convenience.

In many instances, the local medical college may be using PBL in its curriculum. The EMT instructor is encouraged to seek out assistance from these institutions and perhaps even obtain a mentor who can help guide the instructor through course development.

Finally, the University of Delaware, as well as other universities and colleges, offers seminars on problem-based learning. Attending one of these seminars can be extremely valuable to the instructor whose goal is to educate thinking EMTs.

The primary goal of PBL, broadly speaking, is to make EMTs who are "meaning-makers, and not just mere fact-collectors." Students using their analytical skills can be called "thinking EMTs"—students who, in the final analysis, are able to adapt to a rapidly changing medical information/technology environment and remain street-smart.

Hopefully, this chapter has provided just the intellectual nourishment needed to start an EMT instructor using problem-based learning in the classroom.

FURTHER STUDY

Articles

Aspy, D. N., Aspy, C. B., & Quimby, P. M. (1993). What doctors can teach teachers about problem-based learning. *Educational Leadership, 50* (7), 22–24.

Bernstein, P., Tipping, J., Bercovitz, K., & Skinner, H. A. (1995). Shifting students and faculty to a PBL curriculum: Attitudes and lessons learned. *Academic Medicine, 70* (30), 245–247.

Bridges, E. M. (1992). *Problem based learning for administrators* (ERIC Document Reproduction Service No. ED 347 617). Eugene, OR: ERIC Clearinghouse on Educational Management.

Norman, G. R., & Schmidt, H. G. (1992). The psychological basis of problem-based learning: A review of the evidence. *Academic Medicine, 67* (9), 557–565.

Sage, S. M., & Torp, L. T. (1997). What does it take to become a teacher of problem-based learning? *Journal of Staff Development, 18* (4), 32–36.

Savey, J. R., & Duffy, T. M. (1995). Problem based learning: An instructional model and its constructivist framework. *Educational Technology, 35* (5), 31–37.

Vernon, D. T. (1995). Attitudes and opinions of faculty tutors about problem-based learning. *Academic Medicine, 70* (3), 216–223.

Vernon, D. T., & Blake, R. L. (1993). Does problem-based learning work? A meta-analysis of evaluative research. *Academic Medicine, 68* (7), 550–563.

Textbooks

Barrows, H. S. (1985). *How to design a problem-based curriculum for preclinical years.* New York: Springer.

Barrows, H. S., & Tamblyn, R. M. (1980). *Problem-based learning: An approach to medical education.* New York: Springer.

Boud, D., & Feletti, G., eds. (1997). *The challenge of problem-based learning* (2nd ed.). Sterling, VA: Stylus Publishing, Inc.

Waterman, R., Duban, S. L., Mennin, S. T., & Kaufman, A. (1988). *Problem-based learning: A workbook for integrating basic and clinical science.* Albuquerque: University of New Mexico Press.

Woods, D. R. (1994). *Problem-based learning: Helping your students gain the most from PBL.* Hamilton, Ontario, Canada: The Bookstore, McMaster University.

Websites

http://edweb.sdsu.edu/clrit/learningtree/PBL.htm
http://www.biology.iupui.edu/
http://www.edbydesign.org/foundations/pbl.htm
http://www.imsa.edu/team/cpbl/cpbl.html
http://www.ntlf.com/
http://www.pbli.org/pbl/pbl.htm
http:/www.samford.edu/pbl/
http://www.uchsu.edu/CIS/PBL.htm
http://www.udel.edu/pbl/

CHAPTER 1

Introduction to Emergency Medical Services

OBJECTIVES

Upon completion of this chapter, the reader should be able to:

1. Describe the impact of historical events on the evolution of EMS.
2. Describe the evolution of emergency health care.
3. Describe the place of modern EMS in the health care system.
4. List key scientific and position papers that directly influenced EMS systems development.
5. Compare the role of the EMT of the 1960s with that of the EMT today.
6. Identify some organizations that have influenced EMS.
7. List two major professional EMS associations.
8. List the four elements of a good EMS system, as defined by the National Highway Traffic Safety Administration.
9. Compare the evolution of emergency medicine and emergency medical services.
10. Discuss the professional challenges that will face the EMT of the future.

GLOSSARY

9-1-1   The three-digit access number for emergency services in the United States.

ambulances volante   Literal meaning, "flying ambulances"; these vehicles, considered to be the first ambulances, were used by Baron Larrey in the Napoleonic Wars to retrieve injured soldiers.

American National Red Cross (ARC)   Organization founded by Clara Barton in the Civil War era; this relief organization has played a large role in training civilians and rescuers in first aid and CPR.

cardiopulmonary resuscitation (CPR)   A life-preserving technique involving chest compressions and artificial respiration that has been widely taught to both civilians and health care providers since the late 1950s.

certified first responder (CFR)   A person who has completed training for a nationally recognized level of prehospital health care involving simple airway management, oxygen administration, bleeding control, and rescuer CPR.

chain of survival   A concept embraced by the American Heart Association that refers to the multiple elements needed in a first response system in order to have a successful resuscitation. As in a chain, each element is connected with the others and the strength of the entire chain is equally dependent on the strength of each link.

continuous quality improvement(CQI) Process by which an organization monitors and addresses areas in need of improvement.

emergency medical dispatch (EMD) An organized program that allows properly trained providers to take emergency calls, give first aid instructions to callers, and prioritize the responding units.

emergency medical services (EMS) A coordinated network of providers whose function is to provide a variety of medical services to people in need of emergency medical care.

emergency medical technician-basic (EMT-B) A person who has completed primary prehospital medical training. The most common level in the United States. The course at this level includes training in CPR, defibrillation, airway management, and basic medical and trauma care.

emergency medical technician-intermediate (EMT-I) A person who has completed the second level of prehospital medical training beyond that of EMT-Basic. The course at this level includes training in intravenous therapy, advanced airway management, cardiac arrest management, and trauma care.

emergency medical technician-paramedic (EMT-P) A person who has completed the highest level of pre-hospital medical training. This course includes training in advanced airway management, intravenous access techniques, defibrillation, cardiac pacing, and advanced pharmacology.

emergency physician A physician specifically trained to provide care to acutely ill and injured patients in an emergency department setting.

first responder The first person who arrives on the scene of an incident; also may refer to the level of medical training provided to persons who expect to be put in this position during their daily routine, such as firefighters, police officers, and security guards.

Good Samaritan Traditionally, one who would stop and help an injured traveler on the roadside; today Good Samaritan laws provide for the protection of those who would render aid to others freely and out of concern for others' well-being.

National Association of Emergency Medical Technicians (NAEMT) National organization that represents EMTs to the public and the government.

National Highway Traffic Safety Administration (NHTSA) The division of the U.S. Department of Transportation that has taken a leading role in establishing standards for training for emergency services.

star of life A six-pointed star with staff and serpent in the center; recognized as the symbol of EMS. Each point on the star represents a key component of the EMS system: detection, reporting, response, on-scene care, care in transit, and transfer to definitive care.

trauma center A specially designated hospital that is experienced in and capable of caring for patients with severe emergencies.

white paper A detailed or authoritative report on any subject: the National Academy of Sciences article entitled "Accidental Death and Disability: The Neglected Disease of Modern Society," written for President Kennedy, laid the groundwork for EMS legislation.

PREPARATORY

Materials: EMS Equipment: None.

Personnel: Primary Instructor: One EMT-Basic instructor knowledgeable in EMT-Basic course overview, administrative paperwork, certification requirements, Americans with Disabilities Act issues, and roles and responsibilities of the EMT-Basic.

Recommended Minimum Time to Complete: 1.5 hours

STUDENT OUTLINE

I. Chapter Preparation
II. The History of Emergency Medical Services
    A. The Military and Emergency Medical Services
        1. The Napoleonic Wars
        2. The American Civil War
        3. The World Wars
        4. The Korean War
        5. The Vietnam War
    B. The Civilian World
        1. The American Red Cross
        2. Father of EMS
        3. Star of Life
        4. National Association of Emergency Medical Technicians
        5. Public Perception of EMS
III. Modern EMS
    A. Universal Access
    B. Emergency Medical Dispatch
    C. First Responders
    D. Emergency Medical Technician-Basic
    E. Emergency Medical Technician-Intermediate
    F. Emergency Medical Technician-Paramedic
IV. Acute Medical Care
    A. Emergency Medicine
    B. Trauma Centers
    C. Aeromedical Transport
V. The Future of EMS
    A. Aging Americans
    B. Homelessness
    C. Human Resources
    D. Financial Restrictions
    E. Accountability
    F. EMS Research
VI. Conclusion

LECTURE OUTLINE

I. Chapter Welcome
- A. Welcome to EMS
- B. Thirty-Year History
- C. Paradigm Shift
  - 1. Lifesavers
  - 2. Health Care System "Safety Net"

II. The History of Emergency Medical Services
- A. Early Beginnings
  - 1. Good Samaritan
  - 2. Ancient Soldiers
- B. Out-of-Hospital Care
  - 1. Driven by necessity
- C. The Military and Emergency Medical Services
  - 1. The Napoleonic Wars
    - a) The ambulances volante concept
    - b) Bring the wounded to the surgeon
  - 2. The American Civil War
    - a) Formation of the Army Ambulance Corp.
      - (1) General McClellan
    - b) "Treat them where they lie"
      - (1) Clara Barton
        - (a) Founder—American Red Cross
  - 3. The World Wars
    - a) Weapons of Mass Destruction
    - b) Soldiers as First Responders
      - (1) Self-Care
      - (2) Buddy Care
    - c) Field "Paramedics"
    - d) Mechanized Ambulances
      - (1) Ambulance Drivers Born
  - 4. The Korean War
    - a) Developments
      - (1) Aeromedical Evacuation
      - (2) Mobile Field Hospitals
        - (a) Mobile Army Surgical Hospital
          - (i) M*A*S*H
  - 5. The Vietnam War
    - a) Advanced Field Techniques
      - (1) Field IV
- D. The Civilian World
  - a) Paradigm Shift

(1) Out-of-Hospital Care by Nonphysicians
- (a) Formerly—Home Visits
- (b) Transportation
  - (i) "Emergency Room"

1. The American Red Cross
- a) Public Education
  - (1) CPR
  - (2) First Aid
2. Father of EMS
- a) J. D. "Deke" Farrington
  - (1) "Death in a Ditch" article
- b) President Kennedy's White Paper
  - (1) "Accidental Death and Disability"
    - (a) Better survival in Vietnam than on the streets of America
- c) National Highway Safety Act of 1966
  - (1) National Highway and Traffic Safety Administration
  - (2) Lead EMS Agency
- d) EMS Systems Act of 1973
  - (1) Fifteen essential components of EMS system
    - (a) Manpower
    - (b) Training
    - (c) Communications
    - (d) Transportation
    - (e) Emergency Facilities
    - (f) Critical Care Units
    - (g) Public Safety Agencies
    - (h) Consumer Participation
    - (i) Access to Care
    - (j) Patient Transfer
    - (k) Standardized Record-Keeping
    - (l) Public Informa-

tion and Educa-
tion
(m) System Review and
Evaluation
(n) Disaster Manage-
ment
(o) Mutual Aid Agree-
ments
3. Star of Life
a) National EMS symbol
(1) Detection
(2) Reporting
(3) Response
(4) On-scene care
(5) Care in-transit
(6) Definitive care
4. National Association of Emergency
Medical Technicians
a) formed 1975
5. Public Perception of EMS
a) "Emergency"
(1) Jon and Roy
(2) Expert field care
III. Modern EMS
1. Continuum of Care
a) Chain of Survival Depiction
(1) Early Access
(2) Early CPR
(3) Early Defibrillation
(4) Early Advanced Care
A. Universal Access
1. 9-1-1 Designation
2. Computer-Aided Dispatcher
B. Emergency Medical Dispatch
1. First-first aid
2. Medically driven dispatch protocols
a) Prioritization
b) Appropriate use of resources
(1) System-status manage-
ment
C. First Responders
1. Early first aid courses
a) Civil Defense
2. Targeted groups
a) law enforcement officers
(LEOs)
b) fire service
3. Certified First Responders
a) Basic airway control
b) Rescue breathing

(1) Oxygen administration
c) Shock Treatment
(1) Hemorrhage control
d) CPR
D. Emergency Medical Technician-Basic
1. Original—Ambulance Attendants
2. Modern—Basic
a) Professional
(1) entry-level EMS
provider
b) Diverse examples
(1) Ambulance
(2) Soldier
(3) Firefighter
3. Training
a) CFR plus
(1) Defibrillation
(2) Drugs—limited
(3) Medical Emergencies
(4) Intubation (limited)
E. Emergency Medical Technician-Intermediate
1. First—EMT-Basic
2. Second—EMT-Advanced
a) Training
(1) Intubation
(2) IV
(3) Cardiac drugs
3. Cardiac arrest "managers"
F. Emergency Medical Technician-Paramedic
1. First—EMT-Basic
2. Second—EMT-Advanced
a) Health care career professionals
b) Extensive training
(1) College-level education
IV. Acute Medical Care
1. Early "accident" rooms
a) "Moonlighters"
2. Modern emergency department
a) emergency medical center
A. Emergency Medicine
1. Medical specialty
a) American Medical Association recognition
2. American College of Emergency
Physicians
a) Professional organization
B. Trauma Centers

1. Categorization of hospitals
    a) Special care centers
C. Aeromedical Transport
    1. Critical care transportation
V. The Future of EMS
    1. Challenges
A. Aging Americans
    1. America graying
       a) Baby-boomers coming of age
B. Homelessness
    1. Increased economic pressures
    2. Increasing population of mentally ill
       a) The miracle of psychotropic medications
          (1) Deinstitutionalization
C. Human Resources
    1. Volunteerism, an American Tradition
       a) economic pressures
       b) changing ethics

D. Financial Restrictions
    1. Cost of health care
       a) Equipment
       b) Safety
E. Accountability
    1. Consumer demand
       a) Legal Action
    2. Governmental regulation
    3. Continuous Quality Improvement
       a) Accreditation
          (1) Ambulances
          (2) EMS education programs
F. EMS Research
    1. Paradigm shift
       a) Formerly—Practice-driven
       b) Research-driven
VI. Conclusion
    1. EMS has a rich past
    2. Shared future with other health care professionals

TEACHING STRATEGIES

1. Have the students watch the videotape production of *A Brief History of EMS*. Then ask them to create a timeline of events that they observed in the video. The timeline should minimally contain references to the white paper, "Death and Disability: The Neglected Disease of Modern Society," created in 1966; the National Registry of EMTs formed in 1970; and the television show "Emergency," which aired for the first time in 1971.

2. Have the students retrieve and analyze the white paper "Death and Disability: A Neglected Disease of Modern Society." This white paper contained twenty-nine recommendations for improving trauma care, including a dozen pertaining specifically to EMS. Have the students identify each of these recommendations and present a brief remark on how each of these recommendations has or has not been implemented.

3. Obtain a copy of the television show "Emergency." Ask the students to review an episode. They should be able to identify each of the elements that are contained within the six-pointed star of life. Also ask the students to compare and contrast their roles in EMS to those of firefighter/paramedics Johnny Gage and Roy DeSoto. Ask the students if the scope of practice for an EMT has changed over the past thirty years.

4. Have the students view episodes of "Emergency," "Rescue 9-1-1," and "Paramedics." Ask them to prepare a discussion of the similarities and differences between these television programs plus the impacts that each of these television shows had on EMS.

5. Have the students perform a patent search for the following medical devices commonly used in EMS: Thumper® (1962), LifePak® defibrillator/monitor (1965), Jaws of Life® (1967), Hare® cervical collar (1974), Clark® military anti-shock trousers (MAST) (1976), Kendrick® Extrication Device (1981), and Life Support Products Automatic Transport Ventilator (1988),

6. Have the students perform a record search for the most influential papers or articles and legislative acts to impact EMS, including the white paper "Accidental Death and Disability: The Neglected Disease of Modern Society," the Highway Safety Act of 1966, the national standard curriculum for EMT-Ambulance distributed in 1969, the Emergency Medical Services System Act (PL-154) passed in 1973, Omnibus Budget Reconciliation Act of 1981, Emergency Medical Services for Children (EMSC) passed in 1983, "Injury

in America: A Continuing Public Health Problem" printed in 1985, and the Trauma Care Systems Planning and Development Act passed in 1990.

7. Have the students perform a web search for sites that pertain to EMS using the key terms: EMS, EMT, trauma care, search and rescue, rescue, CPR, wilderness EMS, and others of interest. Have the students compare and then compile a common list for distribution. This list of web sites will serve as an excellent resource for the EMT student and the rest of the class.

FURTHER STUDY

Barkley, K. T. (1990). *The ambulance: The story of emergency transportation of sick and wounded through the centuries.* Kiamesha Lake, NY: Load N Go Press.

Clawson, J. J., & Dernocoeur, K. B.(1997). *Principles of emergency medical dispatch* (2nd ed.). Salt Lake City, UT: Medical Priority Consultants.

Page, J. O. (1989). *A brief history of EMS.* 14,S11.

National Association of Emergency Medical Technicians, 408 Monroe Street, Clinton, MS 39056, www.naemt.org.

ANSWERS TO TEST YOUR KNOWLEDGE

1. EMS history can be roughly divided into two categories: military medicine and civilian medicine. In the past, advances in prehospital care were primarily the result of war. Each war brought certain improvements in field care. For example, the Napoleonic Wars brought the advent of the ambulance. More recently, the civilian sector has made advances on two fronts: cardiac care (specifically, sudden cardiac death) and trauma care.

2. Improved health care has led to longevity, increasing the number of elderly patients. Health care management organizations have mandated earlier discharges and more home care in order to decrease the steadily rising cost of health care. As a result of these changes, more patients are sent home "sicker" and more advanced levels of care are being provided within the home.

3. EMS can be simply thought of as the front door to the health care system. While many patients enter the health care system via a network of primary providers, those who are having an emergency enter the system using 9-1-1 and EMS.

4. Two key papers that had a dramatic impact on EMS were the white paper "Death and Disability" and "Death in a Ditch." Both pointed out the deficiencies in American trauma care. Legislation that resulted—the National Highway Safety Act of 1966 and the EMS Systems Act of 1973—served to create the underpinnings of the modern EMS system.

5. An EMT's primary role as health care provider has remained relatively unchanged over the years. However, the education and practice of an EMT have undergone dramatic changes as the result of new technology and advances in medicine and science.

6. The EMT serves as the "safety net" of the health care system, providing immediate and lifesaving care in times of health crisis.

7. The National Association of EMTs serves the broad interests of all EMTs. However, other groups also serve. For example, the International Association of Fire Fighters, the single largest group of EMS providers in the United States, frequently intercedes on issues related to EMS that impact on its consituency. Another powerful group is the American Ambulance Association. This organization represents proprietary EMS providers who are interested in influencing legislation such as reimbursements or standards of care.

8. The star of life's six points each represent a phase of EMS. In order, they are detection, reporting, response, on-scene care, care in-transit, and definitive care. The caduceus, the snake, and the staff, in the middle represent the relation of EMS to medicine.

9. Societal changes, economic pressures, and medical advances have resulted in several challenges to EMS. Homelessness is a national problem. The primary care for many homeless patients is provided by

EMS and the emergency department. Much of EMS in suburban and rural communities is provided by volunteers. Demands of two-income families have reduced the number of volunteers to crisis levels. Finally, Americans are simply living longer. A larger and larger proportion of Americans are elderly as a result of the increased longevity. The care of the elderly patient is frequently more complex and difficult for the EMT.

CHAPTER 2

Medical Responsibilities

OBJECTIVES

Upon completion of this chapter, the reader should be able to:

1. Describe the roles and responsibilities of the EMT-Basic.
2. Differentiate the roles and responsibilities of the EMT-Basic from those of other medical care providers.
3. Describe the roles and responsibilities of the EMT-Basic that are related to personal safety.
4. Discuss the roles and responsibilities of the EMT-Basic toward the safety of the crew, the patient, and bystanders.
5. Describe desirable attributes and conduct of the EMT-Basic.
6. Discuss the EMT code of ethics.
7. Define quality improvement and discuss the EMT-Basic's role in the process.
8. Define medical direction and discuss the EMT-Basic's role in the process.

GLOSSARY

certification Proof of satisfactory completion of the minimum requirements in a curriculum.

continuing education Training beyond the initial certification requirements.

lifelong learning Education that a person continues throughout life by keeping current on new information and maintaining competence in skills.

medical direction Advice provided by a higher medical authority, usually a physician.

medical director A physician who acts as a medical expert, consultant, and educator.

off-line medical control The involvement of a physician in protocol and procedure preparation.

on-line medical control Direct communication between the EMT and the physician while care is being rendered in the field.

personal safety The assurance that no hazards are present that might endanger the EMT.

prehospital health care team A multidisciplinary team composed of medical personnel, firefighters, and law enforcement officers who care for patients before their admittance to the hospital.

professional conduct A caring, confident, and courteous demeanor expected of all health care providers.

prospective quality assessment Evaluation of the quality of care before or during an actual call.

quality improvement Actions taken to improve the quality of care given.

quality management A continual process that involves the planning, execution, assessment, review, and improvement of the plan.

retrospective quality assessment Evaluation of the quality of care given by reviewing documentation after the call has been completed.

PREPARATORY

Materials: None.

Personnel: Primary Instructor: One EMT-Basic instructor knowledgeable in the medical/legal aspects and ethical issues the EMT-Basic will encounter.

Recommended Minimum Time to Complete: 1.5 hours

STUDENT OUTLINE

I. Chapter Overview
II. Roles and Responsibilities of the EMT
    A. Job Description
        1. Procedural Duties
        2. Patient Care Duties
    B. Safety
        1. Personal Safety
        2. Crew, Patient, and Bystander Safety
III. Professional Attributes
    A. Appearance
    B. Skill Maintenance
    C. Physical Preparedness
    D. Personality Traits
IV. Training
    A. Certification and Licensure
    B. Continuing Education—Professional Development
    C. Refresher Training—Competency Assurance
V. Code of Ethics
VI. Current Affairs in EMS
VII. Continuous Quality Improvement
    A. Quality Management Roles
        1. Planning
        2. Execution of the Plan
        3. Assessment of Quality
    B. Quality Improvement
    C. Quality Assurance
VIII. Medical Direction
IX. Conclusion

LECTURE OUTLINE

I. Chapter Overview
II. Roles and Responsibilities of the EMT
    1. Health Care Team
        a) Prehospital Phase
            (1) Communication Specialists
            (2) Law Enforcement Officers (LEOs)
            (3) Firefighters
            (4) EMT
            (5) Paramedics
            (6) Emergency Physician
    A. Job Description
        1. Procedural Duties
            a) Stock emergency response vehicle
            b) Maintain equipment
            c) Respond to emergencies
            d) Render patient care
            e) Transport patient
            f) Report to receiving facility
        2. Patient Care Duties
            a) Airway maintenance
            b) Ventilation of patients
            c) Cardiopulmonary resuscitation
            d) Use of automated external defibrillators
            e) Hemorrhage control
            f) Treatment of hypoperfusion
            g) Bandaging of wounds
            h) Immobilization of extremities
            i) Assisting in childbirth
            j) Management of respiratory, cardiac, diabetic, allergic, behavioral, suspected poisonings, and environmental emergencies
            k) Assisting patients with prescribed medications (nitroglycerin, epinephrine, and bronchodilator inhalers)
            l) Administration of oxygen, oral glucose, and activated charcoal
    B. Safety
        1. Personal Safety
            a) First priority—personal safety
        2. Crew, Patient, and Bystander Safety
            b) Crew—second priority
            c) Public—third priority
            d) Patient—fourth priority
III. Professional Attributes
        a) Professional conduct
    A. Appearance
        a) First impressions
    B. Skill Maintenance
        a) Practice makes perfect
    C. Physical Preparedness
        a) Physical conditioning limits injuries
    D. Personality Traits
        a) Compassion
IV. Training
        a) Professional groups with a vested interest
            (1) National Association of EMS Physicians
            (2) Society for Academic Emergency Medicine
            (3) American Academy of Pediatrics
            (4) American Academy of Orthopedic Surgeons
            (5) National Association of State EMS Directors
            (6) American College of Emergency Physicians
            (7) Emergency Nurses Association
            (8) Joint Review Commission
            (9) National Flight Paramedics Association
            (10) National Registry of EMTs
            (11) International Association of Fire Chiefs
            (12) National Council of State EMS Training Coordinators
            (13) National Association of EMTs
            (14) American Heart Association
    A. Certification and Licensure
        a) Certification
            (1) completion of an examination
                (a) minimal standards met

b) Licensure

    (1) governmental permission to practice

B. Continuing Education—Professional Development

    a) lifelong learning

        (1) changes in medicine

        (2) improvement in methods

C. Refresher Training—Competency Assurance

    a) core content

        (1) defined

    b) maintenance of skills

        (1) irregular skills

V. Code of Ethics

    a) oath of professional conduct

    b) list of moral rules

VI. Current Affairs in EMS

    a) periodicals

    b) Internet

        (1) professional interest bulletin boards

    c) current literature

        (1) research journals

VII. Continuous Quality Improvement

    A. Quality Management Roles

        a) cyclical process

            (1) plan

            (2) execute

            (3) review

            (4) improve

        1. Planning

            a) establish mission

            b) determine overall strategic goals

            c) declare tactical objectives

        2. Execution of the Plan

            a) suitability

            b) functionality

        3. Assessment of Quality

            a) prospective field audit

            b) retrospective

                (1) chart review

                (2) patient survey

    B. Quality Improvement

        a) changes in process/method

    C. Quality Assurance

        a) minimal standards

VIII. Medical Direction

    a) allied health care providers

    b) medical control

        (1) moral/professional responsibility

        (2) legal obligation

    c) extension of the physician

        (1) medical direction

        (2) medical control

            (a) off-line control

                (i) protocols

            (b) on-line control

                (i) telecommunications

IX. Conclusion

    a) EMT is

        (1) specially trained

        (2) health care provider

        (3) unique environment

        (4) professional

        (5) physician guidance

TEACHING STRATEGIES

1. Ask the students to brainstorm about what it is to be an EMT. Have them divide the list into roles and tasks. Then ask the students to assign these roles and tasks to an EMS call, utilizing the six phases described on the star of life. It should be quickly apparent to the students that the job of an EMT is multifaceted and rapidly changes according to the time and situation.

2. Ask the students to, first, investigate the codes of conduct/ethics for other allied health professionals, then to create their own code of ethics for an EMT. Give the students a questionable situation and ask them to defend or criticize the EMT, using the code of ethics as the basis for their argument. The situation should involve questionable, but not illegal, conduct. An example would be an EMT who discusses a child abuse case with his priest or an EMT who is verbally but not physically abusive to an alcoholic.

3. Ask a local medical control physician, perhaps the medical director for the EMT program, to discuss his or her position on the following topics: conduct, appearance, character, and disposition. It may be helpful to ask the physician to discuss the continuing medical education that is required of emergency physicians, emergency nurses, and physician assistants.

4. Distribute the list of national organizations that have a vested interest in EMS. Ask the students to explain how these groups either serviced EMS or are the external customers of EMS and the relationship that an EMT should have with members of these groups.

5. Advise the students that their EMS agency has been tasked by the local government to respond to the alarming rise in pediatric drowning in the community. Following the quality management process, ask the students to describe how they would accomplish each step in the process. When the students have completed their plan, add a "problem" to the situation that impacts one of the steps and ask them how would they respond.

FURTHER STUDY

Polsky, S. (1992). *Continuous quality improvement in EMT.* Dallas: American College of Emergency Physicians.
Emergency Medical Services: The Journal of Emergency Care, Rescue, and Technology. Summer Communications, Inc. 7626 Densmore Avenue, Van Nuys, CA 91406-2042, www.emsmagazine.com
Journal of Emergency Medical Services, JEMS Communications, PO Box 2789, Carlsbad, CA 92018, www.jems.com
National Association of EMS Physicians, PO Box 15945-281, Lenexa, KS 66285-5945, www.naemsp.org
National Highway Traffic Safety Administration, U.S. Department of Transportation, 400 Seventh Street, SW, Washington, DC 20590, www.nhtsa.dot.gov

CASE STUDY   ANATOMY OF A CALL

"Rescue 50, respond to a Priority One motor vehicle collision at the corner of Routes 155 and 20." Deb carefully copied down the information.

Deb and Earl climbed into the ambulance and fastened their seatbelts. Deb started the engine, turned on the emergency lights and siren, and proceeded toward the scene of the call.

Upon arrival at the scene, Deb parked the ambulance in a position that was well out of traffic yet still allowed easy access to the rear compartment and would permit an easy exit from the scene. Deb stayed with the ambulance while Earl donned personal protective equipment and then approached the scene.

Earl quickly scanned the scene and determined that there were three persons involved; one young woman was trapped in her vehicle by a damaged door. He immediately called the dispatcher on the radio and requested additional ambulances to the scene as well as the local fire department for extrication.

Earl briefly assessed each patient to determine which needed his attention first. The entrapped woman was still seatbelted in. Earl assessed her airway and breathing and gave her oxygen, based on her complaint of shortness of breath. Continuing his assessment, he found that she had the physical signs of shock. Earl immediately called for assistance in rapidly removing her from the vehicle.

The woman was quickly removed from the vehicle and placed on a backboard with the help of several firefighters. With continued assistance, Earl maintained spinal immobilization and placed the patient on a stretcher. Then they placed the stretcher into the back of the waiting ambulance.

Deb began driving, lights and sirens on, toward the regional trauma center while Earl continued to assess the patient in the rear of the ambulance.

As soon as he was able, Earl used the mobile radio to call the trauma center to advise them of the woman's condition and of their impending arrival. Receiving no further orders, Earl continued to provide care for the patient and frequently reassessed her condition.

Upon arrival at the hospital, Deb parked the ambulance in the designated ambulance entrance and helped Earl remove the stretcher from the rear of the ambulance. A nurse, who was expecting them, met them at the emergency department's doors.

Earl gave a thorough verbal report of his assessment and treatment as they transferred the woman onto the hospital stretcher. The nurse carefully noted their work.

After quickly cleaning up and placing new sheets on the stretcher, Deb and Earl returned to service. Once they were at the station, they documented the call and cleaned and restocked the ambulance in preparation for another call.

ADDITIONAL CASE STUDY

The bell alarm rang and the loudspeaker blared, "Engine nine, rescue nine, respond to the corner of Eagle Street and Madison. Possible man down, not breathing." Pulling on his pants, then his boots, Earl rolled out of bed and slid down the pole to the truck bay below. Deb, the paramedic on the rescue, was already in the passenger seat when Earl opened the driver's door.

"Only a couple of blocks away. We should get there first," Deb declared as the siren wailed. A small crowd had gathered around the stricken person, a middle-aged man wearing a jogging suit. Citizen CPR was already in progress when the rescue unit pulled up to the scene. The engine company strategically placed the pumper to block the spectacle from passing motorists.

The engine company quickly dismounted and proceeded directly to the patient, with an automated defibrillator in hand. While they prepared the defibrillator, Earl confirmed that the patient was still in arrest and directed the engine company to take over CPR. The engine company's lieutenant thanked the two Good Samaritans for their efforts.

Defibrillator pads were quickly placed on the patient's chest and the machine's mechanical voice calmly stated, "No shock advised." Deb went about securing the airway, looking at the cardiac monitor, starting an IV, and doing various other things that medics do.

After what seemed like hours (it was actually only 8 minutes), the ambulance pulled up. The patient was quickly loaded on the stretcher and into the ambulance. Driving "hot," with all emergency lights activated, the ambulance would occasionally shudder as the vehicle rounded the turn at a light, momentarily throwing the crew off its feet. Quickly bracing themselves against the bulkheads, the crew continued CPR.

In the meantime, Deb had contacted the resource hospital and received further orders for treatment beyond those that she was allowed to perform without consulting medical control. She feverishly pushed one drug after another, but all to no avail. The patient remained flatline.

Arriving at the hospital, the crew rushed the patient into the resuscitation room, where a host of staff was standing by. Immediately the patient was transferred to the hospital's gurney while Deb briefed the medical staff regarding the treatments she had performed while en route.

Walking out of the room, Deb and Earl were passed by pastoral care, Father Nick, and a sobbing woman who may have been the patient's wife. Sitting down, they started to write their patient care report when they saw the team streaming out of the room. "They must've called it," Earl uttered in a hushed tone.

Replacing the drugs they had used on the "code" from the hospital stock, Deb and Earl moved about the rescue unit in silence. "Hey, Earl, when we are done cleaning up and restocking, do you feel like a cup of coffee?" asked Deb.

STOP AND THINK

1. What roles do the EMTs in this case play?
2. What are an EMT's responsibilities in this case?
3. What should be included in an EMT's job description?

ANSWERS TO STOP AND THINK

1. The students should be encouraged to list the various roles that an EMT might play. Examples include:
   a. apprentice
   b. emergency vehicle operator
   c. public safety officer
   d. patient caregiver
   e. healthcare team member
   f. educator
2. The students should be encouraged to list the responsibilities of an EMT, in chronological order.
   a. preparation
   b. response
   c. scene safety
   d. provision of care
   e. transportation
   f. transfer of care

The students should be encouraged to investigate the meaning of the star of life.

3. The students should be encouraged to list the elements of a functional job description for an EMT. The students should be asked to answer the following questions.
   1. What are the basic characteristics of an EMT?
   2. What are the physical demands placed on an EMT?
   3. How well does an EMT need to be able to read?
   4. Does an EMT need to be able to think logically?
   5. Does an EMT need to have good motor coordination?
   6. Does an EMT need to have good manual dexterity?

After the list has been compiled, the students should prepare a written job description. The student functional job description should be compared to the functional job analysis provided in the federal DOT EMT curriculum.

CASE STUDY   FAIR TREATMENT

Dave and Rich respond to a motor vehicle collision involving a pick-up truck and a minivan. The driver of the minivan was killed instantly, and her three children are seriously injured.

EMS command orders Dave and Rich to care for the driver of the pick-up truck. As Dave and Rich approach the driver, they note the odor of alcohol permeating the air inside the vehicle. Glancing around the interior, they see several dozen empty beer bottles on the front seat.

Dave gruffly commands the driver to get out of the vehicle and orders him to lie down on a backboard placed on the stretcher. Rich, a little confused, asks Dave if he should get a cervical collar first.

Dave answers, "Look, Rich, this guy is obviously drunk, and drunks never get hurt in these accidents. Only innocent people, like that mother of three, ever get hurt."

ADDITIONAL CASE STUDY

The engine crew was standing around the patient when Dave and Rich arrive. "What's up?" Dave asked.

"He just got done seizing," the engine company lieutenant replied.

Looking over a firefighter's shoulder, Rich exclaims, "Man, it's Michael, you know, the guy that thinks he's the arch-angel. He fakes seizures all the time so he can ride to the hospital and get a free meal."

"I don't know," responded the lieutenant, "he really whacked his head good on the curb and he's still bleeding." He motioned to an EMT-firefighter to take head stabilization precautions. "Listen, Lieutenant, I know this guy, he's a faker. Let us take it from here and you guys can go back in-service."

STOP AND THINK

1. Was Dave's treatment of the patient appropriate? On what basis can that statement be made?
2. If the care is inappropriate, what mechanism(s) are there to respond to this type of situation?
3. Should the degree of importance linked to an act (important, not immediately significant, or critical, for example) affect the reaction of the EMT?

ANSWERS TO STOP AND THINK

1. The students should be encouraged to differentiate between the legal and ethical responsibilities of an EMT. After various opinions have been elicited, the students should be asked if professionalism is the province of law or ethics.

2. The students should be encouraged to clearly delineate the issue and then the possible mechanisms, formal and informal, for dealing with the issue. Possible mechanisms include informing EMS command, contacting on-line medical control immediately, and reporting the problem to the medical director or writing an incident report.

3. The students should be encouraged to develop a "code of ethics," listing those actions that need immediate reaction and those that are considered significant but can wait.

Asking the students to plot a list of questionable behaviors on a scale can be helpful. One end of the scale should be labeled "hurt the patient." The middle of the scale should be labeled "did not hurt but did not help the patient." The other end of the scale should be labeled "helped the patient."

Underneath the scale the various responses should be listed.

ANSWERS TO TEST YOUR KNOWLEDGE

1. The EMT has an overall professional responsibility to provide compassionate care to sick and injured persons. While specific responsibilities vary from region to region, all EMTs are responsible for preparedness, timely response, thorough patient assessment, competent care on-scene and safe transportation to definitive care.

2. The fact that EMTs care for people in the field, rather than in the structured and controlled environment of a hospital, makes the practice of EMTs unique. Because of the unpredictable nature of pre-hospital care, the EMT must not only be well-grounded in practice, but must also be a creative problem-solver.

3. The EMT's personal safety comes first. An injured EMT only compounds the problems on-scene, rather than resolves them.

4. An EMT should be like a Boy Scout in some aspects. The EMT should be trustworty, clean, brave, and kind, as well as resourceful and intelligent. EMTs who are untrustworthy (i.e., thieves), who are cruel, or who fail to aspire to the qualities of a medical professional should not be allowed to practice.

6. Quality care is a perception of the consumer. In the case of EMS, the consumer is the patient. However, EMTs also share a practice with physicians, as allied health care providers, and therefore the physician is another customer.

7. For the quality of care to be improved it must first be measured. Standards of care must be established and then the care provided must be compared to those standards. When a deficit is noted, the problem must be researched and a solution created that results in improved care.

8. As an allied health care provider, the EMT works under the control, or direction, of a physician. Therefore, the protocols, orders, and practice of an EMT is always under medical direction. Medical direction is usually provided by a medical director or a medical advisor.

CHAPTER 3

The Legal Responsibilities of the EMT

OBJECTIVES

Upon completion of this chapter, the reader should be able to:

1. List the legal responsibilities of the EMT.
2. Describe the EMT's duty to act.
3. List some of the elements in the patient's bill of rights.
4. Discuss the patient's right to confidentiality.
5. Explain what is meant by capacity to refuse care.
6. Identify the important components of the EMT's responsibility when a patient refuses care against medical advice.
7. Discuss and define three types of advance directives.
8. Explain how consent is obtained in different circumstances.
9. Discuss the legal importance of documentation.
10. Identify the circumstances under which resuscitation may be withheld.
11. Discuss the EMT's role in reporting suspected abuse.
12. Identify the most common allegations that may be raised against an EMT in a court of law.
13. Discuss the laws that are in place to help protect EMTs from litigation.

GLOSSARY

abandonment A situation in which a care provider assumes responsibility for an incapacitated person and then leaves the patient unsupervised.

advance directive A document prepared before a life-threatening event that provides direction to family, caregivers, and medical staff regarding end-of-life decisions.

age of majority The age at which a person may act without parental permission and is generally treated as an adult.

assault In civil law, a person in fear of being touched without the person having given consent.

battery In civil law, touching a person without having the person's consent.

breach of confidentiality A situation in which a person divulges information about a patient without having the permission of the patient to do so.

child abuse Physical, sexual, or psychological maltreatment of a child.

competent Able to act in a responsible manner and comprehend the decision at hand.

consent Voluntary agreement by a person to allow something to take place.

domestic violence An act of violence against a partner, spouse, family member, or member of the household.

do not resuscitate order (DNR) A medical-legal order to restrain health care providers from providing invasive procedures and resuscitation such as CPR.

elder abuse An act of violence toward or neglect of an elderly person who is dependent upon the other person.

emancipated minor A person who is under the age of majority but who is no longer under the control of the parent or guardian and is legally responsible for his or her own decisions and any consequences that arise from those decisions.

emergency doctrine A legal principle that allows for emergency treatment of prisoners or children if they are incapable of giving consent.

evidence conscious Aware of the importance of preserving items that may be considered evidence of a crime and conditions that pertain to a crime.

express consent The act of verbally advising a medical provider to proceed with treatment.

false imprisonment The intentional confinement of a patient without the patient's consent and without an appropriate reason.

Good Samaritan laws Laws that protect certain classes of people, such as physicians, who volunteer to assist others; laws vary from state to state.

guardian A person who has authority to act on behalf of another individual and to give consent for medical care.

health care proxy A person who has been properly designated by a person to make health care decisions in the event the person becomes incapable of making such decisions.

immunity statute A law that protects a specific group of people from having to pay civil damages as a result of occurrences during job performance.

implied consent The legal presumption that a patient who is unable to verbally express agreement to treatment would agree to be treated in certain circumstances.

legal duty to act The requirement that an EMT respond to calls as an employee under contract or as a volunteer.

liability The legal responsibility for one's own actions.

living will A document signed by a patient that informs the reader of what types of treatment and under what conditions that patient would want or would not want treatment.

mandated reporter A person whom the law requires to report abuse or neglect.

mechanism of injury The instrument or event that results in harm to a patient.

medical protocols A set of written regulations that specify the proper procedures for patient care.

negligence Delivery of care in a manner that is considered to be below the accepted standard.

parentis loco Someone who has authority to act in place of the parent.

patient's bill of rights The rights and privileges a person enjoys as a patient.

pattern of injury Injuries characteristic of a particular mechanism of injury.

physical restraint The restriction of a patient's freedom by use of ties, cravats, or other means to prevent movement.

scope of practice The extent to which a health care provider is permitted to perform medical procedures.

standard of care The level of care that is recognized as being appropriate for a particular level of training and certification.

PREPARATORY

EMS Equipment: None.

Personnel: Primary Instructor: One EMT-Basic instructor knowledgeable in the medical/legal aspects and ethical issues the EMT-Basic will encounter.

Recommended Minimum Time to Complete: 1.5 hours

STUDENT OUTLINE

I. The Legal Responsibilities of an EMT
    A. Knowledge of Standard of Care
    B. Legal Duty to Act
    C. Respect for Patient's Rights
        1. Right to Confidentiality
        2. Right to Refuse Care
            a) Against Medical Advice
            b) Do Not Resuscitate Orders
    D. Obtaining Patient Consent
        1. Children and Consent
        2. Prisoners and Consent
            a) Documentation
            b) Initiating Resuscitation
            c) Collaborating with Law Enforcement
                (1) Motor Vehicle Collisions
                (2) Threat of Violence On-Scene
            d) Physical Restraint Of Combative Patients
            e) Reporting of Abuse
                (1) Child Abuse
                (2) Domestic Violence
             f) Elder Abuse and Neglect
II. Common Allegations Against EMTS
    A. Ambulance Collisions and Liability
    B. Negligence
        1. Duty
        2. Breach of Duty
        3. Causation of Injury
        4. Damages
    C. Patient Abandonment
    D. Breach of Confidentiality
    E. Assault and Battery
III. Protection Against Lawsuits
    A. Good Samaritan Act
    B. Immunity
    C. Best Practices

LECTURE OUTLINE

I. The Legal Responsibilities of an EMT
  A. Roles
    1. Health care Professional
    2. Physician Extender
  B. Scope of Practice
    1. Medical Limitations
      a) Off-Line Medical Control
      b) On-Line Medical Control
  C. Knowledge of Standard of Care
    1. Defined
      a) Medical Care
      b) Same Or Similar Training
        Standard
    2. Sources
      a) Statute
      b) Ordinance
      c) Regulation
      d) Protocols
      e) Textbooks
      f) Expert Witness
  D. Duty to Act
    1. Parties
      a) Employees
      b) Volunteers On-Call
    2. Duration of Duty
      a) Turned Over to
        (1) Equal or Higher Training
      b) Early Termination
        (1) Abandonment
  E. Respect for Patient's Rights
    a) Right to Consent to or Refuse
      Medical Care
    a) Right to Confidentiality
    1. Right to Confidentiality
      a) Source
        (1) Role as Physician Extender
        (2) Common Courtesy
      b) Privileged Communications
        (1) Other Health Care Professionals
          (a) In the Course of
            Patient Care
      c) Legally Mandated Reporting
        (1) Child Abuse
        (2) Crimes
      d) Failure to Maintain Confidentiality

        (1) Breach of Confidentiality
          (a) Libel
          (b) Slander
    2. Right To Refuse Care
      a) Conditions
        (1) Competent
          (a) Comprehend the
            Situation
            (i) Mentally
              Retarded
            (ii) Dementia
              (1) Guardian
              (2) Health
                Care
                Proxy
            (iii) Medical Condition
              (1) Head
                Injury
              (2) Intoxication
              (3) Mental
                Illness
          (b) Questionable
            (i) Contact Medical Control
              (1) Adult
          (c) Age of Majority
            (i) Eighteen
              Years Of Age
      b) Against Medical Advice
        (1) Differentiation
          (a) Refused Medical
            Advice
            (i) Stable
            (ii) Competent
            (iii) Will Seek
              Health Care
              Later
          (b) Against Medical
            Advice
            (i) Unstable or
              Critical
            (ii) Competent
            (iii) Exercising
              Right
        (2) Approach

(a) Calm

(b) Rational Explana-
tions

(c) Offer of Limited
Service

(i) Step-Wise
Approach to
Goal

c) Conditions of Refusal

(1) Inform

(a) Reasonable Conse-
quences of Refusal

(b) Alternatives to
Reach Health Care

(i) Calling 9-1-1
Again

(2) Attempt Contact with
Medical Control

(a) Patient Advice

(b) Physician Notifica-
tion

(3) Left in Care of

(a) Competent Adult

3. Do Not Resuscitate Orders

a) Utility

(1) Terminal Disease

(2) Medical Futility

b) Patient Right to Refuse Care

(1) Unconscious

(a) Implied Consent

(2) Special Circumstances

(a) Living Will

(i) Attorney And
Patient
Agreement

(b) Do Not Resuscitate
Order

(i) Physician
and Patient
Agreement

c) Limitations

(1) Enforceable at Death
Only

(2) Comfort Measures Per-
missible

4. Health Care Proxy

a) Conditions

(1) Patient Incapacitated

b) Designated Health Care Deci-
sion-Maker

(1) Best Interests

F. Obtaining Patient Consent

1. Definition

a) Voluntary Agreement to
Treatment

2. Types of Consent

a) Expressed

(1) Freely Given

(2) Understands Implica-
tions

b) Implied Consent

(1) Unconscious

(2) Assumption of Consent

G. Children and Consent

1. Standards

a) Fails to Meet Standards

(1) Age of Majority

2. Substituted

a) Parental

b) Guardian

(1) Parentis Loco

(a) Athletic Permis-
sion Slips

c) Emergency Exception

(1) Life- or Limb-Threatening

3. Emancipated Minors

a) Marriage

b) Military Service

c) Independent

(1) Court Declaration
Papers

d) Special Cases

(1) STD Treatment

(2) Child Abuse

H. Prisoners and Consent

1. Prisoners Rights Intact in Some
Cases

a)

2. Special Cases

a) Prisoner/Arrestee Incapable
of Permission

b) Officer Can Consent

3. Court-Ordered Treatment

a) Mental Health Laws

I. Documentation

1. Complete

2. Part of the Medical Record

J. Initiating Resuscitation

1. CPR

a) Absence of Pulse and Breathing

2. No CPR
    a) Signs of Advanced Death
       (1) Lividity
       (2) Rigor Mortis
       (3) Decomposition
    b) DNR
    c) Injuries Incommensurate
      With Life
       (1) Decapitation
K. Collaborating with Law Enforcement
  1. The Criminal as Patient
    a) Nonjudgmental Care
  2. Crime Scene
    a) Disturbing Evidence
       (1) Patient Care First
    b) Proactive EMT Behaviors
       (1) Example: Do Not Touch
          Knives or Guns
       (2) Documentation of Scene
          (a) Sworn Statement
  3. Motor Vehicle Collisions
    a) Observe as Possible Crime
      Scene
    b) Evidence-Conscious
    c) Documentation
  4. Threat of Violence On-Scene
    a) Scene Safety First
    b) Specific Concerns
       (1) Familarity with Local
          Gangs
       (2) Weapons Search
L. Physical Restraint of Combative Patients
  1. Cause of Combativeness
    a) Medical Until Proven Other-
      wise
  2. Safe Restraint
    a) Police Assistance
M. Reporting of Abuse
  1. Privileged Entrance
    a) Special Circumstances
    b) Patient Care First Priority
       (1) Nonjudgmental
  2. Child Abuse
    a) Mandated Reporters
    b) EMT as detective
       (1) Comparision
          (a) Mechanism of
             Injury-to-Injury
             Pattern
  3. Domestic Violence
    a) Empathic Care
    b) Safe Haven

  4. Elder Abuse and Neglect
    a) EMT as Detective
       (1) Comparision
          (a) Mechanism of
             Injury-to-Injury
             Pattern
    b) Social Services Referrals
II. Common Allegations Against EMTs
  A. Ambulance Collisions and Liability
    1. Largest Number of Lawsuits Against
      EMS
  B. Negligence
    1. Defined
      a) Failure to Meet Standard of
        Care
       (1) Same or Similarly
          Trained EMT
    2. Elements of Negligence
      a) Duty
       (1) Legal Obligation to
          Respond/Be Responsive
          (a) Vehicle Mainte-
             nance
          (b) Equipment Pre-
             paredness
      b) Breach of Duty
       (1) Commission
          (a) Performed an Act
       (2) Omission
          (a) Failed to Perform
             an Act
      c) Causation of Injury
       (1) Direct Relationship
          from Breach of Duty
          and Injury
      d) Damages
       (1) Actual Losses
       (2) Compensatory Damages
          (a) Example: Loss of
             Companionship
       (3) Punitive Damages
          (a) Setting an Exam-
             ple
  C. Patient Abandonment
    1. Duty
      a) Transfer of Care
    2. Failure of Proper Transfer of Care
  D. Breach of Confidentiality
    1. Right to Know
  E. Assault and Battery
    1. Fear of Harm
      a) Actual or Implied

2. Nonconsensual Touching
3. Intentional Confinement
III. Protection Against Lawsuits
   A. Good Samaritan Act
     1. Commonly Applies to Health Care Professionals
       a) Lists Protected Classes
     2. Medical Care Rendered
       a) Offered Freely
       b) No Expectation of Compensation
   B. Immunity
     1. Specific Cases
   C. Best Practice
     1. Good Patient Care in a Conscientious Manner
     2. Err in the Patient's Favor

TEACHING STRATEGIES

1. Have the students obtain a copy of the federal patient's bill of rights and ask them to create a similar prehospital patient's bill of rights. If a local or state prehospital bill of rights exists, the students should be asked to compare and contrast the two documents.

2. Ask a local attorney familiar with EMS law to speak to the class specifically about refusals of care and the potential liabilities that can arise. Ask the attorney to present a case of an obviously injured individual who is intoxicated and refusing medical care. It is also useful for the medical director to attend and present his or her perspective on the case.

3. Ask local law enforcement officers (LEOs) to participate in a mock take-down of a violent patient. Emphasize the importance of scene control, personal safety, and concepts such as show-of-force and medical priority. This exercise provides an opportunity for EMTs and LEOs to practice safe restraint practices. A discussion about unsafe restraint and times when EMS should withdraw should also be encouraged.

4. Ask a local judge or justice if he or she will sit for a moot civil trial. The students should be presented with a controversial case and then divided into the defense team and prosecution team. The students should be encouraged to obtain depositions from witnesses and research the law for applicable portions. Examples of interesting cases: a case where CPR was allegedly performed on a patient with a valid DNR (wrongful death) and a patient who was intoxicated and transported against his will (false imprisonment). Be sure that the students review all the elements of a lawsuit.

5. Ask the students to observe a simulation of a person with an obvious injury who is refusing medical care. The students should document the facts surrounding the call. Then they should be asked to write a "death warrant," a refusal of care that indicates the possible harm that may befall the patient if he or she should refuse care, usually up to and including death.

FURTHER STUDY

Cid, D., & Maniscalco, P. (1999). Integrating criminal investigation into major EMS scenes. *Journal of Emergency Medical Services*, 24(68), 9.

Colwell, C. B., Pons, P., Blanchet, J. H., &, Mangino C. (1999). Claims against a paramedic ambulance service: A ten-year experience. *Journal of Emergency Medicine*, 17, 999–1002.

Hall, S. A. (1998). Potential liabilities of medical directors for actions of EMTs. *Prehospital Emergency Care*, 2, 76–80.

Krebs, D. R., Henry, K. C., & Gabriele, M. B. (1990). *When violence erupts: A survival guide for emergency responders*. Philadelphia: Mosby.

Laard, R. A. (1989). *EMS law: A guide for EMS professionals*. Aspen.

Partridge, R. A., Virk, A. Sayah, A., & Antosia, R. (1998). Field experience with prehospital directives. *Annals of Emergency Medicine*, 32, 589–593.

Shanaberger, C. J. (1990). Escaping the charge of false imprisonment. *Journal of Emergency Medical Services*, 58–61.

Weaver, J., Brinsfield, K. H., & Dalphond, D. (2000). Prehospital refusal of transport policies: Adequate legal protection? *Prehospital Emergency Care,* 4, 53–56.

CASE STUDY   CONSENT

After handcuffing the young shoplifter, Officer Barnes took a moment to catch his breath. He knew that the security cameras had caught all the action on tape. The cameras had recorded the kid picking up the jeans and stuffing them into the shopping bag. The cameras had also recorded him being stopped at the door and being asked to open the bag.

Then there was the chase in the parking lot as he ran from store security, all recorded on tape. The security cameras had recorded him running, slipping on the wet pavement, and falling flat on his face, with his hands full of stolen merchandise.

The kid's face was a bloody mess, probably from the cut on his forehead and the bloody nose. He looked like he had been beaten. The cameras would prove that the injuries were from the fall.

"Son, how old are you?" asked Officer Barnes, as he used his portable radio to call for EMS. "Sixteen," the teenager replied, "and I don't need EMS."

ADDITIONAL CASE STUDY

Officer Barnes took a minute to look at the cut. It looked particularly vicious, running across the entire length of the patient's palm. "How did you do this?" Barnes inquired.

"I was running with this ornament when I tripped. I guess I fell and my hand landed on the glass," replied the young man.

The dishcloth made a sloppy but effective dressing. "You really should get this looked at by a doctor. Can you feel your fingers?" asked Barnes.

"I really don't want to go the hospital. I just started work here and I don't have any sick time or insurance yet."

"This cut is really deep. You could lose some function in your hand. You really ought to go to the hospital," implored Barnes. "I'm going to call EMS and you can talk to them about it."

"Look," exclaimed the young man, "I'm sixteen and I know my rights and I don't have to go to the hospital if I don't want to!"

STOP AND THINK

1. Can an adolescent consent to care? Are there any exceptions?
2. Who can consent for an adolescent? What if that person is not available?
3. What is different about consent in this case?
4. Can an adolescent legally refuse care? Are there any exceptions?
5. What duties does the EMT have regarding this teenager?

ANSWERS TO STOP AND THINK

1. An adolescent cannot consent to care, except in some very specific cases. These exceptions vary from state to state; check local statutes. Most states provide adolescents the ability to consent for reproductive medical care, or for medical care due to abuse.

2. Usually a parent or legal guardian consents for treatment. If the child is left in the care of another adult, that adult serving in the capacity of the parent, under the doctrine of parentis loco, can consent for the child.

If no one is available to consent, and the child is in danger of losing life or limb, then EMS can treat and transport under the doctrine of emergency exception. In short, the details will be sorted out later, and the child is treated immediately, before she or he suffers a lifelong affliction or dies.

3. In this case, the adolescent teenager is in custody. Depending on local and state laws, the security officer may be a peace officer, legally entitled to arrest and detain individuals until law enforcement officers arrive. In any case, the child will be turned over to law enforcement for processing. Once the patient is in custody, the officer has the responsibility to care for the individual, including obtaining medical treatment as needed.

4. In order to refuse treatment, one must have the legal capacity to consent to treatment. Capacity, generally speaking, is a combination of the mental ability to understand the consequences of accepting treatment and age. In most states the age of consent is eighteen, although in some it is still twenty-one years of age.

5. While this patient cannot legally accept or refuse treatment, the EMT may not abandon the patient either. Efforts must be made to obtain consent to treat. If all else fails, the child should be given first aid and transported under the emergency exception doctrine.

CASE STUDY   A CLAIM OF NEGLIGENCE

Driving alone late at night, Mr. Miller falls asleep at the wheel and loses control of his truck. The truck runs off the road and crashes into an old oak tree.

Dazed for just a moment, Mr. Miller uses his cell phone to call 9-1-1. After some time Mr. Miller grows tired of waiting for EMS and exits the vehicle. He is intent on walking to the nearest farmhouse for help.

As he stands up, he gets lightheaded, his legs buckle under him, and he collapses to the ground. When Mr. Miller regains consciousness, he is no longer able to feel anything below the waist.

On-duty EMTs from the local volunteer rescue squad respond, from their homes, to the EMS call. Upon arrival, they immediately survey the scene, decide that the situation is a trauma, and immediately go about manually stabilizing Mr. Miller's head and neck.

After completing an initial assessment and a rapid trauma assessment, the EMTs correctly conclude that he may have suffered a neck injury. The EMTs carefully apply a cervical collar to protect his cervical spine, and they log-roll him onto a backboard. Afterwards they assess his extremities for feeling and motion. The assessment is unchanged from the initial assessment.

After turning Mr. Miller over to the emergency department staff, the rescue squad returns to service. Several months later Mr. Miller's attorney serves the rescue squad with an "intent to sue" notice. In the notice it is alleged that the EMTs were negligent in their treatment and that this negligent treatment caused or aggravated Mr. Miller's condition, resulting in permanent paralysis of his legs.

ADDITIONAL CASE STUDY

"Meet the officer by the soldiers monument, Washington Park, for a male acting strangely, possibly intoxicated," the portable radio loudly announced. Putting their half-full coffee cups down, Ernie and Akem turned to Cybil. "See you later. We'll pay you when we get back."

Pulling up to the scene, Ernie surveyed the cast of characters present: a couple of citizens, a police officer standing next to a patrol car with its lights flashing, and an assortment of prostate figures lying around the base of the monument.

"Hey, Ernie, this guy is new!" exclaimed Akem as he performed a quick initial assessment. "Just another drunk," Ernie responded. "Let's get him into the ambulance so we can get back to Cybil." Akem quickly helped package the patient and load him into the ambulance.

The scene of chaos that met Ernie and Akem at the emergency department was reminiscent of a Korean war M*A*S*H unit. Patients lined the hallways, some attended by family, while others tried to turn their backs on the turmoil and sleep. Orderlies and nurses were running to and fro and the din was almost unbearable.

"Akem, I spy an empty stretcher in the back hall. Let's dump our patient there, then give the triage nurse our report." Ernie indicated a stretcher at the far end of the hall. After leaving the patient, on his back, with the side rails up, Ernie stood in line waiting for his turn to report to the triage nurse.

"Ernie, we got to go. Multiple patient MVC up on the interstate," called out Akem. So they both rushed out the doors and into the night.

Months later, Akem and Ernie were called into the supervisor's office. "You've both been named in a lawsuit! Seems some guy with diabetes you picked up near the soldiers monument was allegedly left in the hall unattended. Remember him?"

"Diabetes!" Akem thought to himself. "I didn't know the guy had diabetes!"

STOP AND THINK

1. What are the elements of a civil action necessary to prove a case? Are all of these elements in the case that is presented?
2. What is the weakness in the patient's case against the EMT?
3. What should be included in the EMT's documentation of this call?

ANSWERS TO STOP AND THINK

1. The students should be encouraged to dissect the case study and identify the following elements:
   a. the duty to act
   b. the error that caused injury
   c. the proximate causation
   d. the injury

All of the elements of civil suit, or tort, are present.

2. The students should be encouraged to discuss the case. One group of students may be assigned to be the plaintiff's attorneys while another group may be assigned to be the defendant's attorneys.

The weakness in the plaintiff's case is the proximate causation. From the case study, it appears that the injuries are a direct result of exiting the vehicle when the spinal column was unstable, resulting in paralysis. However, he could argue that the "rough handling" by the EMTs further worsened the injuries, resulting in the paralysis.

3. The students should be encouraged to first outline the elements that should be included in the patient care report, then to write a narrative report describing the care given. Minimally, the following should be included:
   a. The determination of the mechanism of injury
   b. The immediate stabilization of the head and neck
   c. The assessment of the extremities for movement and sensation.
   d. The movement of the patient to the backboard.
   e. The reassessment of the patient's extremities.
   f. The turnover to hospital personnel.

Emphasis should be placed on including all of the elements, in order, and not on the format of the documentation. Documentation format is covered later in the textbook.

ANSWERS TO TEST YOUR KNOWLEDGE

1. An EMT is legally responsible to respond to medical emergencies within his or her jurisdiction, and to care for the patient, following medical protocols in the process.

2. An EMT has a duty to act when a citizen requests aid and EMS is summoned. Once on-scene, the EMT has a further duty to treat the patient within the recognized standards of care. In most states, an EMT does not have a duty to act when off-duty.

3. The patient's bill of rights begins with the patient's right to considerate and respectful care. The patient's bill of rights supports the patient's right to make an informed choice and to reasonably participate in decision-making in his or her care to the limits of his or her capacity. If the patient is incapacitated, the patient's bill of rights provides for an advance directive, such as a living will or health care proxy.

4. The patient's right to confidentiality stems from the physician-patient privilege. The physician-patient privilege establishes confidential communication. An EMT, as a physician extender, is afforded the same privilege of confidentiality.

5. As all patients have a right to consent to care, all patients are also allowed to refuse care as well. To refuse care, from a legal perspective, the patient must be mentally capable of understanding the ramifications of the decision before her or his refusal can be accepted. In other words, the patient must be of sound mind.

6. When a patient refuses care, the EMT is obligated to explain to the patient the foreseeable ramifications of the decision as well as alternatives for medical care, including summoning EMS again. The EMT must also provide the patient medical care to the extent that he or she will accept it.

7. Advance directives include the health care proxy, the living will, and the Do Not Resuscitate (DNR) order. the health care proxy is a concerned person who is designated to make medical decisions for the patient in the case when the patient is incapable of making such decisions for himself or herself. A living

will is a legal document drawn up by a lawyer and client that specifies the patient's wishes in the case where the patient cannot express his or her own wishes. The DNR is a medical order, written by a physician, which instructs health care providers to not initiate CPR and other treatments to a dying patient.

8. A conscious adult, who is of sound mind and is of the age of majority, can give express consent to treatments offered. If the patient is unconscious, a legal assumption is made that the patient would express consent if conscious and therefore the consent is said to be implied. Children are unable to consent, by reason of age and mental capacity. In the case of children, a parent or legal guardian must consent to care on behalf of the child. All of the conditions that are required for an express consent for an adult must be met before an adult can consent for a child. Prisoners, by virtue of their loss of freedom, are necessarily dependent on the law enforcement officer to give consent to treatment.

9. The patient care record, and all forms of documentation in EMS, confirm that the EMT met her or his duty to act, responsibly and in accordance with the medical protocols. Care that is not documented does not exist in the eyes of the law.

10. In most cases an EMT cannot withhold resuscitation or CPR. However, there are certain obvious cases when resuscitation would be fruitless. These cases include decapitation, severe lividity, rigor mortis, decomposition, or any unambiguous signs of death.

11. Whenever a trauma is the result of violence, the trauma is a potential crime. On this type of scene the EMT must work closely with law enforcement officers. Motor vehicle collisions, child abuse, elder abuse, and drug overdoses are examples of some of the scenes where EMTs work together with law enforcement.

12. EMTs are expected to report suspected abuse to the medical professionals at the receiving hospital. In some states the EMT must also make a report to the legal authorities. These legal reporting requirements vary from state to state and therefore an EMT is advised to seek out legal counsel regarding local laws.

13. The greatest number of claims against EMTs made in a court of law involve driving. In terms of patient care, common allegations include abandonment, a failure to properly turn over care, and a breach of confidentiality, where the EMT divulges privileged information to someone who does not have a right to know.

14. The Good Samaritan laws are probably the first and best example of laws that protect an EMT from litigation. Designed to encourage health care providers to assist those injured or ill while outside a health care facility, the Good Samaritan laws protect the EMT from claims of negligence. In some special situations, the law provides an EMT immunity from litigation. Child abuse reporting statues, for example, protect the EMT from litigation for reporting in good faith. However, in most cases the courts would rather have the two parties work it out in court than provide the EMT with an immunity.

CHAPTER 4

Stress in Emergency Medical Services

OBJECTIVES

Upon completion of this chapter, the reader should be able to:

1. Define stress from an EMT's perspective.
2. Identify examples of positive and negative stressors.
3. List several emotions an EMT may experience when exposed to a stressor.
4. List the physical signs and symptoms seen in a stress response.
5. Identify several emotionally charged situations that will likely cause a stress response.
6. Identify several job-specific stressors for EMTs.
7. Identify several home-related stressors for EMTs.
8. List ways an EMT can reduce the effects of stress on the body.
9. Discuss the stress that a patient may perceive.
10. Discuss the possible reactions a patient's family member may exhibit when confronted with illness and injury of a loved one.
11. State the steps an EMT can take to help reduce the stress experienced by patients and their families.
12. Differentiate between an acute stressor and chronic stress.
13. Identify physical, emotional, and behavioral effects of chronic stress.
14. Discuss two general methods for stress management (quantity and quality).
15. Describe a relaxation technique useful for management of an acute stress response.
16. Describe several diversionary tactics useful for management of an acute stress response.
17. Discuss the purpose of debriefing after a critical incident.
18. Identify the key elements of a critical incident stress debriefing (CISD).
19. Identify specific incidents likely to require CISD.

GLOSSARY

acute stress A single event that creates a stress response.

body substance isolation Measures taken to protect oneself from unwanted exposure to potentially infectious body substances.

burnout   The condition that exists when an EMT no longer feels able to perform her or his duties because of the effects of chronic stress.

chronic stress   Repeated stressors that affect an EMT over a period of time.

critical incident stress debriefing (CISD)   Organized discussions that occur after a particularly stressful incident among all involved team members and other key players. Such a debriefing can help participants effectively deal with the stress of the incident.

critical incident stress management team   Specially trained personnel whose job is to prevent or mitigate the negative impact of acute stress on emergency service workers. They also may begin to speed the recovery process after a particularly traumatizing event via a critical incident stress debriefing.

debriefing   The process of gathering the team members involved in an incident and discussing the details of the event.

diversionary techniques   Activities such as physical exercise, deep breathing, or creative imagery that are useful in dissipating the effects of an acute stressful event.

fight or flight response   Reaction of the body to a stressor in which it prepares to fight to defend itself or to run away.

healthy lifestyle   A lifestyle that includes exercise, a balanced diet, and avoidance of unhealthy habits such as smoking.

multiple casualty incident (MCI)   An incident involving multiple injured patients, often overwhelming the initial responding units.

relaxation exercises   Techniques that may be employed during or after a stressful event that can help to dissipate an acute stress response.

scene survey   Procedure used to initially evaluate a situation for potential dangers.

stress   The physical, emotional, and behavioral response of the body to changing conditions.

stress management program   Means of dealing effectively with acute and chronic stress.

stressors   The events that trigger stress.

unwind time   Time that is designated in an EMT's personal life to relax and participate in hobbies, sports, or exercise.

PREPARATORY

EMS Equipment: None.

Personnel: Primary Instructor: One EMT-Basic instructor knowledgeable in stress and stress management, critical incident stress debriefing, and identifying child/elderly abuse, stages of death and dying, and aspects of scene safety.

Recommended Minimum Time to Complete: 1.5 hours

STUDENT OUTLINE

I. Chapter Overview
II. Stress Defined
    A. The Stress Response
        1. Emotional Response
        2. Physical Response
III. Call-Related Stress
    A. Death
    B. Trauma
    C. Family, Friends, Co-workers as Patients
    D. Abuse
    E. Disasters
IV. Stress Related to Job Dynamics
    A. Training
    B. Work Hours
    C. Pay
    D. Poor Sleeping and Eating Opportunities
    E. Lack of Formal Rewards
V. Stress Related to the Home Environment
    A. Time Issues
    B. Social Life
VI. Managing Personal Stress
    A. Personal Well-Being
        1. Healthy Lifestyle
        2. Immunizations
        3. Body Substance Isolation
        4. Scene Safety
    B. Recognizing Stress
        1. Acute Stress
        2. Chronic Stress
    C. Stress Management Programs
        1. Critical Incident Stress Debriefing
        2. Recognizing the Need for Further Help
        3. Suicide in EMS
VII. Managing Stress of Patients and Families
VIII. Conclusion

LECTURE OUTLINE

I. Chapter Overview
II. Stress Defined
      a) Stressors
  A. The Stress Response
     1. Emotional Response
        a) Overwhelming Feelings
     2. Physical Response
        a) Sympathetic Nervous System
           (1) Fight or Flight Syndrome
III. Call-Related Stress
      a) Special Situations
  A. Death
      a) Positive Impacts of Stress
         (1) Looking for the Good
  B. Trauma
      a) Press to Perform
      b) Carnage
  C. Family, Friends, Co-workers as Patients
  D. Abuse
      a) Child Abuse
      b) Elder Abuse
  E. Disasters
      a) Enormity
IV. Stress Related to Job Dynamics
      a) Inherent in the Job
      b) Harsh Working Environment
  A. Training
      a) Lifelong Learning
  B. Work Hours
      a) 24-7 Schedule
      b) Irregular Hours
  C. Pay
      a) Financial Hardship
  D. Poor Sleeping and Eating Opportunities
      a) Importance of Regular Sleep
      b) Importance of Good Nutrition
  E. Lack of Formal Rewards
V. Stress Related to the Home Environment
      a) Lack of Understanding
  A. Time Issues
      a) On-Call
      b) Family-Work Conflicts

  B. Social Life
      a) Hobbies
      b) Sports
VI. Managing Personal Stress
  A. Personal Well-Being
      a) Stress Decreases Resistance
      b) Long-Term Health Risks
     1. Healthy Lifestyle
        a) Regular Exercise
        b) Balanced Diet
        c) Elimination of Unhealthy Habits
           i) Smoking
           ii) Excessive Caffeine
           iii) Alcohol
     2. Immunizations
        a) Standard Vaccinations
           i) Tuberculosis Testing
     3. Body Substance Isolation
        a) Handwashing
        b) Barrier Devices
     4. Scene Safety
  B. Recognizing Stress
     1. Acute Stress
        a) Symptoms
     2. Chronic Stress
        a) Burnout
          (1) Signs
  C. Stress Management Programs
     1. Critical Incident Stress Debriefing
        a) The Process
          (1) Fact Phase
          (2) Symptoms Phase
          (3) Reentry Phase
     2. Recognizing the Need for Further Help
     3. Suicide in EMS
VII. Managing Stress of Patients and Families
      a) Dignity
      b) Privacy
      c) Sense of Control
      d) Comfort
VIII. Conclusion

TEACHING STRATEGIES

1. Have the students think back to a first romantic encounter or a try-out for a sports event. Have them describe the tension and the feelings that existed during those anxious moments. Then review the systemic effects of stress on the body. Ask the students if they have ever experienced any of those symptoms. Ask them if they have any of those symptoms now after describing the event. Relate how certain memories can trigger a stress response in a person, both consciously and unconsciously.

2. Describe to the students a scene where a saber-toothed tiger is about to attack his human prey. System by system, ask the students how they would want their body to react to this threat. For example, would they want less blood flow to the skin to reduce bleeding? Would they want more blood flow to their large muscles for flight?

3. Ask the students to list those stresses that are directly related to the job of being an EMT. Then ask them the usual manner in which they deal with stresses, such as examinations. Discuss the healthiness of these stress management techniques.

4. Ask the local critical incident stress debriefing team to come to the class. The team should be prepared to describe how the team is activated, the role of the CISD team, the nature and format of a CISD meeting, and employee assistance/mental health resources available.

FURTHER STUDY

Angle, J. (1999). *Occupational safety and health*. Albany, NY: Delmar.

Appelbaum, S. (1981). *Stress management for health care professionals*. Rockville, MD: Aspen Publishing.

Boudreaux, E., Mandry, C., & Brantley, P. J. (1997). Stress, job satisfaction, coping, and psychological distress among emergency medical technicians. *Prehospital Disaster Medicine, 12*, 242–249.

Christie, A. M. (1997). Balancing stress in work and at home. *Emergency Medical Services, 26*, 52–55.

DeLaune, S., & Ladner, P. (1998). *Fundamentals of nursing: Standards and practice*. Albany, NY: Delmar.

Neely, K. W., & Spitzer, W. J. (1997). A model for a statewide critical incident stress debriefing program for emergency services personnel. *Prehospital Disaster Medicine, 12*, 114–119.

Van Stralen, D., & Perkin, R. M. (1999). Stress reactions. Understand and accept their appearance. *Journal of Emergency Medical Services, 24*, 50–52.

Welser, C. F., & Holmes, J. G. (1997). With EMS: The rest of the story . . . caring for those close to the patient. *Journal of Emergency Medical Services. 22*, 62–63, 65–69.

CASE STUDY   A DREADED CALL

Just as Dan and Kris sat down to eat, the alert tones sounded. As they hastily left the restaurant, Dan wondered if he would get to eat at all that day.

Dan gingerly slid into the front seat, remembering that his back was still sore from this morning's rescue. He fastened his seatbelt and acknowledged the call on the mobile radio.

The dispatcher advised, "Car fire, possible persons entrapped, fire-rescue dispatched, corner of Palma Boulevard and Gipp Road, time out 13:40."

This was a call that Dan dreaded. His brother had died from burns due to a fire, and he remembered how much pain his brother had been in before he died. This memory caused his stomach to become instantly queasy.

Attempting to put the painful memory out of his mind, Dan tried to concentrate on the task at hand. "Focus on the basics. Remember critical trauma patients are extricated in less than 10 minutes, stick to the ABCs." He could almost picture his EMT instructor over his shoulder. His heart was pounding, and his back was getting stiff.

Arriving on-scene, Dan and Kris found that the car had crashed into the side of a tractor-trailer. The gas tank on the truck had ruptured and caught fire.

The fire was quickly extinguished by fire-rescue, but through the smoke the hands of the driver could be seen thrashing around. Fire-rescue was already busy cutting the car apart as Dan donned his protective gear.

"Will I remember what to do?" Dan thought as he entered the car. The palms of his hands were already slick with sweat as he thought, "Airway. Airway is always first." In the meantime, Kris had climbed in the backseat. She yelled out over the loud din of the power tools, "Hey, do you want me to take head stabilization first?" Frustrated, Dan thought to himself, "I know that I am supposed to take manual stabilization first. How could I forget!" Wondering if Kris could see how red his face was, Dan quickly checked the driver for breathing and a pulse.

ADDITIONAL CASE STUDY

He had never felt so helpless in his life. The smoke and flames rolled out of the front cab of the truck and he could still see the form of a man thrashing around inside. But the fire was just too intense to approach the cab and firefighters were forced to stand back and just watch.

While Dan stood there, grinding his teeth, he remembered how his brother, also a firefighter, had died in a house fire just a year ago. The ceiling had collapsed and a cross-beam fell across his back and pinned him to the ground. Despite the fact that a team of firefighters rushed to his aid, the beam was too heavy and there was nothing that they could do to save him. Soon the fire engulfed the room and all hope was lost.

Dan thought to himself, "And history repeats itself." As he stood there, his back started to ache. On the off chance that the driver did survive the fire (not likely), Dan prepared his equipment. "Airways, check, BVM, check, oxygen, crack the tank, what?!" Dan looked at disbelief at the gauge. The tank was empty. In a rage, he picked up the tank and threw it, while uttering a few expletives. "What's wrong with you people?" he yelled at the crew. "Can't you do anything right!"

STOP AND THINK

1. What stressors is Dan experiencing?
2. What are Dan's physical and emotional responses to those stressors?

ANSWERS TO STOP AND THINK

1. The memory of Dan's brother dying in a fire could trigger the same physiological response now that it did then. The back pain adds another physical component to Dan's stress response. Finally, the real threat of fire on-scene can trigger fears of pain, suffocation, and disability.

2. The mere memory of Dan's brother's death has already triggered the stress response, as indicated by his queasy stomach. Further evidence of the stress response is seen in both the sweaty palms and the disorganized thinking.

CASE STUDY   STRESS AND YOUR HEALTH

It was the end of another busy night at engine 10. Jim laughed to himself, "Who said EMS means earn money sleeping!" Jim had been counting on getting at least a few hours of sleep that night so he could go to his day job and be somewhat productive. He felt exhausted and hadn't been sleeping well lately.

As Jim was changing uniforms, he suddenly had another stomach cramp. The pain was sharp and stabbing. Usually he would have diarrhea afterward. However, this pain was more severe than usual. He called for the supervisor, Nanci, to come into the locker room.

After a quick examination, Nanci advised Jim to go to the hospital, but Jim refused. As a compromise, Jim did allow Nanci to call the company's physician for an appointment later that day.

At the doctor's office, Jim related that he had been having trouble sleeping, seemed to catch more colds lately, and couldn't sleep, even when he had the chance. Asking to speak to the physician confidentially, he related that he felt he was drinking too much lately and that he was more irritable than usual with both his co-workers and his patients.

ADDITIONAL CASE STUDY

"Jim, Jim. Wake up. It's your wife." Jim, bleary-eyed looked up at the dispatcher holding a phone in his face and then at the clock. "For crying out loud, I only got one hour of sleep!" Jim bellowed as he grabbed the phone from the dispatcher's hand.

"Hello, yes, yes, yes, I'll be home at eight. Bye." Jim mumbled into the phone. The baby was coming down with the flu that he had just gotten over and his wife had been up all night trying to comfort his son.

Jim was just coming off his third 24-hour shift this week, was working two full-time jobs, and hadn't had 4 straight hours of sleep in almost a week. Exhausted, Jim felt his head start to pound again. The headaches were new. His partner had checked his blood pressure repeatedly over the past week, and it was getting dangerously high. Jim knew he had to see a doctor, but there simply was no time in his schedule.

"OK, OK," Jim answered. "I've only got time for one beer." Jim felt guilty about going out for one beer but he didn't want the guys to think he was hen-pecked. He knew that he would have to pay for that decision later.

STOP AND THINK

1. What are Jim's stressors?
2. Which of Jim's symptoms could be stress-related?
3. What can be done to relieve the stress?

ANSWERS TO STOP AND THINK

1. Jim has many stressors, including lack of sleep, pressure from two jobs, and guilt from being irritable.

2. All of Jim's symptoms can be stress-related. Coronary vascular disease, hypertension and chronic upper respiratory infections are just a few of the more common illnesses that are impacted by stress.

3. There are a number of actions Jim can take to relieve his stress and generally improve his health. First, he should replace his maladaptive behaviors with enabling behaviors. For example, while socialization can be beneficial, excessive alcohol consumption is destructive behavior. He could consider inviting the crew to go bowling, play darts, go to softball games, and the like. Jim should also carefully weigh the financial gains he realizes from holding down two jobs versus the negative impact that this behavior is having on his health. Essentially, it's a risk/benefit analysis and his present health would seem to indicate he made a bad decision to try to hold down two jobs.

ANSWERS TO TEST YOUR KNOWLEDGE

1. Stress is the body's reaction to stimulus in the envrionment. Stress is a two-edged sword. It is necessary for the body to maintain alertness. Too much stress, however, can overwhelm the body, causing an imbalance in the body's homeostasis, leading to fatigue and illness.

2. Personal stresses typically revolve around family obligations, emotional relationships, and financial problems. EMS can add to this stress by either compounding these problems or by layering other stresses, such as injury, pain, and disability on top.

3. While the gamut of emotions can be wide, the body's response is fairly regular and predictable. Some reasonable reactions to a baby's death might include sadness, anger at lost opportunities, guilt over performance, or behavior and confusion. The reactions to a partner's death may be similar.

4. The fight or flight reaction is the body's response to sudden stress.

The physical impact of the fight or flight reaction include tachycardia, tachypnea, nausea, vomiting, and diarrhea as well as hyperalertness and tunnel vision.

Continuous bombardment of stress on the body can lead to maladaptive physical responses. For example, during acute stress the heart races (tachycardia). During chronic stress, the patient's resting heart rate may remain elevated in a persistent tachycardia, which can lead to cardiovascular complications later.

5. The first response that an EMT should have to excessive stress is to remove himself or herself from the stressful environment. While this may not be reasonably possible in a day-to-day situation, it is important for an EMT to take time out for vacation, rest and relaxation. Next, the EMT should not engage in or should attempt to replace any maladaptive responses to stress, like chronic or excessive alcohol consumption or use of tobacco products. Instead, the EMT should practice healthy living habits, including exercise and a proper diet, especially when off-duty.

6. Certain events, such as the death of an infant, are attended by a host of emotions that every crew member faces. By coming together in a confidential meeting, these EMTs and other emergency services providers can share these emotions with one another, reaffirming that no one is out of line for feeling depressed or angry.

7. The typical high-profile calls should be debriefed (for example, the death of an infant or child, the serious injury of a crew mate, or the in-the-line-of-duty death of a crew mate). Each case must be looked at individually and a decision made, based on the observation of the crew, whether stress-debriefing is needed. However, it is good policy to have certain calls designated, in a protocol, for CISD.

CHAPTER 5

Anatomy and Physiology

OBJECTIVES

Upon completion of this chapter, the reader should be able to:

1. Define the term anatomy.
2. Describe and demonstrate the standard anatomical position.
3. List and define the main directional terms.
4. Describe a location of injury using the directional terms.
5. Describe and demonstrate typical patient positions.
6. List the functions of the skin.
7. Describe several important muscles.
8. List the bones in the axial skeleton and describe their function.
9. List the bones of the spinal column and describe their function.
10. List the bones in the appendicular skeleton and describe their function.
11. Describe nervous system function.
12. Describe the physical orientation of the heart.
13. Describe the four chambers of the heart.
14. Describe the heart's conduction system.
15. Compare the locations of the pulmonary and systemic circulation circuits.
16. Define what blood is.
17. Differentiate between the main types of blood vessels in the body.
18. List the functions of the mucous membranes of the respiratory system.
19. Name the structures of the upper respiratory system.
20. Name the structures of the lower respiratory system.
21. Name the organs of the digestive tract.
22. Describe the location of the major organs within the abdominal cavity.
23. Describe the parts of the urinary system.
24. Name the male and female gonads.m

GLOSSARY

abdominal cavity   The space between the chest and the pelvis that holds the organs of digestion and elimination.

abduction   Movement away from the body.

acetabulum   The socket in the pelvis where the proximal femur meets the pelvis.

adduction   Movement toward the body.

alveoli   Tiny air sacs in the lungs that allow exchange of carbon dioxide and oxygen.

anatomy   The study of the structure of an organism.

angle of Louis The bony ridge where the manubrium meets the body of the sternum; also called the sternal angle.

anterior A directional term referring to a location toward the front.

anus The end of the digestive tract; it allows for exit of solid wastes.

aorta The largest artery in the body; it carries the blood from the left ventricle of the heart out to the rest of the body.

apex The point of a triangle; a directional term used to describe the top of the lungs or the bottom tip of the heart.

appendicular skeleton The bony extremities composed of the shoulder girdle, arms, pelvic girdle, and legs.

appendix A small saclike portion of the large intestine that may become inflamed in a condition called appendicitis.

arachnoid The weblike middle protective membrane covering the brain and spinal cord.

arteries Vessels that carry blood away from the heart. With the exception of the pulmonary artery, they carry oxygenated blood.

atlas The first cervical vertebra.

atrium A small receiving chamber, one on each side of the heart, which empties blood into its corresponding ventricle to be pumped out of the heart; plural, atria.

autonomic nervous system A collection of nerves that originate in the brainstem and transmit impulses to many organs in the body to allow for many basic body functions.

atrioventricular (AV) node Node of specialized cardiac conduction fibers that slow the electrical impulse as it moves from the atria to the ventricles to allow for the mechanical contraction of the heart to catch up to its electrical activity.

axial skeleton Bony skeleton that forms the axis of the support structure of the body; includes the skull, spinal column, and thoracic cage.

axilla The armpit.

axis The second cervical vertebra around which the atlas sits and may rotate.

base A directional term used to describe the bottom of an object, such as a triangle.

biceps muscle The widely known muscle that allows flexion of the arm at the elbow; antagonist to the triceps muscle.

bilateral A directional term used to describe points on both sides of the body.

bladder The organ in the pelvis that stores urine as it is made by the kidneys.

blood Made of several types of cells, this fluid carries fuels and wastes around the body for distribution and removal as appropriate.

blood vessels The structures that carry the blood around the body.

brainstem The most basic part of the human brain that acts as a junction box from the body to the rest of the brain structures and back.

bronchi Cartilaginous tubes that carry air into the lungs; singular, bronchus.

bronchioles Small muscular tubes with cartilaginous rings that carry air from bronchi into smaller air spaces in the lungs.

bundle branches Part of the heart's specialized conduction system; they receive electrical impulses from the bundle of His and transmit them to the Purkinje fibers in the ventricles.

bundle of His Part of the heart's specialized conduction system; it receives an electrical impulse from the AV node and transmits it to the bundle branches.

calcaneus The largest bone in the foot; commonly known as the heel bone.

capillaries Tiny blood vessels that receive blood from arteries and pass it into adjacent veins.

carina Point at which the trachea ends and the right and left bronchi begin.

carpal bones The eight bones of the wrist.

central A directional term used to describe points toward the center of the body.

central nervous system Consists of the brain and spinal cord; is involved in the initiation and transmission of all control-oriented messages throughout the body.

cerebellum The part of the brain that controls muscular coordination and complex actions; sometimes called the athletic brain.

cerebro spinal fluid (CSF) Liquid that bathes the brain and spinal cord, bringing it nutrients and removing wastes.

cerebrum The largest and most highly evolved area of the brain.

cervical spine The uppermost section of the spinal column; made up of seven vertebrae in the neck, it protects the cervical spinal cord.

circulation The action of blood flowing in the circuitry of blood vessels and the heart.

clavicle The collarbone located at the very top of the chest, connecting the shoulder to the sternum.

coccyx The tailbone, or last portion of the spinal column.

costal arch The umbrella-appearing arch at the lower portion of the front of the thoracic cage.

costovertebral angle The angle formed by the tenth rib as it meets the thoracic spine.

cranium The bony skull.

deep Term used to describe an injury that extends far into an injured structure.

deltoid muscle The triangular muscle covering the shoulder and upper arm. A site commonly used for intramuscular injections.

dermis The layer of skin just beneath the surface, or epidermal, layer. Contains capillaries and specialized nerve endings.

diaphragm The specialized muscle that separates the chest from the abdomen and is the main muscle of breathing.

distal A directional term used to describe points farther from the core of the body trunk.

dorsal A directional term referring to the top or back surface of a structure such as the hand.

dura mater The outermost membrane covering the spinal cord and brain.

endocrine system Assists the nervous system in maintaining control over the body by producing hormones that act on certain organs.

epidermis The outermost layer of skin.

epiglottis Located above the larynx, a cartilaginous structure that protects the trachea from foreign bodies.

esophagus A collapsible muscular tube that directs food from the mouth into the stomach.

eversion An outward movement, such as when the foot twists outward and strains the ankle; the opposite of inversion.

extension A movement that widens the angle at the joint between two bones; the opposite of flexion.

fallopian tube Tiny muscular tube that allows an egg to travel from the ovary to the uterus.

false ribs The eighth through tenth ribs, which are not attached directly to the sternum; rather, they are attached anteriorly to the seventh rib by cartilage.

femur The single bone in the thigh; it is the longest and strongest bone in the body.

fibula The laterally placed bone in the lower leg.

flexion A movement at a joint that decreases the angle between the two bones on either side of it; opposite of extension.

floating ribs The last two pairs of ribs in the thoracic cage; they are unattached anteriorly.

fontanels Soft, flexible, fibrous regions in an infant's skull that allow for skull growth; also known as soft spots.

foramen magnum Large opening at the base of the skull through which the spinal cord passes.

Fowler's position Position in which a person is sitting at a 45-degree to 60-degree angle.

frontal bone The strong anterior-most bone in the skull that makes up the forehead.

gallbladder A small pouchlike organ that lies underneath the liver and stores bile to be used in digestion.

gastrocnemius muscle The muscle in the back of the calf that enables a person to stand on his or her toes.

glands Specialized organs that respond to and produce the hormones of the endocrine system.

gluteus muscles Strong muscles in the buttocks that are important in allowing proper leg movement.

gonads Organs of reproduction; testes (male) and ovaries (female).

hard palate The bony structure that forms the roof of the mouth.

heart Four-chambered muscular pump that provides the body with nutrient-rich blood.

hemostasis The process of controlling bleeding.

high-Fowler's position   Position in which a person is sitting upright at a 90-degree angle.

hormones   Chemicals that are excreted into the bloodstream by specialized organs called glands.

humerus   The single long bone of the upper arm.

iliac bones   The main component of the bony pelvis; the hip bones are sometimes described as "wings" because of their shape.

inferior   Lower than the reference point.

insulin   A hormone produced by the pancreas that allows glucose utilization by the body.

integumentary system   The skin and skin structures that cover and protect the body.

intervertebral disc   The fibrous pad that cushions each vertebra from the others.

inversion   Turning something inward; opposite of eversion.

ischium   The portion of the bony pelvis that supports our weight as we sit.

jugular vein   A large vein in the neck that is situated close to the surface of the skin.

kidney   A solid organ in the retroperitoneal space that filters toxins from the blood and makes urine to dispose of such toxins and excess salts or water.

knee   The joint that joins the upper leg and the lower leg.

large intestine   Hollow organ that encircles the abdominal cavity and receives digested food from the small intestine.

larynx   A cartilaginous structure in the midline of the neck that contains the vocal cords and is the beginning of the trachea, or windpipe.

lateral   A directional term used to describe the side of a structure; points farther from the midline.

left lateral recumbent position   Position in which the person is lying on the left side; also known as the recovery position.

liver   Large solid organ in the right upper abdomen that creates bile for digestion, produces special factors to help in blood clotting, and filters specific toxins from the blood.

lower   extremities A term used to refer to the legs.

lumbar vertebrae   The five vertebrae that make up the lower back and support the weight of the entire upper body.

malleolus   The bony prominences at the medial and lateral aspects of the ankles.

mandible   The bony lower jaw.

manubrium   The upper section of the bony sternum.

mastoid sinus   Air-filled space within the mastoid bone, behind the ears.

maxillae   The two fused bones forming the upper jaw.

medial   A directional term used to describe points closer to the midline of the body.

meninges   Protective membranes covering the brain and spinal cord.

menstruation   The monthly flow that rids the uterus of its lining when fertilization of an egg does not occur.

metabolism   The use of fuels by the body.

metacarpals   The five bones that connect the carpal bones in the wrist to the phalanges in the fingers.

midaxillary line   An imaginary line drawn from the center of the armpit down the side of the chest.

midclavicular lines   Imaginary lines drawn from the middle of each clavicle, or collarbone, down the front of the chest.

midline   An imaginary line drawn down the center of the body, splitting it equally into right and left halves.

mitral valve   A bicuspid valve that prevents blood flow backward from the left ventricle into the left atrium.

modified   Trendelenburg position Position in which a person is lying supine with legs elevated 12 to 16 inches; also known as the shock position.

nasopharynx   The back of the throat that is immediately behind the nose; the nasal passage.

nervous system   The body system made up of the brain, spinal cord, and nerves that controls and coordinates all body functions.

occipital bone   The most posterior bone in the skull.

orbit   The bony cavity that houses the eyeball.

oropharynx   The section of throat that is visible from the mouth.

ovary   The primary female gonad, located in the pelvis. Produces female sex hormones.

palmar   A directional term used to describe the palm of the hand.

pancreas   An important organ located in the retroperitoneal space that produces both digestive enzymes and hormones such as insulin.

parietal bone   The largest of the bones in the skull, located in the lateral part of the cranium.

parietal pleura   The thin covering adhering to the inside of the chest wall.

patella   The small bony island over the knee joint, known as the kneecap.

pectoralis muscles   Muscle that cover the upper part of the anterior chest and helps to lift the sternum and upper ribs.

penis   The male organ that serves as a conduit for the passage of urine and semen.

perfusion   The term describing the supply of blood with oxygen and nutrients to the organs of the body.

peripheral   A directional term used to describe points farther from the core of the body trunk.

peripheral nervous system   Composed of nerves that originate in the spinal cord and transmit messages to and from the body's organs and tissues.

phalanges   Fingers and toes.

physiology   The study of the function of an organism.

pia mater   The innermost membrane covering the spinal cord and brain.

plantar   A directional term used to describe the bottom surface of the foot.

posterior   A directional term that refers to a location toward the back.

posterior tibial pulse   An easily palpable pulse created by blood flow through the posterior tibial artery behind the medial malleolus of the ankle.

pressure points   pecific areas over major arteries where compression can halt bleeding from that artery.

pronation   The action of turning something, such as the hand, downward.

prone   Position in which a person is lying face down.

prostate gland   Male organ that produces a fluid that assists in the transport of sperm.

proximal   A directional term used to describe points on the body that are closer to the core of the body trunk.

pubis   The front of the bony pelvis.

pulmonary artery   The large artery that transfers blood from the right ventricle to the pulmonary circulation for oxygenation.

pulmonary circuit   The blood vessels that pass through the lungs and allow oxygenation and removal of carbon dioxide.

pulmonary valve   A semilunar valve that prevents the backflow of blood from the pulmonary artery into the right ventricle.

pulmonary vein   The large vessel that takes oxygenated blood from the pulmonary criculation and delivers it to the left atrium.

pulse   The palpable feeling of blood flow through a superficial artery; count of the heartbeat.

Purkinje fibers   Specialized cardiac conduction fibers within the ventricles.

quadriceps muscle   The strong muscle in the anterior thigh that permits leg extension.

radius   The more lateral of the two bones in the forearm.

recovery position   Position in which the person is lying on the side; also known as left lateral recumbent position.

rectum   The end of the large intestine where stool is stored before it is eliminated via the anus.

red blood cells   Hemoglobin-carrying blood cells that deliver oxygen to tissues.

respiration   The exchange of gases, such as oxygen and carbon dioxide, at the capillary level.

retroperitoneal cavity   The most posterior section of the abdomen, containing organs, such as the kidneys, and the pancreas and the aorta.

ribcage   The bony ribs that surround the organs of the chest like a protective cage.

sacral vertebrae   Five strong bony vertebrae that close the pelvic ring posteriorly.

scapulas   Strong bony prominences on the back, also known as the shoulder blades.

scrotum   The externally located sac that encloses the male testes.

shock position   Position in which a person is lying supine with legs elevated 12 to 16 inches; also known as modified Tredelenburg position.

sinoatrial (SA) node   Specialized cardiac conduction fibers that serve as the primary pacemaker of the heart.

small intestine   Very long, hollow organ that takes up much of the abdominal cavity and is responsible for much of the absorption of nutrients from food.

sperm   Male reproductive material responsible for fertilization of the female egg.

spinal column   The series of bones that support the back and protect the spinal cord.

spinal cord   The collection of nerves that run from the brain through the spinal column and branch out to body organs and tissues.

spinous process   The centrally palpable posterior element of each vertebrae.

standard   anatomical position Facing forward, legs slightly apart with feet pointing forward, arms straight and extended a few inches away from the side with palms facing forward.

sternal angle   The bony ridge where the manubrium meets the body of the sternum; also called the angle of Louis.

sternal body   The largest center piece of the bony sternum, or breastbone.

sternocleidomastoid muscle   An important accessory muscle of respiration; it is a triangular muscle that connects the sternum with the clavicle and the mastoid process; also called the strap muscle.

sternum   The bony island in the center of the chest, also known as the breastbone.

subcutaneous tissue   The fatty tissue beneath the dermis of the skin; connects the skin to the underlying muscle.

superficial   Term used to describe something at or close to the top or surface.

superior   A directional term referring to a location toward the top of an object.

supination   The action of turning something, such as the hand, upward.

supine   Position in which a person is lying face up with the spine to the ground.

suprasternal notch   The notch formed where the clavicles meet the manubrium.

sutures   Immovable joints composed of connective tissues; in the skull, where the different cranial bones meet. These joints begin to fuse as a child gets older and are completely fused in an adult.

symphysis pubis   The joint at the center of the front of the pelvis where the two pubis bones meet.

systemic circuit   Refers to the circuit of blood vessels providing blood to the body's many systems; includes all of the vessels from the aorta through to the vena cava.

target organs   Specific organs that hormones are intended to work on.

tarsals   Small bones within the foot, corresponding to the carpal bones of the wrist.

temporal bone   The cranial bone that forms the base of the skull, behind and at the sides of the face.

terminal bronchioles   The smallest tubular airways leading to the alveoli.

testes   The male gonads.

thoracic cavity   The space enclosed within the ribcage, bordered inferiorly by the diaphragm; otherwise known as the chest cavity.

thoracic vertebrae   The twelve vertebrae that are found below the cervical spine and above the lumbar spine attached to the twelve sets of ribs.

tibia   The larger of the two bones in the lower leg; the shinbone.

topographic anatomy   The study of the relationship of one body part to another.

trachea   The cartilaginous tube that is the passageway for air to get from the upper airway to the lungs; also known as the windpipe.

trapezius muscle   Triangular muscle that covers the upper back and helps to lift the shoulders.

triceps muscle   The muscle in the back of the upper arm that allows elbow extension; the antagonist to the biceps muscle.

tricuspid valve   The three-cusped valve between the right atrium and right ventricle that prevents back-flow of blood.

true ribs   The first seven pairs of ribs, which attach directly to the sternum anteriorly.

ulna   The more medial bone in the forearm.

unilateral   A directional term used to describe a point to only one side of the body.

upper extremities   A term used to refer to the arms.

ureters   The muscular tubes that carry urine from the kidneys to the bladder.

uterus The female muscular organ that is commonly known as the womb. It is within this organ that a fertilized egg implants and matures into a fetus.

vagina A part of the female genitalia; it allows passage of menstrual flow or a baby during labor and serves as the conduit for the acceptance of the male penis during coitus.

veins Vessels that carry blood back to the heart, usually with deoxygenated blood.

vena cava The largest vein in the body.

ventilation Movement of air into and out of the lungs.

ventral A directional term used to describe points located in the front of the body.

ventricles The primary pump chambers of the heart.

vertebrae The individual bones of the spine.

vertebral foramen A canal formed by a ring of bone that houses the spinal cord.

visceral pleura The membrane lining the surface of the lungs.

xiphoid process The inferior portion of the sternum.

zygomatic bone The facial bone that extends anteriorly from the temporal part of the skull on each side to form the prominence of the cheeks.

PREPARATORY

Materials: AV Equipment: Utilize various audiovisual materials relating to the human body. The continuous design and development of new audiovisual materials relating to EMS requires careful review to determine which best meet the needs of the program. Materials should be edited to assure the objectives of the curriculum are met.

EMS Equipment: Anatomy models.

Personnel: Primary Instructor: One EMT-Basic instructor knowledgeable in human body systems and topographical terminology.

Recommended Minimum Time to Complete: 2.5 hours

STUDENT OUTLINE

I. Chapter Overview
II. Topographic Anatomy
    A. Lines of Reference
    B. Directional Terms
III. Anatomic Positions
IV. Range of Motion
V. The Integumentary System
VI. The Muscular System
VII. The Skeletal System
    A. The Axial Skeleton
        1. The Skull
        2. The Spinal Column
        3. The Thoracic Cage
    B. The Appendicular Skeleton
        1. The Shoulder Girdle
        2. The Arms
        3. The Pelvic Girdle
        4. The Legs
        5. The Lower Leg
        6. The Joints
VIII. The Nervous System
    A. The Central Nervous System
        1. The Brain
        2. The Spinal Cord
    B. The Peripheral Nervous System
    C. The Autonomic Nervous System
IX. The Endocrine System
X. The Circulatory System
    A. The Heart
        1. Cardiac Function

        2. Direction of Blood Flow
        3. Electrophysiology
    B. The Blood Vessels
        1. The Arteries
        2. The Veins
    C. The Blood
XI. The Respiratory System
    A. The Upper Airway
        1. The Larynx
    B. The Lower Airway
    C. The Pleura
    D. The Diaphragm
        1. Ventilation
XII. The Digestive System
    A. The Abdominal Cavity
    B. The Digestive Organs
        1. The Appendix
        2. The Liver
        3. The Pancreas
    C. The Retroperitoneal Cavity
        1. The Kidneys
XIII. The Reproductive System
    A. Male Reproductive Organs
        1. The Testes
        2. The Penis
    B. Female Reproductive Organs
        1. The Ovaries
        2. The Uterus
        3. The Vagina
XIV. Conclusion

LECTURE OUTLINE

I. Chapter Overview
    1. Anatomy is foundation of medicine
        a) Learn normal to understand
           abnormal
    2. Anatomy refers to structure
    3. Physiology refers to function
II. Topographic Anatomy
    1. Standard Anatomical Position
    2. Reference Points
        a) Landmarks
  A. Lines of Reference
    1. Imaginary Lines
    2. Reference Points
        a) Midclavicular Line
        b) Midaxillary Line
  B. Directional Terms
    1. Common Terminology
    2. Descriptive Terms
        a) Superior—Inferior
        b) Anterior—Posterior
        c) Lateral—Medial
        d) Unilateral—Bilateral
        e) Proximal—Distal
        f) Central—Peripheral
        g) Ventral—Dorsal
        h) Palmar—Plantar
        i) Apex—Base
        j) Superficial—Deep
III. Anatomic Positions
    1. Standard Positions
        a) Prone
        b) Supine
        c) Fowler's Position
        d) Modified Trendelenburg
        e) Left Lateral Recumbent
           (1) Recovery Position
IV. Range of Motion
    1. Limb Movement
        a) Extension—Flexion
        b) Abduction—Adduction
        c) Supination—Pronation
        d) Eversion—Inversion
V. The Integumentary System
    1. Skin Layers
        a) Epidermis
        b) Dermis
        c) Subcutaneous
    2. Skin Functions
        a) Protection
        b) Sensation
VI. The Muscular System
    1. Muscle Groups
        a) Chest
           (1) Sternocleidomastoid
           (2) Trapezius
           (3) Pectoralis
        b) Arm
           (1) Deltoid
           (2) Biceps
           (3) Triceps
        c) Abdomen
           (1) Diaphragm
        d) Legs
           (1) Gluteus
           (2) Quadriceps
           (3) Gastrocnemius
VII. The Skeletal System
    1. Divisions
        a) Axial
        b) Appendicular
  A. The Axial Skeleton
    1. Divisions
        a) Skull
        b) Spinal Column
        c) Thoracic
    2. The Skull
        a) Divisions
           (1) Face
               (a) Mandible
               (b) Maxillae
               (c) Zygoma
               (d) Orbits
           (2) Cranium
               (a) Frontal
               (b) Temporal
                  (i) Mastoid
                     Process
               (c) Occipital
                  (i) Foramen
                     Magnum
               (d) Parietal
           (3) Sutures
               (a) Fontanel
    3. The Spinal Column
        a) Vertebrae
           (1) Spinous Process
           (2) Intervertebral Disc
           (3) Vertebral Foramen

b) Divisions
   (1) Cervical
      (a) Atlas (C-1)
      (b) Axis (C-2)
   (2) Thoracic
      (a) Ribcage
   (3) Lumbar
      (a) Back Injury
   (4) Sacrum
      (a) Pelvis
   (5) Coccyx
      (a) Tailbone
4. The Thoracic Cage
   a) Divisions
      (1) Bony Ribs
         (a) True Ribs
            (i) Liver/Spleen
         (b) False Ribs
            (i) Costal Arch
            (ii) Costoverte-
               bral Arch
      (2) Carilage
      (3) Sternum
         (a) Body
         (b) Manubrium
            (i) Suprasternal
               Notch
            (ii) Sternal Angle
         (c) Xiphoid Process
B. The Appendicular Skeleton
   1. Divisions
      a) Shoulder Girdle
      b) Pelvic Girdle
      c) Extremities
   2. The Shoulder Girdle
      a) Clavicles
      b) Scapulas
   3. The Arms
      a) Humerus
         (1) Brachial Artery
      b) Radial
         (1) Radial Artery
      c) Ulna
      d) Hand
         (1) Carpals
         (2) Metacarpals
         (3) Phalanges
   4. The Pelvic Girdle
      a) Form
         (1) Bowl-like
      b) Function

         (1) Protection
            (a) Bowels
            (b) Bladder
      c) Divisions
         (1) Ilium
            (a) Illiac Crests or
               Wings
         (2) Ischium
            (a) Ischial Tuberosity
         (3) Pubis
            (a) Symphysis Pubis
               (i) Bladder
5. The Legs
   a) Femur
      (1) Acetabulum (hip)
   b) Patella
      (1) Dislocation
   c) Tibia
      (1) Malleolus
         (a) posterior tibial
            pulse
   d) Fibula
   e) Foot
      (1) Tarsals
         (a) Calcaneus
7. The Joints
   a) Range of Motion
VIII. The Nervous System
   1. Divisions
   A. The Central Nervous System
      1. The Brain
         a) Brainstem
            (1) Life Functions
         b) Cerebellum
            (1) Athletic Brain
         c) Cerebrum
            (1) Higher Functions
         d) Meninges
            (1) Pia Mater
               (a) Epidural
                   (i) Arteries
            (2) Dura Mater
               (a) Subdural Space
                   (i) Veins
            (3) Arachnoid
               (a) Subarachnoid
      2. The Spinal Cord
         a) Message Conduit
   B. The Peripheral Nervous System
      1. Sensation
      2. Motor Activity

3. Reflex Arc
C. The Autonomic Nervous System
  1. Automatic Functions
    a) Vital Signs
IX. The Endocrine System
  1. Equilibrium
    a) Hormones
      (1) Insulin
X. The Circulatory System
  1. Functions
    a) Transportation
    b) Elimination
  A. The Heart
    1. Cardiac Function
      a) Pump
        (1) Systemic Circulation
        (2) Pulmonary Circulation
      b) Chambers
        (1) Atrium
        (2) Ventricles
    2. Direction of Blood Flow
      a) Valves
        (1) Right/Pulmonary
          (a) Tricuspid Valve
          (b) Pulmonary Valve
        (2) Left/Systemic
          (a) Mitral
          (b) Aortic Valve
    3. Electrophysiology
      a) Conduction System
        (1) Sinoatrial (SA) Node
        (2) Internodal Pathways
        (3) Atrioventricular (AV) Node
        (4) Bundle of His
        (5) Purkinje Fibers
  B. The Blood Vessels
    1. The Arteries
      a) Away from the heart
        (1) Oxygenated Blood
          (a) Exception: Pulmonary Vein
      b) Aorta
        (1) Thoracic then abdominal
      c) Terminology
        (1) Bone Designations
    2. The Veins
      a) Toward the heart
        (1) Deoxygenated Blood
          (a) Exception: Pulmonary Artery

b) Vena Cava
  (1) Superior
    (a) Upper Body
  (2) Inferior
    (a) Lower Body
      (i) Iliac Veins—Legs
      (ii) Renal Veins—Kidneys
      (iii) Hepatic Vein—Liver
      (iv) Mesenteric—Intestines
  3. The Capillaries
    a) Bridge veins and arteries
      (1) Cellular Exchange
        (a) Oxygen–Carbon Dioxide
C. The Blood
    a) Functions
      (1) Transport
        (a) Oxygen
        (b) Glucose
      (2) Defense
        (a) White Blood Cells
      (3) Hemostasis
        (a) Coagulation
    b) Perfusion
      (1) To pour through
      (2) Hypoperfusion
        (a) Shock
XI. The Respiratory System
  A. Components
    1. Ventilation
      a) Mechanical Act
    2. Respiration
      a) Chemical Act
        (1) Diffusion of Gases
          (a) Oxygen
          (b) Carbon Dioxide
  B. Divisions
    1. The Upper Airway
      a) Functions
        (1) Filtration
        (2) Humidification
        (3) Warmth
        (4) Conduit
      b) Structures
        (1) Pharynx
          (a) Oral
          (b) Nasal

TEACHING STRATEGIES

1. Ask the students to use sticky notes and label all the bones of a skeletal model. Ask them to use any lay terms as well as the medical terms for the bones. This cross-reference will improve the ability of the EMT student to use correct terminology when describing an injury to a medical professional that was previously described by a lay person and vice versa.

2. Ask the students to take notes while watching the autopsy series in the Emergency medical update. Afterwards have the students discuss or research any unfamiliar terms.

3. Ask the students to identify the structures of the heart of a cow. A local butcher will be able to supply a cow's heart for dissection. The cow's heart is analogous to the human heart.

4. Ask the students to research a fire engine's pumping system, then compare and contrast the pumper's system to the human circulatory system. Reference the importance of fluid levels, system integrity, and the mechanical and electrical soundness of the pump itself.

5. Ask the students to mark, with nonpermanent markers, the placement of the vital organs on a model wearing a full-body stocking/suit. The accurate identification of organ location is important.

6. Ask the students to attend an autopsy at a local morgue. When the body is dissected, have the students identify the organs as well as their functions.

FURTHER STUDY

Scott, A. S., & Fong, E. (1998). *Body structures and functions* (9th ed.). Albany, NY.: Delmar/Thomson Learning.

ANSWERS TO TEST YOUR KNOWLEDGE

1. A person in the standard anatomical position is standing upright, feet slightly apart with toes pointing forward, arms slightly away from the body with the palms of the hand forward, and the body is looking forward.

2. The midline should divide the sternum into two portions along the axis of the body, creating a right and a left. To each side of the midline, the midclavicular line should divide the clavicle and divide the right and left into two equal halves. Using the lower ribcage margin as the top of the space and the pelvic floor as the bottom and the two flanks as the two sides respectively, an imaginary box should be created. Using the umbilicus as the center, the box should be divided into four equal sections, or quadrants and labels left or right and lower or upper quadrant accordingly.

3. The wrist injury is on the dorsal surface of the arm proximal to the wrist and distal to the elbow.

4. The most important function of the skin is protection from the environment.

5. The bones of the cervical spine are named according to their place from top to bottom, that is, C-1,C-2, etc. The first cervical vertebra is called the atlas and the second vertebra is called the axis.

6. The bones of the appendicular skeleton are the bones of the pelvic girdle and shoulder girdle and the limbs attached to them. The shoulder girdle consists of the scapula and the clavicle. The upper extremity attaches to the shoulder girdle. Starting from the shoulder, there is the humerus, the radius, the ulna, the carpals, the metacarpals, and the phalanages. The pelvic girdle consists of the ischium, the illium, and pubis, which together create a ring. Inserted into the pelvic ring is the femur, at the hip. Below the femur are the tibia and fibula. In front of the joint created by the joining of these three bones is the patella, also known as the kneecap. Finally, the feet are like the hands and have tarsals, metatarsals, and phalanges.

7. The nervous system provides the muscles and organs control and coordination, permitting such vital life functions as breathing and heartbeat as well as mobility.

8. The upper airway is called the pharnyx, which is composed of three portions, the nasopharynx (the

nose), the oropharynx (the mouth), and the hypopharnyx (the back of the throat). The pharynx becomes the trachea (windpipe) at the larynx (voicebox). Below the larynx is sometimes referred to as the mainstem bronchus. The mainstem bronchus is the start of the lower airway. The mainstem bronchus divides into the right and left mainstem bronchi, then keeps dividing into smaller sections until the terminal bronchioles become the alveoli. It is at the alveoli that oxygen and carbon dioxide exchange occurs.

9. Insulin is the hormone that is responsible for the metabolism of sugar.

10. Starting at the heart, all blood vessels leaving the heart are called arteries. The arteries subdivide into smaller vessels, called arterioles, until they become capillaries. The single-cell-layer-thick capillary allows oxygen and carbon dioxide to exchange. As capillaries start to rejoin they become venules, which eventually become veins and return the blood to the heart.

11. The central organs of digestion include the pharnyx, the esophagus, the stomach, the small intestine, and the large intestine. Accessory organs of digestion include the pancreas and liver, which store their secretions in the gallbladder.

12. The kidneys filter waste and excess fluid from the circulation, creating urine in the process.

13. The male gonads are the testes, which create sperm and the hormone testosterone. The female gonads are the ovaries, which contain the eggs and create the hormones estrogen and progesterone.

CHAPTER 6

Infection Control

OBJECTIVES

Upon completion of this chapter, the reader should be able to:

1. Explain the importance of infection control.
2. List a few of the elements of OSHA 1910.1030.
3. List five of the more common infectious illnesses an EMT may encounter.
4. Explain the different modes of disease transmission.
5. Explain what is meant by the term portal of entry.
6. List possible personal defenses against infectious disease transmission.
7. Define what is meant by the term personal protective equipment.
8. Define the term standard precautions.
9. Describe the methods of infection control used for typical medical procedures performed by EMTs.
10. List the different levels of disinfection.
11. Explain what an infection control plan is and where it can be found.
12. Explain the importance of documenting a potential infectious disease exposure.
13. Describe how notification laws affect the EMT.
14. Describe what is proper medical follow-up for an infectious disease exposure.

GLOSSARY

antibody   Specialized defense particle within the blood that helps to protect against foreign material.

biohazard   Short for "biological hazard," this term refers to any material that is considered unsafe because of contamination with body fluids.

body substance isolation   Protecting oneself from unnecessary exposure by avoiding direct contact with any body substance that may be infectious.

carrier   Someone who carries an infectious microorganism; she or he does not necessarily become ill from it, but can transmit it to someone else.

contagious   The state of an illness when the affected person can transmit it to others.

decontamination   Removal of potentially hazardous substances by either chemical or physical means.

designated officer (DO)   A specific person within an EMS agency who is responsible for receiving notifications of potential exposures and following up as appropriate.

direct contact   Actually coming into direct contact with the infectious material on a person.

immunity   Insusceptibility to a specific illness, usually as a result of prior exposure or immunization.

immunization   The process of exposing the body to or inoculating it with weakened pathogens in order to allow it to create specific antibodies.

immunocompromise   Lack of disease resistance.

indirect contact   Exposure to an infectious agent that is on a nonhuman surface.

infection control   Taking preventive measures to lessen the likelihood of disease transmission in the workplace.

microorganism   A tiny living creature that is visible only by microscope.

mucous membranes   A porous tissue lined with blood vessels that creates a liquid that serves to wash away foreign material. The surfaces of the respiratory and gastrointestinal tracts that are regularly in contact with the outside environment are examples of mucous membranes.

Pathogen   A disease-causing organism, such as a virus or a bacterium.

personal protective equipment (PPE)   Gear that may be used by a health care provider to protect against exposure or injury.

portal of entry   The route that an organism uses to enter the body.

prophylaxis   Doing something to prevent an unwanted outcome.

risk management   Actions geared toward protection from hazard.

risk profile   The likelihood of the presence of a disease in a person or group of people.

Ryan White law   States that a hospital is required to notify an EMS agency if its staff identifies an infectious illness that the agency's employees may have been exposed to.

safety officer (SO)   A designated person who is charged with knowledge of relevant CDC, OSHA, and NFPA regulations and standards regarding safety.

sharps   Instruments with a sharp point such as needles, syringes, and sharp blades.

sharps container   A puncture-proof container used to dispose of needles and other sharp instruments; usually red with a biohazard sign.

standard precautions   Refers to the personal protective equipment used routinely in certain circumstances.

sterilization   Thorough cleaning of an item so that all microorganisms are completely removed.

transmission   The transfer of an infectious agent from one source to another.

vector   An organism that carries a disease from one source to another, where it can result in infection.

PREPARATORY

Materials: EMS Equipment: None.

Personnel: Primary Instructor: One EMT-Basic instructor knowledgeable in infection control and related safety issues as well as the roles and responsibilities of the EMT-Basic.

Time: Recommended Minimum Time to Complete: 1.5 hours

STUDENT OUTLINE

I. Infection Control
    A. Personal Safety
    B. Patient Safety
    C. Family Safety
II. Legal Obligations
    A. The Safety Officer
III. Causes of Disease
IV. Disease Transmission
    A. Contact Transmission
    B. Vehicle Transmission
    C. Vector-Borne Transmission
V. Portal of Entry
VI. Susceptibility to Disease
    A. Defense Against Disease
    B. Handwashing
    C. Personal Protective Equipment
    D. Barrier Devices
        a) Gloves
        b) Goggles
        c) Masks
        d) Pocket Mask
        e) Gowns
        1. Donning and Removing Protective Apparel
VII. Preparing for Infection Control
    A. House Rules
    B. Responding to a Call
    C. Arrival On-Scene
        1. Needle Disposal
        2. Waste Disposal
    A. After the Call
        1. Documentation
        2. Cleaning Up
            a) Emergency Equipment Cleanup
            b) Cleaning Areas
        3. Cleaning The Ambulance
X. Reporting Exposure
XI. Notification by Employer
XII. Conclusion

LECTURE OUTLINE

I. Infection Control
    A. Personal Safety
        1. Risk Management
        2. Risk Profile
    B. Patient Safety
        1. Immunocompromised Patient
    C. Family Safety
        1. Carrier States

II. Legal Obligations
        1. CDC Guidelines
        2. OSHA Mandates
        3. NFPA Recommendations
    A. The Safety Officer
        1. Designated by Command

III. Causes of Disease
        1. Microorganisms
            a) Fungus
            b) Bacteria
            c) Virus

IV. Disease Transmission
        1. Direct Contact
        2. Indirect Contact
    A. Contact Transmission
        1. Airborne Droplets
        2. Surfaces
    B. Vehicle Transmission
        1. Water Carrier
        2. Food Carrier
    C. Vector-Borne Transmission
        1. Vector
            a) Ticks

V. Portal of Entry
        1. Mucous Membrane
        2. Broken Skin

VI. Susceptibility to Disease
        1. Virulence
        2. Resistance
        3. Infection
            a) Contagion
               (1) Isolation
    A. Defense Against Disease
        1. Host Defenses
            a) Intact Skin
            b) Mucous Membranes
            c) Health
               (1) Immunizations
    B. Handwashing
        1. Single Best Personal Protection

            a) Before and After Patient Contact
    C. Personal Protective Equipment
        1. Dress Up Philosophy
            a) Body Substance Isolation
               (1) Potentially Infectious Materials
            b) Standard Precautions
    D. Barrier Devices
        1. Gloves
            a) Sterile versus Non-sterile
            b) Fitting
            c) Latex Allergies
        2. Goggles
            a) Contact by Splash
            b) Eye Protection
               (1) Splash Guards
        3. Masks
            a) Inhalation exposure
            b) N95 Masks
        4. Pocket Mask
            a) Shields
            b) Pocket Mask
        5. Gowns
            a) Splash Protection
               (1) Limited use for special cases
            b) Paper versus Cloth
    E. Donning and Removing Protective Apparel
        1. Practice

VII. Preparing for Infection Control
        1. Infection Control Plan
        2. PPE Supply Check
    A. House Rules
        1. Good health practices
    B. Responding to a Call
    C. Arrival On-Scene
        1. Complaint-based PPE
        2. Task-oriented PPE
            a) Needle Disposal
               (1) Sharps
               (2) Sharps Container
        3. Disposal of Waste
               (1) Biohazardous waste
                  (a) Red Bags
    A. After the Call
        1. Documentation
        2. Cleaning Up

a) Decontamination
    (1) Sterilization
a) Emergency Equipment
    Cleanup
    (2) Disinfection
    b) Cleaning Areas
    3. Cleaning the Ambulance
VIII. Reporting Exposure

A. OSHA Regulations
B. Medical Examination
    1. Prophylaxis
IX. Notification by Employer
    A. Ryan White Law
      1. Designated Officer
X. Conclusion

TEACHING STRATEGIES

1. Contact the local county health department or a local hospital and ask the epidemiologist to speak to the class. The epidemiologist should have information on current outbreaks of disease as well as efforts to control them. Ask the epidemiologist to explain the services of either the infection control department or the health department. Last, ask the how the designated officer works with the county or hospital epidemiologist to protect the EMT.

2. Have the students pretend there is an outbreak of "Arctic flu" in the community. Have the students describe, in writing or via flowchart, how they would be notified if they were exposed and how they would notify authorities if they felt they had an exposure.

3. Have the students create a chart that lists typical EMS tasks and the personal protective equipment (PPE) that would be worn while performing that task.

4. Invite a surgical nurse to demonstrate scrubbing and gowning. Ask the nurse to explain aseptic techniques. Ask the nurse what personal protective equipment would be used in the operating room for similar tasks in the field.

FURTHER STUDY

Angle, J. S. (1999). *Occupational safety and health in the emergency services.* Albany, NY: Delmar-Thomson Learning.

A curriculum guide for public safety and emergency response workers. (1989). Washington, DC: U.S. Department of Health and Human Services.

Silent war, infection control for emergency responders. (1992). On guard: training for life. Fort Collins, CO.

Guide to developing and managing an emergency service infection control program. (1992). Emmitsburg, MD: U.S. Fire Administration.

CASE STUDY WORKPLACE EXPOSURE

"It was when we were transferring the patient over to the hospital stretcher that I got the blood on me," Don explained to the emergency physician Dr. Bosco.

The patient had cut his wrists in an apparent suicide attempt. The first responding engine company had bandaged the wrists securely before the ambulance arrived and helped the crew secure the combative patient to the gurney. The patient was then transported to the local hospital for a medical evaluation. Sam, Don's partner, rode with the patient while Don drove. Don took off his gloves before he started to drive.

When they arrived at the hospital, the crew unloaded the stretcher and took the patient to the triage area. She advised them isolation room 1-A was prepped and ready.

As they rolled the gurney into the room, the patient immediately started to buck and pull at his restraints. It took an orderly, a nurse, and the two EMTs to move him over to the stretcher.

That's when it happened. Don was holding the patient's wrists when the bandages slipped. Blood started spurting all over the place and all over Don's bare arms. They quickly finished restraining the patient, and the nurse reinforced the original bandages to control the bleeding.

Don immediately washed his hands and then went out to the desk to speak with the doctor.

STOP AND THINK

1. Why is this EMT concerned?
2. What could he have done to prevent this from happening?

ANSWERS TO STOP AND THINK

1. The EMT could be potentially exposed to and could acquire a bloodborne disease.
2. A barrier device, such as gloves, could have limited or eliminated his exposure to the infectious source, in this case, the blood.

CASE STUDY POTENTIAL FOR EXPOSURE

The call was for a "woman in labor." This was the fourth pregnacy for this mother, and she was telling the crew that she was "ready." The question that the crew had was, were they ready?

Helping the mother to an overstuffed chair, an EMT confirmed that the baby was "crowning" and they had better prepare to deliver the infant right there.

Following local protocols, one EMT contacted medical control via the telephone, another prepared the birthing kit, and still another donned personal protective equipment. A paramedic had to be requested to the scene in the event the delivery became complicated or the infant needed advanced-level care.

Everyone was ready, and the delivery went naturally. It was a baby girl. The mother and child were transported, without lights or siren, to the birthing center, and the crew went back into service.

Back at the station, as the crew cleaned up, the captain came out and affixed a pink stork emblem to the front quarter panel of the ambulance.

STOP AND THINK

1. What body substances might an EMT encounter during childbirth? Are they potentially infectious?
2. What protective equipment should be utilized for this type of call?
3. What postcall activities must occur?
4. How would an EMT report a suspected infectious disease exposure?

ANSWERS TO STOP AND THINK

1. The EMT might encounter blood, amniotic fluid, urine, feces, sputum, and vomitus. Each fluid is capable of harboring an infection.

2. The EMT attending the patient should be wearing a gown, mask, eye protection, and gloves.

3. All of the disposable supplies should be placed in a container marked for biohazardous materials. The scalpel used to cut the umbilical cord should be placed in a sharps container. The rest of the soiled equipment should be washed and decontaminated.

4. If EMTs suspects they may have an infectious disease exposure, they should follow the instructions found in the infection control manual. The EMTs should then contact their designated officer, or safety officer, as soon as possible.

ANSWERS TO TEST YOUR KNOWLEDGE

1. Infection control helps prevent the spread of disease from the patient to the EMT, from the EMT to the patient, from the EMT to the community, and from the EMT to the EMT's family.

2. EMTs typically are exposed to childhood diseases, such as chicken pox and measles, as well as dermatological conditions like scabies and lice. If blood or body fluids are spilled on the EMT, the EMT may contract human immunodeficiency virus (HIV), hepatitis B (HBV), hepatitis C (HCV), or syphilis.

3. The three major modes of disease transmission are contact, vector, and vehicle. Direct contact with contaminated surfaces can transmit some diseases. Mosquitoes are the vectors that transmit diseases like malaria. Airborne and water droplets are the most common modes of disease transmission.

4. A portal of entry is an entrance for disease into the body that is not protected by skin or mucous membranes.

5. Personal protective equipment, for infectious disease prevention, should include a gown, mask, gloves, and protective eyewear or goggles.

6. Standard precautions assume that all body substances are potentially infectious and therefore personal protective equipment must be worn to prevent contact with these substances.

7. The lowest level of disinfection is low-level disinfection, typically accomplished with soap and water. Intermediate and high-level disinfection is used for gross contamination. Sterilization is the highest level of disinfection, killing all microorganisms as well as their spores.

8. An infection control plan is a strategy to decrease or eliminate disease transmission to an EMT. Every EMS agency should have an infection control plan that is readily available at all times.

9. Reporting a potential disease exposure ensures that the EMT will have prompt medical care now and in the future.

10. Notification laws, such as the Ryan White law, protect EMTs by ensuring their prompt notification in cases of potential infectious disease exposure.

11. Medical follow-up, whether with a private physician or employee health services, should follow the guidelines provided by the federal Centers for Disease Control in Atlanta. Typically, there is a notification of suspected exposure, an investigation that may include blood tests, and a follow-up phase where the EMT is either discharged or entered in the health care system as a patient.

Student Name: _____ Date: _____

Skill: Handwashing
Equipment Needed:
1. Liquid Soap
2. Paper Hand Towels
3. Sink

YES: _____   RE-TEACH: _____   RETURN: _____   INSTRUCTOR INITIALS _____

Step 1: Turn on the water and adjust it to a comfortable temperature. The water should flow freely

YES: _____   RE-TEACH: _____   RETURN: _____   INSTRUCTOR INITIALS _____

Step 2: Liberally apply the liquid soap. Bar soap should be avoided because this type of soap harbors bacteria.

YES: _____   RE-TEACH: _____   RETURN: _____   INSTRUCTOR INITIALS _____

Step 3: Scrub vigorously, rubbing hands together to create friction. Particular attention should be paid to the space in between the fingers and the area under the nails. Skin underneath rings and watches should also be cleaned. Scrub for at least one minute.

YES: _____   RE-TEACH: _____   RETURN: _____   INSTRUCTOR INITIALS _____

Step 4: Rinse from wrists, allowing soap and water to drip off fingertips.

YES: _____   RE-TEACH: _____   RETURN: _____   INSTRUCTOR INITIALS _____

Step 5: Dry hands with either a paper towel or air blower.

YES: _____   RE-TEACH: _____   RETURN: _____   INSTRUCTOR INITIALS _____

Step 6: Turn off faucet with clean towel.

YES: _____   RE-TEACH: _____   RETURN: _____   INSTRUCTOR INITIALS _____

Student Name: _____   Date: _____

Skill: Donning Gloves
Equipment Needed:
1. Nonsterile Gloves
2. Hazardous Waste Container

YES: _____   RE-TEACH: _____   RETURN: _____   INSTRUCTOR INITIALS _____

Step 1: Choose an appropriate size and type of glove for the task at hand.

YES: _____   RE-TEACH: _____   RETURN: _____   INSTRUCTOR INITIALS _____

Step 2: Arrange one glove so that the thumb is aligned with the thumb of the hand it is intended to go on.

YES: _____   RE-TEACH: _____   RETURN: _____   INSTRUCTOR INITIALS _____

Step 3: Grasp the front of the cuff with one hand, while sliding the other hand into the glove. Be sure to place each finger in the appropriate finger section.

YES: _____   RE-TEACH: _____   RETURN: _____   INSTRUCTOR INITIALS _____

Step 4: Pull at the cuff to ensure that the glove is completely applied to the hand.

YES: _____   RE-TEACH: _____   RETURN: _____   INSTRUCTOR INITIALS _____

Step 5: Repeat the process for the other hand.

YES: _____   RE-TEACH: _____   RETURN: _____   INSTRUCTOR INITIALS _____

Student Name: _____   Date: _____

Skill: Removal of Contaminated Gloves

Step 1: Grasp the palm of the left glove with the gloved right hand.

YES: _____   RE-TEACH: _____   RETURN: _____   INSTRUCTOR INITIALS _____

Step 2: Pull the left glove toward the fingertips. The glove should turn inside out as it is removed.

YES: _____   RE-TEACH: _____   RETURN: _____   INSTRUCTOR INITIALS _____

Step 3: Hold the removed glove in the still gloved right hand.

YES: _____   RE-TEACH: _____   RETURN: _____   INSTRUCTOR INITIALS _____

Step 4: Place two fingers of the ungloved left hand under the cuff of the right glove, carefully avoiding any contaminated areas.

YES: _____   RE-TEACH: _____   RETURN: _____   INSTRUCTOR INITIALS _____

Step 5: Pull the right glove toward the fingertips, turning it inside out as it is removed.

YES: _____   RE-TEACH: _____   RETURN: _____   INSTRUCTOR INITIALS _____

Step 6: Completely remove the right glove, with the balled up left glove remaining inside the right glove as it is removed.

YES: _____   RE-TEACH: _____   RETURN: _____   INSTRUCTOR INITIALS _____

Step 7: Dispose of the gloves in an approved biohazard container.

YES: _____   RE-TEACH: _____   RETURN: _____   INSTRUCTOR INITIALS _____

Step 8: Wash hands thoroughly.

YES: _____   RE-TEACH: _____   RETURN: _____   INSTRUCTOR INITIALS _____

Student Name: _____   Date: _____

Skill: Donning a Gown and Mask

Equipment Needed:

1. Gown
2. Disposable Mask
3. Hazardous Waste Container/Laundry Bin

YES: _____   RE-TEACH: _____   RETURN: _____   INSTRUCTOR INITIALS _____

Step 1: Select an appropriate mask and eye protection for the task at hand.

YES: _____   RE-TEACH: _____   RETURN: _____   INSTRUCTOR INITIALS _____

Step 2: Fit the top of the mask to the bridge of the nose by squeezing on the flexible metal nosepiece within the mask.

YES: _____   RE-TEACH: _____   RETURN: _____   INSTRUCTOR INITIALS _____

Step 3: Pull the remainder of the mask to cover the chin. Assure that the mask covers the nose and mouth with no gaps anywhere around the face and that the eyes are not covered except by the transparent eye shield.

YES: _____   RE-TEACH: _____   RETURN: _____   INSTRUCTOR INITIALS _____

Step 4: Tie the mask ties at the top of the head and at the base of the skull to assure a snug fit of the mask.

YES: _____   RE-TEACH: _____   RETURN: _____   INSTRUCTOR INITIALS _____

Step 5: If not a part of the chosen mask, apply appropriate eye protection.

YES: _____   RE-TEACH: _____   RETURN: _____   INSTRUCTOR INITIALS _____

Step 6: Select an appropriate gown for the task at hand.

YES: _____   RE-TEACH: _____   RETURN: _____   INSTRUCTOR INITIALS _____

Step 7: Hold the gown up with the inside facing you and the top of the gown up.

YES: _____   RE-TEACH: _____   RETURN: _____   INSTRUCTOR INITIALS _____

Step 8: Place one arm, then the other, into the gown, pulling the neck of the gown up against your neck.

YES: _____   RE-TEACH: _____   RETURN: _____   INSTRUCTOR INITIALS _____

Step 9: Reach around behind your neck and tie the neck ties snugly.

YES: _____   RE-TEACH: _____   RETURN: _____   INSTRUCTOR INITIALS _____

Step 10: Reach around behind your waist and tie the waist ties snugly. If this is not feasible, ask a partner to tie the waist ties for you.

YES: _____   RE-TEACH: _____   RETURN: _____   INSTRUCTOR INITIALS _____

Student Name: _____   Date: _____

Skill: Removal of Contaminated Mask and Gown

Step 1: After removal of contaminated gloves, the EMT should untie (or break if a paper gown) the waist and neck ties of the gown. If the gown is grossly contaminated, the EMT should ask a partner to do this to avoid contamination of ungloved hands.

YES: _____   RE-TEACH: _____   RETURN: _____   INSTRUCTOR INITIALS _____

Step 2: With the left hand, grasp the right neckline of the gown, as close to the shoulder as can be done without contamination, and pull the gown off the front of the body.

YES: _____   RE-TEACH: _____   RETURN: _____   INSTRUCTOR INITIALS _____

Step 3: As the gown is pulled forward, it should be removed from the right arm.

YES: _____   RE-TEACH: _____   RETURN: _____   INSTRUCTOR INITIALS _____

Step 4: The ungloved right hand can then grasp the uncontaminated inner surface of the gown and pull it off the left arm.

YES: _____   RE-TEACH: _____   RETURN: _____   INSTRUCTOR INITIALS _____

Step 5: Being careful to touch only the uncontaminated inner surface of the gown, the EMT should roll the gown up and dispose of it in the appropriate hazardous waste container.

YES: _____   RE-TEACH: _____   RETURN: _____   INSTRUCTOR INITIALS _____

Step 6: Reaching behind the head, the EMT should untie, or tear, the ties from the mask.

YES: _____   RE-TEACH: _____   RETURN: _____   INSTRUCTOR INITIALS _____

Step 7: The mask should be held by the uncontaminated ties and pulled away from the face.

YES: _____   RE-TEACH: _____   RETURN: _____   INSTRUCTOR INITIALS _____

Step 8: The contaminated mask should be disposed of in the proper hazardous waste container.

YES: _____   RE-TEACH: _____   RETURN: _____   INSTRUCTOR INITIALS _____

CHAPTER 7

Basic Airway Control

OBJECTIVES

Upon completion of this chapter, the reader should be able to:

1. Name and label on a diagram the major structures of the respiratory system.
2. Describe the steps in performing the head-tilt, chin-lift.
3. Relate mechanism of injury to methods of opening the airway.
4. Describe the steps in performing the jaw-thrust.
5. State the importance of having a suction unit ready for immediate use when providing emergency care.
6. Describe the technique of suctioning.
7. Describe how to measure and use an oropharyngeal (oral) airway.
8. Describe how to measure and use a nasopharyngeal (nasal) airway.

GLOSSARY

airway   The passageway for air movement into and out of the lungs.

apnea   Lack of breathing; breathlessness.

cyanosis   A bluish discoloration to the skin seen with poor oxygen content of the blood.

epiglottis   A cartilaginous structure at the base of the tongue that helps to protect the airway during swallowing.

esophagus   The muscular tubelike structure that passes food from the mouth to the stomach.

French catheter   A flexible suction catheter used when suctioning through an endotracheal tube or via the nasopharynx.

gag reflex   The protective response that a person has when the back of the throat is stimulated by the presence of a foreign substance.

head-tilt, chin-lift   Method used to open the airway involving tilting the head back and lifting the jaw up; used only in nontrauma patients.

jaw-thrust   A technique that lifts the mandible and tongue up and away from the pharynx, often effective in opening the airway; is used on trauma patients with suspected spinal injury.

larynx   The voicebox or sound-producing portion of the throat.

mandible   The lower jawbone.

maxilla   The upper jawbone.

nasal flaring   Widening of the nostrils during breathing; a sign of increased respiratory effort commonly seen in children.

nasopharyngeal airway (NPA)   A flexible tube passed through the nose into the pharynx that can help to hold the tongue off the back of the throat and keep the airway open; also called a nasal airway.

occlusion   A blockage.

oropharyngeal airway (OPA)   A plastic device placed in the mouth to assist in keeping the tongue off the back of the throat and keeping the airway open; also called an oral airway.

pharynx   Back of the throat.

recovery position   The position in which the patient is on her or his side so that secretions may spontaneously drain from the airway; also known as the coma position.

saliva   Normally occurring secretions from the mouth.

sputum   Secretions formed in the airways.

sublingual   Under the tongue.

tonsils   Pillars of soft tissue on each side of the back of the throat.

trachea   The windpipe.

uvula   A small piece of tissue that is seen hanging off the roof of the mouth in the pharynx.

ventilation   The process of moving air into and out of the lungs; breathing.

Yankauer catheter   A rigid suction catheter that has a curvature that is meant to follow the pharyngeal curve and a large open suction tip.

PREPARATORY

Materials: AV Equipment: Utilize various audiovisual materials relating to airway management. The continuous design and development of new audiovisual materials relating to EMS requires careful review to determine which best meet the needs of the program. Materials should be edited to assure the objectives of the curriculum are met.

EMS Equipment: Pocket mask, bag-valve mask, flow-restricted, oxygen-powered ventilation device, oral airways, nasal airways, suction units, suction catheters, oxygen tank, regulator, nonrebreather mask, nasal cannula, tongue blade, and lubricant.

Personnel Primary Instructor: One EMT-Basic instructor knowledgeable in airway management.

Assistant Instructor: The instructor-to-student ratio should be 1:6 for psychomotor skill practice. Individuals used as assistant instructors should be knowledgeable in airway techniques and management.

Recommended Minimum Time to Complete: 4 hours

STUDENT OUTLINE

I. Chapter Overview

II. Anatomy Review

III. Physiology

    A. Personal Protective Equipment

IV. Open

    A. Signs of an Obstructed Airway

    B. Proper Positioning

        1. Head-Tilt, Chin-Lift

        2. Jaw-Thrust

V. Assess

VI. Suction

    A. The Suction Machine

        1. The Catheter

        2. Setup

        3. The Procedure

VII. Secure

    A. The Oropharnygeal Airway

        1. Using the OPA

    B. The Nasopharyngeal Airway

VIII. Conclusion

LECTURE OUTLINE

I. Airway Control
   A. Truly Lifesaving
   B. Most Common Obstruction
      1. Tongue
   C. Procedure Simple
      1. Open
      2. Assess
      3. Suction
      4. Secure

II. Anatomy Review
   A. Oropharnyx
      1. Teeth
      2. Mandible
      3. Maxilla
   B. Pharynx
      1. Uvula
      2. Tonsils
      3. Tongue
         a) Sublingual area
   C. Hypopharynx
      1. Esophagus
      2. Larynx
         a) Epiglottis

III. Physiology
   A. Airway as a Part of Respiration
      1. Ventilation necessary
         a) Oxygenation of blood
      2. Patent airway is start of ventilation
   B. Personal Protective Equipment
      1. Eye protection important
         a) Airborne droplets
      2. Mask
         a) Airborne droplets

IV. Open
   A. Proper Positioning
      1. Passive control
         a) Recovery Position
      2. Active control
         a) Head-Tilt, Chin-Lift
            (1) Rule out spinal injury
         b) Jaw-Thrust
            (1) Tongue attached to mandible

V. Assess
   A. Signs of an obstructed airway
      1. Snoring
      2. Apnea
      3. Cyanosis
   B. Causes

      1. Dentures
         a) Platform for mask seal
      2. Foreign body airway obstruction
         b) Heimlich Maneuver
            (1) Adults only

VI. Suction
   A. Manual
      1. Two-finger sweep
         a) Biteblock
            (1) Oral airway between molars
   B. Mechanical
      1. Machine categories
         a) manual
            (1) Hand-powered
            (2) Foot-powered
         b) electric
            (1) Portable
            (2) On-board
      2. Machine parts
         a) collection chamber
         b) tubing
         c) catheter
            (1) Yankauer
            (2) French
   C. Setup
      1. Assemble equipment
      2. Bowl of water at standby
         a) Clear tip of debris
   D. The Suction Procedure
      1. Preoxygenate
      2. Premeasure insertion depth
         a) Center of the jaw to the angle of the jaw
      3. Insert with suction off
         a) Only as far as can be seen
      4. Withdraw with suction applied
         a) No longer than 10 to 15 seconds

VI. Secure
   A. Oral Airway
      1. Styles
         a) Guedel
         b) Berman
      2. Measure
         a) Center of jaw to angle of jaw
      3. Insertion
         a) Standard
            (1) Start upside down

                     (2) Rotate 180 degrees dur-
                         ing insertion
                 b) Trauma or Pediatric
                     (1) Use tongue blade to
                         push tongue down
                     (2) Insert straight
        B. Nasal Airway
            1. Styles
                 a) Clear plastic
                 b) Rubber
            2. Measure
                 a) Nostril to earlobe
            3. Insertion

                 a) Examine nares for patency
                     (1) Left usually used
                 b) Lubricate nasal airway
                     (1) Water-soluble gel
                 c) Insert straight into skull
                     (1) Stop
                         (a) pain
                         (b) resistance
                     (2) Retry other nostril
    VII. Conclusion
        A. Airway control is first priority
        B. Adjuncts do not replace manual control
        C. Procedure is Open, Assess, Suction,
            Secure

TEACHING STRATEGIES

1. Have the students use an AMBU™ cut-away airway model to demonstrate the measurement and placement of the oropharyngeal and nasophyaryngeal airways.

2. Have the students pair off and demonstrate a head-tilt, chin-lift airway maneuver on each other. Have the students then perform a jaw-thrust maneuver. When a jaw-thrust maneuver is properly performed on a conscious patient it should create some discomfort for the student-patient.

3. Assign the students to research a mechanical suction device (either an electrical, manual, or oyxgen-powered machine) using the Internet. Then ask the students to defend the use of that device in the field, including pros and cons.

4. Have the students research the history of the Berman and the Geudel oral airways. The students should be prepared to discuss the pros and cons of each airway.

FURTHER STUDY

American Red Cross. (1993). *Cardiopulmonary resuscitation for the professional rescuer.*
Metcalf, W., & McSwain, N. (1999). *Professional rescuer CPR.* Jones & Bartlett.
Scott, A., & Fong, E.,(1998). *Body structures and functions.* (9th ed.). Albany, NY: Delmar-Thompson Learning.

CASE STUDY   HE'S NOT BREATHING

The phone rang, and a frantic voice at the other end cried, "Come quick! Brian's not breathing!" Dan, the resident adviser for the dorm, quickly called campus public safety and reported a possible medical emergency in room 951.

Dan was an EMT back in his hometown of Spring Valley, so he knew that he could help. He grabbed his first aid bag and ran up the nine flights of stairs.

Stopping long enough to catch his breath, Dan looked into the room. He saw Brian, a freshman, lying unconscious on the floor next to the couch. Looking around the room he quickly concluded that there had been a dorm party. Dozens of empty beer bottles were scattered on the floor, and a couple of half-empty whisky bottles were on the table. Everyone was huddled against the far wall.

Brian had obviously been laid on the floor. His head had been propped up on a pillow, and he was making a loud snoring sound. As Dan approached Brian, donning gloves in the process, he was suddenly struck by the smell of vomit.

STOP AND THINK

1. Why is Brian snoring? What are the implications of smelling vomit?
2. What can Dan do, alone, to help Brian?
3. Assume that Brian was semiconscious. Would his being semiconscious change how Dan would manage the patient?

ANSWERS TO STOP AND THINK

1. The most likely source of Brian's snoring is a partially occluded airway. The most likely source of that partial occlusion is Brian's tongue. The smell of vomitus raises the possibility that Brian has vomited and may have aspirated into his lungs.

2. Assuming no spinal injury, Dan should roll Brian onto his side, in left lateral recumbent or recovery position, and allow his airway to drain by gravity.

3. A semiconscious patient cannot tolerate an oral airway. The oral airway stimulates the gag reflex and the patient could potentially vomit and aspirate. If Brian was semiconscious, Dan should consider the use of a nasal airway instead.

ADDITIONAL CASE STUDY

"Come quickly, hurry! People are hurt!" cried the caller over the telephone. The 9-1-1 dispatcher calmly advised the cell phone caller that help was on the way. Even as she spoke, the tones were being sent out to activate pagers for the local volunteer rescue squad.

"Ambulance 24, medic fifteen, and Milford fire department, reported motor vehicle collision on old Route 57 near the Parson's place. Persons reported trapped, one man unconscious. Time 15:40."

Jennifer ran into the bay and grabbed the mike to announce, "Medcom, ambulance 24 acknowledging the call." Knowing it was a motor vehicle collision, Jennifer quickly grabbed the turnout gear off the rack.

An unconscious patient, Jennifer thought, needs airway control. What do I need for equipment?

STOP AND THINK

1. How does the fact that the patient is unconscious impact on the state of the airway?
2. What equipment will be needed?
3. What personal protective equipment will be needed?
4. Can an airway be controlled without equipment?

ANSWERS TO STOP AND THINK

1. An unconscious patient is unable to control his or her airway without positioning and/or manual support.

2. Minimally, Jennifer should have personal protective equipment, portable suction, a complete set of airways, including both oral and nasal airways, and a tongue blade.

3. Because of the risk of projectile vomiting, Jennifer should be minimally wearing eye protection, a mask, and gloves.

4. All airway equipment should be considered as an adjunct for, not a replacement of, manual airway techniques. In this case, because of the potential of cervical spine injury due to trauma, the EMT should perform a jaw-thrust maneuver.

ANSWERS TO TEST YOUR KNOWLEDGE

1. After donning appropriate personal protective equipment, the EMT would position himself beside the supine patient's head and place the ulnar surface of the palm against the forehead. Next the EMT would grasp the patient's chin with the thumb and index finger of the other hand in a pincer movement. The EMT would apply a downward pressure to the forehead while simultaneously lifting the chin up, thereby changing the axis of the head and opening the airway.

2. The jaw-thrust is the preferred manual airway maneuver whenever there is suspicion of cervical spine injury.

3. After donning appropriate personal protective equipment, the EMT would position herself at the top of the supine patient's head and place her index finger at the angle of the jaw and then line her other fingers along the jaw's line. The EMT would then place her thumbs on the corresponding cheekbone. Using a pincer type of movement, the EMT would lift the jaw upwards, opening the airway in the process.

4. Some EMTs, as a matter of routine, do not bring the portable mechanical suction, either electric or oxygen-powered, into a residence. As a result, when the patient unexpectedly vomits, the EMT is faced with a possible aspiration risk without the benefit of portable mechanical suction.

5. Prolonged suctioning can lead to hypoxia.

6. An oral airway is measured from the angle of the jaw to the tip of the chin.

7. Using the cross-finger technique and gently rotating the airway into position, direct insertion via tongue blade.

8. The nasal airway does not stimulate the patient's gag reflex whereas the oral airway can, thereby creating an aspiration risk.

9. The nasal airway is measured from the nostril to the earlobe.

Student Name: _____ Date: _____

Skill: Head-Tilt, Chin-Lift Maneuver
Equipment Assembled:
1. Gloves
2. Goggles
3. Mask

YES: _____   RE-TEACH: _____   RETURN: _____   INSTRUCTOR INITIALS _____

Step 1: After donning the appropriate PPE, the EMT positions himself at the side of the patient's head.
YES: _____   RE-TEACH: _____   RETURN: _____   INSTRUCTOR INITIALS _____

Step 2: The palm of one hand is placed on the patient's forehead and the fingertips of the other hand on the patient's jaw.
YES: _____   RE-TEACH: _____   RETURN: _____   INSTRUCTOR INITIALS _____

Step 3: The patient's head is tilted back using firm pressure on the forehead. Care should be taken not to push backward on the jaw, as this will only force the patient's mouth closed.
YES: _____   RE-TEACH: _____   RETURN: _____   INSTRUCTOR INITIALS _____

Step 4: The jaw is then gently lifted up to pull the tongue off the back of the throat.
YES: _____   RE-TEACH: _____   RETURN: _____   INSTRUCTOR INITIALS _____

Student Name: _____ Date: _____

Skill: Jaw-Thrust Maneuver
Equipment Assembled:
1. Gloves
2. Goggles
3. Mask

YES: _____   RE-TEACH: _____   RETURN: _____   INSTRUCTOR INITIALS _____

Step 1: After donning appropriate PPE, the EMT positions herself above the patient's head.
YES: _____   RE-TEACH: _____   RETURN: _____   INSTRUCTOR INITIALS _____

Step 2: The EMT places her middle and index fingers on the angles of the patient's jaw and her thumbs on the cheekbones.
YES: _____   RE-TEACH: _____   RETURN: _____   INSTRUCTOR INITIALS _____

Step 3: The middle and index fingers lift the jaw and the tongue up off of the back of the throat while avoiding any movement of the neck.
YES: _____   RE-TEACH: _____   RETURN: _____   INSTRUCTOR INITIALS _____

Student Name: _____   Date: _____

Skill: Oral Suctioning
Equipment Assembled: Gloves
1. Goggles
2. Mask
3. Suction Machine
4. Tubing
5. Catheter
5. Water
YES: _____   RE-TEACH: _____   RETURN: _____   INSTRUCTOR INITIALS _____

Step 1: After donning appropriate PPE, the EMT assembles the suction equipment and tests it by placing a finger over the distal end of the tubing or kinking the tubing to generate suction. Most portable suction machines should generate between 200 and 300 mm Hg of suction.
YES: _____   RE-TEACH: _____   RETURN: _____   INSTRUCTOR INITIALS _____

Step 2: Select the appropriate catheter and attach it firmly to the distal end of the tubing.
YES: _____   RE-TEACH: _____   RETURN: _____   INSTRUCTOR INITIALS _____

Step 3: The distance from the corner of the mouth to the angle of the jaw is measured as an estimate of the distance the catheter should be placed in the patient's mouth. The EMT should never suction beyond where he or she can see.
YES: _____   RE-TEACH: _____   RETURN: _____   INSTRUCTOR INITIALS _____

Step 4: The EMT uses the cross-finger technique to open the patient's mouth. Start by crossing the thumb under the index finger and placing the thumb against the lower teeth and the index finger against the upper teeth.
YES: _____   RE-TEACH: _____   RETURN: _____   INSTRUCTOR INITIALS _____

Step 5: Spread the thumb and index finger apart to open the patient's mouth.
YES: _____   RE-TEACH: _____   RETURN: _____   INSTRUCTOR INITIALS _____

Step 6: The suction catheter is guided into the patient's mouth, taking care to follow the curvature of the tongue and only advancing as far as can be easily seen (or as far as measured in advance).
YES: _____   RE-TEACH: _____   RETURN: _____   INSTRUCTOR INITIALS _____

Step 7: A finger is then be placed over the whistle port on the catheter to generate suction. Suction should be applied while the catheter is being removed from the mouth and should never be allowed to remain constant for more than 10 to 15 seconds.
YES: _____   RE-TEACH: _____   RETURN: _____   INSTRUCTOR INITIALS _____

Step 8: The patient is reassessed, and oxygen is reapplied. The procedure should be repeated as necessary.
YES: _____   RE-TEACH: _____   RETURN: _____   INSTRUCTOR INITIALS _____

Student Name: _____   Date: _____

Skill: Insertion of the Oropharyngeal Airway
Equipment Assembled:
1. Gloves
2. Goggles
3. Mask
4. Assortment of OPA Sizes

YES: _____   RE-TEACH: _____   RETURN: _____   INSTRUCTOR INITIALS _____

Step 1: After donning the appropriate PPE, the EMT measures the patient for an OPA. The appropriate size OPA reaches from the corner of the mouth to the bottom of the earlobe.

YES: _____   RE-TEACH: _____   RETURN: _____   INSTRUCTOR INITIALS _____

Step 2: Using the cross-finger technique, the EMT opens the patient's mouth.

YES: _____   RE-TEACH: _____   RETURN: _____   INSTRUCTOR INITIALS _____

Step 3: The proper size OPA is initially guided into the patient's mouth with the curvature facing the tongue and the tip against the top of the mouth.

YES: _____   RE-TEACH: _____   RETURN: _____   INSTRUCTOR INITIALS _____

Step 4: At about the halfway point, the OPA is then turned in a 180 degree arc and passed the rest of the way into the mouth, following the curvature of the tongue.

YES: _____   RE-TEACH: _____   RETURN: _____   INSTRUCTOR INITIALS _____

Step 5: The OPA should rest with the flange against the patient's lips.

YES: _____   RE-TEACH: _____   RETURN: _____   INSTRUCTOR INITIALS _____

Student Name: _____   Date: _____

Skill: Insertion of the Nasopharyngeal Airway
Equipment Assembled:
1. Gloves
2. Goggles
3. Mask
4. Assortment of NPA Sizes
5. Water-Soluble Lubricant

YES: _____   RE-TEACH: _____   RETURN: _____   INSTRUCTOR INITIALS _____

Step 1: After donning appropriate PPE, the EMT measures an NPA for size. The proper size NPA will reach from the nostril to the tip of the earlobe.

YES: _____   RE-TEACH: _____   RETURN: _____   INSTRUCTOR INITIALS _____

Step 2: The NPA is generously lubricated with a water-soluble lubricant to ease placement.

YES: _____   RE-TEACH: _____   RETURN: _____   INSTRUCTOR INITIALS _____

Step 3: The EMT selects the nostril that is the largest, usually the right.

YES: _____   RE-TEACH: _____   RETURN: _____   INSTRUCTOR INITIALS _____

Step 4: The lubricated NPA is placed into the nostril with the bevel facing the nasal septum (middle of the nose) to minimize trauma to this vascular area.

YES: _____   RE-TEACH: _____   RETURN: _____   INSTRUCTOR INITIALS _____

Step 5: The NPA is smoothly advanced straight back into the nose until the flange rests against the nostril. Note that the direction of advancement is posterior toward the pharynx, not up into the vascular structures of the nose.

YES: _____   RE-TEACH: _____   RETURN: _____   INSTRUCTOR INITIALS _____

CHAPTER 8

Respiratory Support

OBJECTIVES

Upon completion of this chapter, the reader should be able to:

1. List the signs of adequate breathing.
2. List the signs of inadequate breathing.
3. Define the components of an oxygen delivery system.
4. Identify a nonrebreather mask and state the oxygen flow requirements needed for its use.
5. Describe the indications for using a nasal cannula versus a nonrebreather mask.
6. Identify a nasal cannula and state the flow requirements needed for its use.

7. Describe how to artificially ventilate a patient with a pocket mask.
8. Describe the steps in performing the skill of artificially ventilating a patient with a bag-valve mask while using the jaw thrust.
9. Describe the steps in performing the skill of artificially ventilating a patient with a bag-valve mask for one and two rescuers.
10. Describe the steps in artificially ventilating a patient with a flow-restricted, oxygen-powered ventilation device.

GLOSSARY

accessory muscle breathing   Neck, chest, and abdominal muscles that can be used to assist in respiration in times of distress.

air hunger   The feeling a person may have if his or her oxygen level is low or he or she is unable to breathe effectively; indicated by mouth breathing.

artificial ventilation   A method of providing oxygen to a patient who is not effectively breathing; also known as rescue breathing.

ausculate   Term that means to listen.

bag-valve-mask device (BVM)   A device consisting of a refilling bag, a one-way valve, and a mask that is used to ventilate a patient.

contraindication   A reason not to do something.

cricoid pressure   A technique of applying pressure to the cricoid ring during ventilation to occlude the esophagus and prevent regurgitation.

dead space   The space in the respiratory tract that is not in contact with pulmonary capillaries and cannot participate in gas exchange with the blood.

dentures   False teeth.

dyspnea   The feeling or appearance of respiratory distress; difficulty breathing.

flow-restricted, oxygen-powered ventilation device (FROPVD)   A device that delivers oxygen to a patient at restricted flow rates.

humidification   The process of adding moisture to the inspired air.

hydrostatic testing   Safety testing of oxygen tanks to be sure that they can tolerate the required pressures without danger.

hypoventilation   Breathing more slowly than normal or less effectively than usual.

hypoxic   Lack of oxygen in the body.

indication   A reason to do something.

nasal cannula (NC)   A device that is placed in the patient's nose and can deliver between 25% and 44% oxygen.

nonrebreather mask (NRB)   A device that when used with oxygen at 10–15 lpm can deliver up to 100% oxygen.

onboard oxygen   The large oxygen tank that is kept on an ambulance for purposes of administering oxygen to a patient in the ambulance.

palpate   To feel with one's hands.

pocket mask (PM)   A portable mask for mouth-to-mask ventilation.

pursed lip breathing   Exhaling past partially closed lips.

regulator   The device placed on an oxygen tank to regulate the flow of the gas.

resuscitate   To revive a patient by way of artificial respiration.

stoma   The surgically created hole at the base of the neck to allow patients with severe upper airway disease to breathe.

tachypnea   Respiratory rate faster than normal.

tracheostomy   The surgical creation of a hole in the anterior neck into the trachea that allows more effective ventilation in patients with upper airway problems or chronic lung disease.

tripod position   The three-legged position maintained by a person with severe difficulty breathing: sitting upright with the upper body leaning slightly forward with the arms straight and hands supporting the upper body by resting on the upper legs.

PREPARATORY

Materials: None

Personnel: Primary Instructor: One EMT-Basic instructor knowledgeable in airway management.

Assistant Instructor: The instructor-to-student ratio should be 1:6 for psychomotor skill practice. Individuals used as assistant instructors should be knowledgeable in airway techniques and management.

Recommended Minimum Time to Complete: 4 hours

STUDENT OUTLINE

I. Breathing
II. Assessment
    A. Quick Check
    B. Look
        1. Position
        2. Color
        3. Respiratory Rate
        4. Effort
        5. Level of Consciousness
        6. Pulse Oximetry
    C. Listen
        1. Speech
        2. Obvious Noise
        3. Breath Sounds
        4. Feel
III. Oxygen Therapy
    A. Indications
    B. Contraindications
    C. Oxygen Delivery Systems
        1. Anatomy of an Oxygen Delivery System
    D. Oxygen Delivery Devices
        1. The Partial Nonrebreather Mask
        2. Tracheostomy Mask
        3. The Nasal Cannula
    E. Oxygen Humidification
    F. Putting It All Together
IV. Artificial Ventilation
    A. Use of a Barrier Device
    B. The Pocket Mask
    C. The Bag-Valve Mask
        1. Anatomy of a Bag-Valve Mask
    D. Ventilation Technique
        1. Air Volume
        2. Two-Person Ventilation
            a) Cricoid Pressure
        3. Oxygen-Powered Ventilation Device
        4. Single-Person BVM Ventilation
        5. Ventilation of the Breathing Patient
        6. Ventilation of the Surgical Airway

LECTURE OUTLINE

I. Breathing
- A. Fundamental Life Activity
  - 1. Life-Giving
  - 2. Resuscitation
    - a) Revived from Dead
- B. Respiratory Failure
  - 1. Oxygenation
    - a) Oxygen-Poor
      - (1) Hypoxia
  - 2. Ventilation
    - a) Work of Breathing

II. Assessment
- A. Procedure
  - 1. Look
  - 2. Listen
  - 3. Feel
- B. Quick Check
  - 1. Determination of Cardiac/Respiratory Arrest
- C. Look
  - a) View from Doorway
  - b) Level of Consciousness
    - (1) Alert = Good Respiration
    - (2) Lethargic = Poor Respiration
  - 1. Position
    - a) Tripoding
  - 2. Color
    - b) Cyanosis
  - 3. Respiratory Rate
    - a) Rapid, Ineffectual Breathing
      - (1) Tachypnea
        - (a) Dead Space
    - b) Slow, Ineffectual Breathing
      - (1) Bradypnea
        - (a) Hypoventilation
  - 4. Effort
    - a) Signs
      - (1) Nasal Flaring
      - (2) Mouth Breathing
        - (a) Air Hunger
      - (3) Pursed Lip Breathing
      - (4) Accessory Muscles of Respiration
        - (a) Shoulder and Neck Muscles (Strap Muscles)
        - (b) Abdominal Muscles
          - (i) Seesaw Respiration
        - (c) Intercostal Muscles
        - (d) Sternal Retractions
          - (i) Pediatric
  - 5. Level of Consciousness
    - a) Confused
    - b) Combative
    - c) Lethargic
  - 6. Pulse Oximetry
    - a) Percent Oxygen Saturation
    - b) Range
      - (1) 95-100% Normal
      - (2) >96% Hypoxia
        - (a) Oxygen Administration
- D. Listen
  - a) Chief Complaint
  - b) Catch Phrases
    - (1) Short of Breath
    - (2) Trouble Breathing
  - c) Dyspnea
  - 1. Speech
    - a) Conservation of Speech
    - b) Monosyllabic Answers (Yes-No)
  - 2. Obvious Noise
    - a) Normal Breathing
      - (1) Quiet
    - b) Abnormal Breathing
      - (2) Noisy
  - 3. Breath Sounds
    - a) Ausculate
      - (1) Bilateral
      - (2) Anterior
        - (a) Proximal to Clavicle
      - (3) Lateral
        - (a) Axilla at Nipple Line
    - b) Findings
      - (1) Normal
      - (2) Diminished
      - (3) Absent
- E. Feel
  - 1. Palpation
    - a) Tenderness
    - b) Deformity
    - c) Equality

III. Oxygen Therapy
    1. Most Commonly Administered EMS Drug
  A. Indications
    1. Primary
      a) Reverse Hypoxia
    2. Patient Presentation
      a) Chief Complaint
        (1) Shortness of Breath
        (2) Trouble Breathing
    3. Physical Signs of Hypoxia
      a) Anxiety
      b) Confusion
      c) Tachypnea
      d) Tachycardia
      e) Cyanosis
  B. Contraindications
    1. Effectively—None in the Field
    2. Follow Protocols
  C. Oxygen Delivery Systems
    1. Fixed
      a) Onboard Oxygen
        (1) Large Tank
    2. Portable
      a) Carrying Case
        (1) Lighter Tank
    3. Anatomy of an Oxygen Delivery System
      a) Oxygen Tank (Bottle)
        (1) Steel or Aluminum
        (2) Unique Pin System
          (a) National Standard Pin Index
        (3) Green Color
      b) Tank Valve
        (1) Right Turn to Tighten, Left Turn to Loosen
      c) Regulator (Flowmeter)
        (1) Washer (Critical)
        (2) Flow Control
          (a) Liters per Minute
          (b) Flow Control
            (i) Constant Settings
            (ii) Variable Control
  D. Oxygen Delivery Devices
    1. The Partial Nonrebreather Mask
      a) High-Concentration Oxygen Delivery

      b) Bag Reservoir System
        (1) One-Way Valve on Bag
    2. Tracheostomy Mask
      a) Special Use On Tracheostomy Patients
    3. The Nasal Cannula
      a) Low-Concentration Oxygen Delivery
      b) Claustrophobia
      c) Rule of Sixes
  E. Oxygen Humidification
    1. Purpose
      a) Moisturizes
    2. Delivery System
      a) Sterile Water
      b) Large Tubing
  F. Putting It All Together
IV. Artificial Ventilation
  A. Indications
    1. Apnea
  B. Use of a Barrier Device
    1. Personal Protection
      a) Potentially Infectious Body Fluids
  C. The Pocket Mask
    1. Anatomy
      a) Clear Dome
      b) Soft Face Seal Cushion
      c) Ventilation Port
        (1) Chimney
      d) Oxygen Inlet/Port
  D. The Bag-Valve Mask
    1. Anatomy of a Bag-Valve Mask
      a) Self-Inflating Bag
      b) Oxygen Inlet/Port
      c) Reservoir
        (1) Safety Valve
          (a) Inflates with Room Air When Reservoir Fails
      d) Delivery Valve
        (1) One-Way Valve
        (2) Exhalation Port
        (3) Standard Fitting for Mask
      e) Mask
        (1) Different Sizes
        (2) Clear Dome
        (3) Soft Face Cushion
  E. Ventilation Technique

1. Air Volume
   a) Overventilation
      (1) Rupture (Pneumothorax)
   b) Underventilation
      (1) Hypoxia
F. Two-Person Ventilation
   a) Team Approach
      (1) Airway Control
         (a) Cricoid Pressure
            (i) Prevents Regurgitation
            (ii) Prevents Air in Stomach
      (2) Ventilation
         (a) Chest Expansion
1. Oxygen-Powered Ventilation Device (Demand Valve)
   a) Easy Operation—One Person
   b) Uses
      (1) Nonbreathing Patient—Ventilation
      (2) Breathing Patient—Oxygen Administration
      (a) Oxygen Conservation
2. Single-Person BVM Ventilation
   a) Rescuer Fatigue
      (1) Poor Mask Seal
3. Ventilation of the Breathing Patient
   a) Patient Cooperation
   b) Timed Respiration
   c) Preparation for Apnea
4. Ventilation of the Surgical Airway
   a) Tracheostomy
      (1) Surgical Incision in Neck
         (a) Stoma Created
   b) Tracheostomy Tube
      (1) Standard 15mm BVM Fitting
   c) No Tracheostomy Tube
      (1) Ventilation with Pediatric Mask
   d) Bedside Ventilators
      (1) Similar to FROPVD

TEACHING STRATEGIES

1. Have one student run a 100 yard sprint. Then ask the class to describe, in medical terms, her or his breathing effort. Be sure that the students use ample medical terms.

2. Have students form groups of four. First, have them practice basic manual airway maneuvers on one another, including the jaw-thrust and head-tilt, chin-lift. Then ask them to ventilate one another. To accomplish this, the student-patient must be gently introduced to the mask. Once the student-patient is comfortable with the mask, the bag-valve assembly is attached and again the student-patient is encouraged to "breathe through the bag." Once this has been accomplished, the student at the bag can start to gently ventilate the student-patient, taking note of inspiration and gently ventilating at that moment. The students rotate through the roles of airway, mask, bag, and student-patient.

3. With a recording Resusci-Annie™, have the students practice ventilation for 5 minutes with a pocket mask, one-person BVM, and two-person BVM. Record only the final minute of ventilation. Attention should be given to depth of respiration as well as timing (frequency).

4. Arrange to meet with the respiratory therapist at a local hospital to tour the department. Ask the respiratory therapist to demonstrate humidification of oxygen as well as ventilation of the tracheotomy. A superficial review of the mechanical ventilator's settings can help the students apply physiological parameters such as force of ventilation and volume of ventilation to clinical practice.

FURTHER STUDY

Menegazzi, J. J., & Winslow, H. J. (1994). In-vitro comparison of bag-valve-mask and the manually triggered oxygen-powered breathing device. *Academic Emergency Medicine*, 1(1), 29–33.

Terndrup, T. E., & Warner, D. A. (1992). Infant ventilation and oxygenation by basic life support providers: comparison of methods. *Prehospital Disaster Medicine, 7*(1), 35–40.

CASE STUDY   TROUBLE BREATHING

Grandma Smith had been having trouble breathing for the past several days. When asked why, she would quickly dismiss her grandchildren by saying, "It's just old age."

Tonight was different. Grandma had gone to bed at her usual bedtime, which was nine o'clock. Not more than 3 hours had passed when she called out to her grandson Todd.

Todd rushed to the room. Grandma was standing at the open window, her arms bracing herself on the window ledge. "I can't catch my breath," she said.

Todd, not sure what to do, called 9-1-1.

STOP AND THINK

1. What are the signs and symptoms of difficulty breathing?
2. What abnormal breath sounds would typically be heard in this case?

ANSWERS TO STOP AND THINK

1. The signs of difficulty breathing are limited in this case. The patient standing at an open window trying to catch her breath is a sign. The fact the patient is bracing herself in a tripod position is another sign. Finally, the timing of this episode (paroxysmal nocturnal dyspnea) is suggestive of congestive heart failure.

2. If this patient is in fact experiencing congestive heart failure, then crackles would be heard in the bases and raise up the lung fields according to the degree of severity.

CASE STUDY   A TUMBLE DOWNSTAIRS

Thud. Everyone in the family heard it. Even the baby was startled. Ahmed was first to investigate. The sound had come from the kitchen. Stepping into the center of the room, Ahmed saw the open door to the basement. Then he heard a faint voice. "I'm down here!"

The voice that he heard was Uncle Hameed's. Uncle Hameed, who frequently had bouts of confusion, had apparently opened the wrong door. He had fallen down a dozen stairs to the landing in the basement.

Ahmed ran down the stairs while the family stood in the doorway. Kneeling next to his uncle, he noticed that his uncle was splinting his ribs with one arm and straining to breathe.

Ahmed called upstairs to his mother. "Call the ambulance, I think Uncle Hameed is hurt, maybe some broken ribs."

Using the Buddycare he had been taught in the Army, Ahmed helped his uncle lie down and told him not to move until the ambulance arrived.

Ahmed noticed that his uncle's breathing was getting much worse.

STOP AND THINK

1. What is the primary respiratory problem in this case?
2. What can be done to assist the patient?
3. What can one EMT do? Two EMTs?

ANSWERS TO STOP AND THINK

1. The patient's primary problem is possible rib fractures that are impairing his breathing. His compromised ventilation will eventually lead to hypoventilation, hypoxia, and problems with respiration.

2. The patient's spine should be immobilized, then the patient's head should be elevated a few inches and he should be turned onto his injured side, to allow the uninjured lung to inflate maximally. The patient's respiration needs to be monitored closely and the EMT needs to be ready to assist the patient's breathing.

3. One EMT stabilizes the patient's c-spine and, with the patient's head between his knees, starts to administer oxygen. The EMT can offer verbal encouragement to the patient as well as communicating the patient's condition to responding EMS.

CASE STUDY   RESPIRATORY COMPROMISE

After riding six floors, Tamesha got off the elevator and proceeded to apartment 604. The call had come in as "a man having trouble breathing." The name on the door said "Fish, Ron."

"Hello, Mr. Fish? It's the ambulance," Tamesha called out, while knocking on the door. After getting an invitation to come in, Tamesha stepped into the doorway. She was immediately aware of the acrid smell of cigarette smoke.

Mr. Fish was in the kitchen, sitting upright in a chair at the table, wearing only a T-shirt and briefs. In front of him was an ashtray overflowing with cigarette butts and a half-full cup of coffee.

As Tamesha introduced herself, she noted the oxygen cannula he was wearing. Mr. Fish was a frail, elderly man. Now he was hunched over, hands on his knees. His breathing was rapid and shallow. He was blowing out air through pursed lips.

While assessing his airway, Tamesha noted that his lips were a pale blue, as were his fingernail beds. She quickly listened to his lungs.

He was moving air, but the lung sounds were muffled. Tamesha quickly checked her stethoscope to see that it was adjusted properly.

Mr. Fish's chest was barrel-shaped and did not expand very much with each breath. Tamesha also noticed that the skin between his ribs was retracting every time he took a breath.

Tamesha quickly applied the pulse oximeter, remembering that a high reading may be misleading because of carbon monoxide.

Suddenly, Mr. Fish appeared to be having more trouble breathing. He reached out and grabbed Tamesha by the shirt sleeve. All he could say was "I . . . can't . . . breathe!"

STOP AND THINK

1. What indications (signs and symptoms) of respiratory compromise is this patient displaying?
2. What treatments are indicated in this case? Is one treatment more desirable than another?
3. If these initial treatments are unsuccessful, what actions can the EMT reasonably expect to take?

ANSWERS TO STOP AND THINK

1. The patient's environment offers clues to his condition. The ashtray overflowing with cigarettes as well as the hardback chair that permits the patient to sit upright are clues. The patient has assumed a tripod position to aid his breathing. The pursed lip breathing is a technique used by patients to encourage a longer exhalation phase. Finally, the blue tinge of cyanosis is evident on the patient's fingernails and lips.

2. This patient is in need of a breathing treatment. If the patient has an inhaler, the EMT could

consider assisting the patient with his medication. The EMT should also be calling for an ALS backup, if available. If ALS would be delayed or is not immediately available, the EMT needs to transport this patient immediately.

3. If initial treatments with the patient's breathing medication are unsuccessful, the EMT may have to assist the patient's ventilation.

ANSWERS TO TEST YOUR KNOWLEDGE

1. Physical signs of shortness of breath can be grouped by assessment method, that is, findings can be classified as either look, listen, or feel. Visible signs of respiratory distress or "shortness of breath" include tripod positioning, nasal flaring, open-mouthed breathing, accessory muscle use (strap muscles, intercostal muscles), and abdominal breathing. Auditory signs of shortness of breath include noisy respiration (wheezes or grunts) and speech (monosyllabic or short answers). Palpation of the chest wall of the patient having trouble breathing may reveal unequal or asymmetrical chest rise as well as point tenderness and deformity.

2. Hypoxia is the lack of oxygen in the blood. Anoxia is the complete absence of oxygen in the blood. The signs of hypoxia include increased respiratory rate (tachypnea), increased heart rate (tachycardia), and central cyanosis.

3. Cyanosis is a descriptive term for the color that deoxygenated blood produces. Typically this color is a bluish or gray tinge. Peripheral cyanosis may be due to problems of respiration, but is more commonly due to problems of circulation. Central cyanosis (around the lips, for example), is generally related to problems of respiration.

4. The parts of the oxygen delivery system: tank, washer, regulator, oxygen tubing, oxygen mask.

5. The rule of sixes dictates that all masks must have a minimal flow rate of 6 liters per minute (lpm) and that nasal cannulas have a flow rate no greater than 6 liters per minute (lpm).

6. A nasal cannula is preferred over a nonrebreather mask when (a) the patient is on home oxygen and the EMT is just continuing the previous treatment; (b) the patient is claustrophobic and cannot wear a mask.

7. If an EMT is alone, he should start with mouth-to-mask ventilation. If a flow-restricted, oxygen-powered ventilation device is immediately available it may be used. The EMT should only resort to a bag-valve mask (BVM) when neither of the first two devices are available and additional rescuers are expected in a short period of time. The optimal number of rescuers to perform CPR is three.

8. The first step of properly ventilating the apneic patient is always opening the airway, whether by head-tilt, chin-lift or by jaw-thrust. The next step would be to obtain an adequate mask seal by using a proper-sized mask and applying it to the cleft of the chin first.

9. All ventilation devices have the same risk: inflation of the stomach. The flow-restricted, oxygen-powered ventilation device may have a somewhat greater risk of creating gastric distention because the operator-EMT is incapable of "feeling" the resistance of the filled lungs, which causes oxygen to "spillover" into the stomach.

Student Name: _____   Date: _____

Skill: Oxygen Tank Assembly
Equipment Needed:
Oxygen Tank
Regulator with Washer
Oxygen Wrench or Key
YES: _____   RE-TEACH: _____   RETURN: _____   INSTRUCTOR INITIALS _____

Step 1: After assuring that there is no risk of fire hazard in the area, the EMT confirms that the contents of the tank at hand are oxygen. (These tanks are green in color and have pins that match the oxygen regulator for safety.)
YES: _____   RE-TEACH: _____   RETURN: _____   INSTRUCTOR INITIALS _____

Step 2: Using an oxygen wrench, the EMT quickly opens and closes the oxygen tank by turning the device at the top of the tank counterclockwise, then clockwise. This procedure, called "cracking the tank," blows out any dirt and dust in the outlet.
YES: _____   RE-TEACH: _____   RETURN: _____   INSTRUCTOR INITIALS _____

Step 3: The EMT then mates the regulator to the oxygen tank, being sure to tightly seat the regulator. Often a plastic washer is needed for an airtight fit.
YES: _____   RE-TEACH: _____   RETURN: _____   INSTRUCTOR INITIALS _____

Step 4: The oxygen tank may now be safely opened by again turning the device at the top of the tank counterclockwise as far as it allows, then back one quarter-turn. The pressure within the tank should be noted at this time.
YES: _____   RE-TEACH: _____   RETURN: _____   INSTRUCTOR INITIALS _____

Step 5: The tank is now ready to be used in oxygen delivery. To adjust the liter flow rate, the EMT can turn the flow adjusting knob on the regulator in a counterclockwise motion until the desired liter flow appears.
YES: _____   RE-TEACH: _____   RETURN: _____   INSTRUCTOR INITIALS _____

Student Name: _____   Date: _____

Skill: Application of Nonrebreather Oxygen Mask
Purpose: To provide the patient with high-flow oxygen.
Standard Precautions:
Icon-Handwiashing-Gloves
Equipment: Oxygen Tank, Regulator, Nonrebreather Oxygen Mask
Step 1: The EMT ensures that the oxygen tank and oxygen regulator are correctly assembled. The oxygen tank should have sufficient pressure to provide continuous oxygen flow.

YES: _____   RE-TEACH: _____   RETURN: _____   INSTRUCTOR INITIALS _____

Step 2: The EMT chooses the correct oxygen administration device. A nonrebreather oxygen mask is used when high concentrations of oxygen are desired.

YES: _____   RE-TEACH: _____   RETURN: _____   INSTRUCTOR INITIALS _____

Step 3: To use the nonrebreather oxygen mask, the EMT attaches the oxygen tubing to the regulator and turns on the regulator. The regulator should never be turned below 6 liters per minute.

YES: _____   RE-TEACH: _____   RETURN: _____   INSTRUCTOR INITIALS _____

Step 4. The EMT then places his thumbs over the valve between the bag and the mask, permitting the bag to fill completely.

YES: _____   RE-TEACH: _____   RETURN: _____   INSTRUCTOR INITIALS _____

Step 5. Grasping the mask in one hand and the elastic band in the other, the EMT seats the mask firmly on the bridge of the nose and drapes the elastic band around the head. The EMT pinches the metal strap around the nose.

YES: _____   RE-TEACH: _____   RETURN: _____   INSTRUCTOR INITIALS _____

Step 6. The EMT then adjusts the liter flow to ensure that the oxygen bag is always filled at least one-half.

YES: _____   RE-TEACH: _____   RETURN: _____   INSTRUCTOR INITIALS _____

Student Name: _____   Date: _____

Skill: Application of a Nasal Cannula

Purpose: To provide the patient with oxygen

Standard Precautions:

Icon-Handwashing-Gloves

Equipment: Oxygen Tank, Regulator, Nasal Cannula

Step 1: The EMT ensures that the oxygen tank and oxygen regulator are correctly assembled. The oxygen tank should have sufficient pressure to provide continuous oxygen flow.

YES: _____   RE-TEACH: _____   RETURN: _____   INSTRUCTOR INITIALS _____

Step 2: The EMT chooses the correct oxygen administration device. A nasal cannula is used when the patient cannot tolerate the nonrebreather oxygen mask, or when low concentrations of oxygen are desired.

YES: _____   RE-TEACH: _____   RETURN: _____   INSTRUCTOR INITIALS _____

Step 3: To use the nasal cannula the EMT attaches the oxygen tubing to the regulator and turns on the regulator. As a rule, 4 to 6 liters per minute is sufficient. The regulator should never be turned above 6 liters per minute.

YES: _____   RE-TEACH: _____   RETURN: _____   INSTRUCTOR INITIALS _____

Step 4: The nasal prongs whould be gently introduced into the nostrils, so that they appear to be lying on the floor of the nostril.

YES: _____   RE-TEACH: _____   RETURN: _____   INSTRUCTOR INITIALS _____

Step 5: The tubing should be draped over the ears and the tubing cinched loosely under the chin with the ring. The nasal cannula should not be draped over the neck like a necklace, as the danger of strangulation is too great.

YES: _____   RE-TEACH: _____   RETURN: _____   INSTRUCTOR INITIALS _____

Step 6: The EMT adjusts the liter flow to ensure that the patient is receiving an adequate amount of oxygen.

YES: _____   RE-TEACH: _____   RETURN: _____   INSTRUCTOR INITIALS _____

Student Name: _____   Date: _____

Skill: Use of a Pocket Mask
Equipment Needed:
Pocket Mask with Oxygen Outlet
One-way Valve
Oxygen Tubing
Oxygen Tank
Oxygen Regulator

YES: _____   RE-TEACH: _____   RETURN: _____   INSTRUCTOR INITIALS _____

Step 1: After donning appropriate PPE and properly managing the nonbreathing patient's airway, the EMT assembles the pocket mask by attaching the one-way valve to the pocket mask itself.

YES: _____   RE-TEACH: _____   RETURN: _____   INSTRUCTOR INITIALS _____

Step 2: The pocket mask should be applied over the patient's mouth and nose, with the narrower nose-piece placed over the bridge of the nose.

YES: _____   RE-TEACH: _____   RETURN: _____   INSTRUCTOR INITIALS _____

Step 3: Situated above the patient's head, the EMT places his thumbs facing toward the patient's feet on either side of the mask, using the length of each to hold the mask on the patient's face. The fingers of each hand are then placed under the angle of the jaw, which is raised up to bring the face snugly against the mask while the head is extended backward to maintain an open airway.

YES: _____   RE-TEACH: _____   RETURN: _____   INSTRUCTOR INITIALS _____

In the case of suspected spinal injury, the fingers of both hands will grasp under the angle of the jaw and lift up toward the mask with care taken not to extend the neck at all. While this requires a tighter grip on the mask and jaw than the maneuver that is done without spinal injury, it is important the EMT take care not to worsen any potential spinal injury by extending the neck.

YES: _____   RE-TEACH: _____   RETURN: _____   INSTRUCTOR INITIALS _____

An airtight mask seal is crucial to effective ventilation via this method. The sound of air leaking means that air is not getting into the patient's lungs.

YES: _____   RE-TEACH: _____   RETURN: _____   INSTRUCTOR INITIALS _____

Step 4: Next, in order to ventilate the patient, the EMT seals his lips around the ventilation port on the one-way valve and blows steadily into the port for 1 _ to 2 seconds, or until the patient's chest is seen to rise. This should be repeated every 5 seconds for an adult, every 4 seconds for a child, and every 3 seconds for an infant. Keep in mind that when ventilating smaller adults, children, and infants, the volumes of air necessary to result in chest rise (and lung inflation) are much smaller. It is important to avoid causing overdistension of the lungs.

YES: _____   RE-TEACH: _____   RETURN: _____   INSTRUCTOR INITIALS _____

Step 5: Once the EMT has ventilated the patient for around a minute, it is important to recheck the status of pulse and respirations as in the quick check. At this time the EMT can also quickly turn on the oxygen tank, attach oxygen tubing to the pocket mask inlet and run the oxygen at 15 lpm to deliver supplemental oxygen with each ventilation.

YES: _____   RE-TEACH: _____   RETURN: _____   INSTRUCTOR INITIALS _____

Step 6: With the supplemental oxygen attached, the EMT can return to ventilating the patient as previously described, rechecking the patient's status every few minutes.

YES: _____   RE-TEACH: _____   RETURN: _____   INSTRUCTOR INITIALS _____

Student Name: _____   Date: _____

Skill: Ventilation with a Bag-Valve-Mask Assembly

Equipment Needed:

Appropriate PPE (gloves, mask, goggles)

Bag-Valve-Mask Assembly (BVM)

Oxygen Tubing

Oxygen Regulator

Oxygen Tank

YES: _____   RE-TEACH: _____   RETURN: _____   INSTRUCTOR INITIALS _____

Step 1: After applying appropriate PPE, the EMT ensures that the oxygen tank and oxygen regulator are correctly assembled. The oxygen tank should have sufficient pressure to provide continuous oxygen flow.

YES: _____   RE-TEACH: _____   RETURN: _____   INSTRUCTOR INITIALS _____

Step 2: The EMT chooses the correct oxygen administration device. A bag-valve mask is used when an apneic patient needs to be ventilated by two EMTs.

YES: _____   RE-TEACH: _____   RETURN: _____   INSTRUCTOR INITIALS _____

Step 3: To use the BVM, the EMT first attaches the oxygen tubing to the regulator and turns on the regulator. As a rule, 10 to 15 liters per minute are sufficient.

YES: _____   RE-TEACH: _____   RETURN: _____   INSTRUCTOR INITIALS _____

Step 4: The EMT chooses a properly fitting face mask. The face mask should fit securely over the bridge of the nose and extend to the cleft of the chin.

YES: _____   RE-TEACH: _____   RETURN: _____   INSTRUCTOR INITIALS _____

Step 5: Assuring that the airway has been opened, and an oral airway is in place, the EMT places the mask over the apneic patient's face, maintaining the airway in an open position with either the jaw-thrust or the head-tilt, chin-lift.

YES: _____   RE-TEACH: _____   RETURN: _____   INSTRUCTOR INITIALS _____

Step 6: One EMT should hold the mask in place, assuring a good seal, while another EMT compresses the bag with two hands until chest rise is seen. The patient should be ventilated every 5 seconds.

YES: _____   RE-TEACH: _____   RETURN: _____   INSTRUCTOR INITIALS _____

Student Name: _____ Date: _____

Skill: Ventilation with an Flow-Restricted, Oxygen-Powered Ventilation Device
Equipment Needed:
Appropriate PPE
Flow-Restricted, Oxygen-Powered Ventilation Device (FROPVD)
Oxygen Regulator
Oxygen Tank

YES: _____   RE-TEACH: _____   RETURN: _____   INSTRUCTOR INITIALS _____

Step 1: The EMT first ensures that the oxygen tank and oxygen regulator, with the FROPVD, is correctly assembled. The oxygen tank should show sufficient pressure to provide continuous oxygen flow.

YES: _____   RE-TEACH: _____   RETURN: _____   INSTRUCTOR INITIALS _____

Step 2: The EMT chooses the correct oxygen administration device. A FROPVD is used when an apneic patient needs to be ventilated by an EMT.

YES: _____   RE-TEACH: _____   RETURN: _____   INSTRUCTOR INITIALS _____

Step 3: The EMT chooses a properly fitting face mask. The face mask should fit securely over the bridge of the nose and extend to the cleft of the chin.

YES: _____   RE-TEACH: _____   RETURN: _____   INSTRUCTOR INITIALS _____

Step 4: Assuring that the airway has been opened, and an oral airway is in place, the EMT places the mask over the apneic patient's face, maintaining the airway in an open position with either the jaw-thrust or the head-tilt, chin-lift.

YES: _____   RE-TEACH: _____   RETURN: _____   INSTRUCTOR INITIALS _____

Step 5: The EMT then holds the mask in place while compressing the trigger of the FROPVD for about 2 seconds, or until the chest rises. The patient should be ventilated every five seconds.

YES: _____   RE-TEACH: _____   RETURN: _____   INSTRUCTOR INITIALS _____

CHAPTER 9

Advanced Airway Control

OBJECTIVES

Upon completion of this chapter, the reader should be able to:

1. Identify advantages of endotracheal intubation.
2. Identify indications and contraindications for endotracheal intubation by the EMT-Basic.
3. List equipment needed to perform endotracheal intubation.
4. Describe the necessary steps involved in endotracheal intubation.
5. Describe the proper use of both the Miller and the Macintosh laryngoscope blades.
6. Identify advantages of cricoid pressure during endotracheal intubation.
7. Describe at least four methods to confirm tracheal tube placement.
8. Identify at least four parameters to monitor on the intubated patient.
9. Identify at least four problems that would cause the intubated patient to deteriorate.
10. Describe the most common complications associated with endotracheal intubation and identify how to avoid them or manage them.
11. Describe the procedures involved in intubating a trauma patient and how they differ from the procedures for a nontrauma patient.
12. Identify the indications for intubation of the pediatric patient.
13. Describe the advantages of endotracheal intubation in the pediatric patient.
14. Identify at least four unique anatomic features of the pediatric airway.
15. Identify the proper size for a laryngoscope blade and an endotracheal tube for an infant or a child based on age.
16. Describe why uncuffed endotracheal tubes are used in children under age eight.
17. Identify at least four complications of endotracheal intubation that are more commonly seen in pediatric patients than in adults.
18. Describe the procedure for deep endotracheal suctioning.
19. Identify the indications for and benefits of orogastric tube placement.
20. Describe the procedure for orogastric tube placement.
21. Identify a management plan for the patient with a difficult airway.

GLOSSARY

aspiration A term meaning "to draw into"; refers to foreign material being inadvertently drawn into the airway during inspiration.

D.O.P.E. Acronym to help remember causes of deterioration in the intubated patient: **D**isplaced tube, **O**bstructed tube, **P**neumothorax, **E**quipment failure.

eirect laryngoscopy Using a laryngoscope to directly visualize the airway structures.

end tidal CO_2 detector A device that indicates the presence of carbon dioxide in exhaled air.

endotracheal intubation Placement of a plastic tube in the trachea to allow for ventilation of the lungs.

hyperventilate To breathe faster and more deeply than usual.

MacIntosh blade The name for a type of curved laryngoscope blade.

Miller blade A name for a type of straight laryngoscope blade.

Murphy eye The opening on the side of the distal end of the endotracheal tube.

nasogastric tube Small-diameter flexible plastic tube that is placed through the nose and the esophagus and into the stomach.

orogastric tube Small-diameter flexible plastic tube that is placed through the mouth and the esophagus and into the stomach.

pneumothorax Air in the pleural space potentially causing collapse of the lung.

right mainstem bronchus The right branch off the trachea; is more easily entered than the left because of its steep position and wide diameter.

stylet The rigid guide placed in an endotracheal tube to help guide it during orotracheal intubation.

syringe/bulb aspirator A device that may be used to confirm proper endotracheal tube placement. When the tube is in the trachea, the syringe/bulb will easily withdraw air. When the tube is in the esophagus, the syringe/bulb will not easily withdraw air.

tension pneumothorax Air in the pleural space under tension, causing complete collapse of the affected lung and shift of the heart and other intrathoracic structures.

vallecula The space posterior to the base of the tongue, anterior to the epiglottis.

PREPARATORY

Materials: AV Equipment: Utilize various audiovisual materials relating to airway management. The continuous design and development of new audiovisual materials relating to EMS requires careful review to determine which best meet the needs of the program. Materials should be edited to assure they meet the objectives of the curriculum. EMS Equipment: Exam gloves, eye protection, basic airway adjuncts, adult, infant, and child intubation manikins, stethoscopes (1:6), laryngoscope blades (0–4) (1:6), laryngoscope handles (1:6), stylets, endotracheal tubes in various sizes, "C" batteries, spare laryngoscope bulbs, lubricant, suction units, oxygen cylinders, bag-valve masks (1:6), oxygen supply tubing, adult, infant, and child throat models showing anatomy to include trachea and vocal cords, face masks.

Personnel: Primary Instructor: One EMT-Basic instructor knowledgeable in basic and advanced airway management techniques.

Assistant Instructor: The instructor-to-student ratio should be 1:6 for psychomotor skill practice. Individuals used as assistant instructors should be knowledgeable in basic and advanced airway management techniques.

Recommended Minimum: Time to Complete: 12 hours

STUDENT OUTLINE

I. Endotracheal Intubation
- A. Advantages
  - 1. Indications
  - 2. Contraindications
- B. The Procedure
  - 1. Equipment Preparation
    - a) Sizes of Blades and Tubes
  - 2. Patient Preparation
    - a) Cricoid Pressure
  - 3. Laryngoscopy and Tube Placement
  - 4. Confirmation of Tube Placement
    - a) Direct Visualization
    - b) Auscultation
    - c) Right Mainstem Placement
    - d) Esophageal Placement
    - e) Syringe/Bulb Aspirator
    - f) End Tidal CO_2 Detector
    - g) Patient Improvement
  - 5. Secure the Tube
  - 6. Reassessments
- C. Complications
  - 1. Soft Tissue Trauma
  - 2. Dental Trauma
  - 3. Unrecognized Improper Placement
  - 4. Unique Pediatric Complications
    - a) Bradycardia
    - b) Difficulty in Auscultation
    - c) Easy Movement of Tube
    - d) Smaller Lung Volumes

II. Trauma Considerations

III. Adjuncts to Advanced Airway Management
- A. Deep Suctioning
  - 1. Indications
  - 2. Procedure
- B. OPA Placement
- C. Orogastric Tube
  - 1. Advantages
  - 2. Indications
  - 3. Contraindications
  - 4. Procedure
  - 5. Complications

IV. The Difficult Airway
- A. Basic Airway Maneuvers

LECTURE OUTLINE

I. Endotracheal Intubation
   A. Description
   B. Advantages
      1. Direct ventilation
      2. Prevention of aspiration
      3. Single rescuer ventilation
      4. Indications
         a) inability to control airway
         b) ventilatory assistance
         c) patient condition
            (1) Cardiac Arrest
            (2) Respiratory Arrest
            (3) Drug Overdose
            (4) Persistent Seizures
            (5) Severe Head Injury or Facial Injuries
            (6) Traumatic Arrest
      5. Contraindications
         a) intact gag reflex
         b) insufficient manpower
         c) insufficient skill
            (1) training mandate
   C. The Procedure
      1. familiarity
         a) procedure
         b) equipment
      2. Equipment Preparation
         a) Personal Protective Equipment
            (1) gloves
            (2) mask
               (a) inhalation of infection
            (3) goggles
               (a) vomitus
         b) Sizes of Blades and Tubes
      3. Patient Preparation
         a) Cricoid Pressure
      4. Laryngoscopy and Tube Placement
      5. Confirmation of Tube Placement
         a) Direct Visualization
         b) Auscultation
         c) Right Mainstem Placement
         d) Esophageal Placement
         e) Syringe/Bulb Aspirator
         f) End Tidal CO_2 detector
         g) Patient Improvement
      6. Secure the Tube
      7. Reassessments
   D. Complications
      1. Soft Tissue Trauma
      2. Dental Trauma
      3. Unrecognized Improper Placement
      4. Unique Pediatric Complications
         a) Bradycardia
         b) Difficulty in Auscultation
         c) Easy Movement of Tube
         d) Smaller Lung Volumes
II. Trauma Considerations
III. Adjuncts to Advanced Airway Management
   A. Deep Suctioning
      1. Indications
      2. Procedure
   B. OPA Placement
   C. Orogastric Tube
      1. Advantages
      2. Indications
      3. Contraindications
      4. Procedure
      5. Complications
IV. The Difficult Airway
   A. Basic Airway Maneuvers

TEACHING STRATEGIES

1. Starting from the basics the students should be encouraged to ventilate an airway model, then proceed to intubation of the manikin in a slow and calculating manner. Repeated efforts should eventually instill confidence in the EMT student. BLS teams, two EMTs for ventilation, and ALS teams, two EMTs for intubation, should be combined to make an effective treatment team.

Once the students have demonstrated that they can slowly intubate an airway model competently, they should be encouraged to increase their speed. Complications, such as vomiting and cervical spine injury, should be introduced to the students when they are ready to handle the difficulties of intubation.

2. Students should be asked to watch the "airway cam" video. The video provides the students an opportunity to witness live intubations.

3. Make arrangements with a local veterinarian to permit students to intubate dogs and other small mammals. The anatomy of a dog or goat is remarkably similar to that of an adult and the anatomy of a cat is remarkably similar to that of an infant. (Check local, state, and federal regulations.)

4. Make arrangements for the students to make clinical rotations through the operating room of a local hospital. Students should be encouraged to observe, then participate in, intubation of patients. A local paramedic program may be of assistance in getting these students the experience that they need. (Check insurance regulations.)

FURTHER STUDY

Nordberg, M. (1995). Safe passage: Should basic EMTs be allowed to intubate? *Emergency Medical Services, 24* (9), 39, 42–48.

Bradley, J. S., et al. (1998). Prehospital oral endotracheal intubation by rural basic emergency medical technicians. *Annals of Emergency Medicine, 32* (1), 26–32.

Spaite, D. (1998). Intubation by basic EMTs: Lifesaving advance or catastrophic complication? *Annals of Emergency Medicine, 31* (2), 276–277.

Sayre, M. R., et al. (1998). Field trial of endotracheal intubation by basic EMTs. *Annals of Emergency Medicine, 31* (2), 228–233.

CASE STUDY   OVERDOSE

The tones awoke Bill, an EMT, from a sound sleep. "Cherry Valley Fire and Rural Medical Transport respond to a possible overdose, 420 Possum Road, the Delaney residence, County Fire Control Clear at zero hundred hours." Bill thought to himself, "Possum Road, that's clear on the other end of the district, maybe 25 miles."

Bill could see the flashing lights of the sheriff's patrol car up ahead when he pulled the department's first response truck onto Possum Road. As he pulled up to the house, the deputy yelled from the front porch, "Better bring your suction!"

Once inside Bill could see a thirty-something male, covered in vomit, lying on his back and as blue as his shirt. The deputy was holding a frantic woman who was yelling, "Do something!"

The patient, despondent over his wife's decision to divorce him, had taken a handful of pills and had drunk a fifth of whisky.

Bill donned his goggles, mask, and gloves, and with the assistance of the sheriff, log-rolled the patient onto his side. After placing a large airway between the patient's upper and lower molars, Bill proceeded to scoop out chunks of half-digested meat and potatoes.

When Bill was finished, and after he had used the suction to clear the secretions, Bill prepared to ventilate the barely breathing patient. But every time Bill had the patient on his back for more than a few minutes he would vomit and Bill would have to log-roll him again. The patient's color was not improving and the ambulance, with the paramedic, was still 20 miles out.

STOP AND THINK

1. Why is this patient's airway at risk? What can be done to protect it?
2. What can an EMT do to assist another EMT, or an advanced EMT, who is intubating?

ANSWERS TO STOP AND THINK

1. The presence of vomit indicates that this patient is at risk for aspiration and potential airway obstruction. Starting with basic life support maneuvers, the EMT should open the airway, assess the airway for the

presence of foreign materials, and suction as needed. Once the airway has been cleared, the EMT should proceed to secure the airway with an oral airway while maintaining continuous manual airway control. Provided the EMT is trained, the patient should be ventilated manually using a bag-valve mask and then orally intubated immediately.

2. To assist another EMT who is intubating, the first EMT would first bag-valve-mask ventilate the patient for several minutes while the EMT intubating prepares his equipment. On command, the first EMT would stop bagging the patient and apply cricoid pressure to help the intubating EMT visualize the vocal cords and the glottic opening. If the patient has a large tongue, or the EMT is having trouble visualizing the airway, the second EMT can retract the cheek to improve the field of vision.

CASE STUDY   MOTOR VEHICLE CRASH

Tom and Barb arrive on the scene of a motor vehicle crash to find a mid-sized car that had apparently struck the back of a flatbed truck. The bed of the truck came through the windshield and into the passenger compartment.

After ensuring that they were in no danger of injury from power lines or other hazards resulting from the crash, the two EMTs approached the vehicle. They noted a significant amount of damage, including a broken windshield and pieces of blue cloth caught in the windshield.

Wearing appropriate personal protective gear, Tom entered the car and undertook manual stabilization of the woman's head and neck.

Upon initial assessment, Barb found that the woman was responsive only to painful stimuli. She had multiple bruises and lacerations to her head and face, and bloody drainage was noted from her nose and mouth.

Barb quickly suctioned her mouth as Tom counted respirations. Tom noted that she was barely breathing. The patient tolerated the oral airway Barb inserted into her mouth.

Realizing that the seriously injured woman could not maintain her own airway and needed ventilatory assistance, Barb called for a rapid extrication.

As the firefighters assisted Tom with the rapid extrication, Barb assembled the bag-valve mask.

STOP AND THINK

1. What will be first priority for this patient after she is extricated?
2. What special considerations have to be taken into account for a trauma patient?
3. What can Tom do to assist?

ANSWERS TO STOP AND THINK

1. After the patient is extricated, and while continuous manual stabilization of her neck is being maintained, her airway must be protected. Initially, basic life support measures should be taken. If the patient remains unconscious, then the patient should be orally intubated.

2. The cervical spine of the trauma patient must be held in strict alignment and no movement of the cervical spine should be permitted, including during intubation. It may be necessary for one EMT to take manual stabilization anteriorly while the patient is being intubated.

3. To assist another EMT who is intubating, the first EMT would first bag-valve-mask ventilate the patient for several minutes while the EMT intubating prepares his equipment. On command, the first EMT would stop bagging the patient and apply cricoid pressure to help the intubating EMT visualize the vocal cords and the glottic opening. If the patient has a large tongue, or the EMT is having trouble visualizing the airway, the second EMT can retract the cheek to improve the field of vision.

ADDITIONAL CASE STUDY   BABY NOT BRAETHING

Laura was hanging clothes out to dry in her backyard when she realized that she no longer heard her two-year-old daughter's chatter from the porch. She called out her daughter's name. "Amanda." There was no answer, just a disquieting silence. She walked over to the porch to investigate.

She found her two-year-old lying on the deck. Her face was blue. She immediately picked her up and ran into the house to call 9–1-1. The dispatcher instructed Laura to provide mouth-to-mouth resuscitation and advised her that the ambulance was en route. Each breath failed to go in. The dispatcher changed instructions and told Laura how to perform abdominal thrusts.

The first responder on-scene was Officer Lee. He quickly assessed the child and confirmed that she was not breathing but did have a pulse. He was continuing his series of abdominal thrusts when the rescue squad pulled up. EMT Kelly assessed the situation as she donned her gloves. She could see that Officer Lee's efforts were fruitless.

STOP AND THINK

1. What would be the next step in the care of this child?
2. How are pediatric airways different then adult airways?
3. What special precautions must be taken, or equipment used, when intubating a child?

ANSWERS TO STOP AND THINK

1. Provided that basic life support measures have failed, the EMT could use the larygnoscope and attempt to directly visualize the airway. If she sees the offending object, she can reach in, using a pair of McGill forceps, and remove the object. If she is unable to remove the object after several attempts, it may be necessary to push the object deeper into one mainstem bronchus with an endotracheal tube, permitting ventilation of the unobstructed lung.

2. A pediatric airway is smaller and the tongue is relatively larger then an adult's. The narrowest portion of the airway is not at the vocal cords, as in an adult, but at the level of the cricoid ring. Also, the epiglottis of the child is omega-shaped.

3. Intubating a child is similar to intubating an adult except smaller equipment is used. Special uncuffed endotracheal tubes and typically a straight, or Miller, blade are used.

ANSWERS TO TEST YOUR KNOWLEDGE

1. The most direct advantage of endotracheal intubation is direct access and control of the airway. This helps to prevent aspiration from regurgitation as well as provide a means of ventilation with a decreased incidence of gastric distension.

2. Endotracheal intubation is indicated whenever the patient is unconscious and unable to maintain an independent airway. Endotracheal intubation is contraindicated when the patient has an intact gag reflex.

3. The Macintosh blade indirectly lifts the glottis into view by lifting adjunct structures whereas the Miller blade directly visualizes the structures of the larynx.

4. Cricoid pressure helps prevent regurgitation by pressing the complete cricoid ring down onto the esophagus, effectively occluding it. Gentle downward pressure on the Adam's Apple, or voice box, is applied with the fingers of one hand.

5. The best confirmation of endotracheal tube placement, the so-called gold standard, is visualization of the endotracheal tube passing through the vocal cords. Indirect methods include equal bilateral breath sounds, expansion of the lungs, and absence of sounds in the epigastrium.

6. The EMT needs to reassess all respiratory signs, including cyanosis and pulse oximetry, as well as vital signs.

7. The worse-case scenario is an esophageal intubation. With the endotracheal tube in the stomach and not in the lungs, the patient is denied any oxygen and hypoxia quickly occurs. In some cases, the endotracheal tube may be in the trachea but pushed too far down into one of the mainstem bronchi, resulting in incomplete inflation of the lungs and a risk of a pneumothraox, or ruptured lung.

8. While the medical patient's neck may be manipulated to align the airway for better visualization of all tracheal structures, the trauma patient's neck must remain essentially neutral. This position makes intubating a trauma patient extremely difficult.

9. The pediatric airway is different from the adult airway in some important ways. Starting at the outside, the teeth are fragile, the tongue is relatively larger, and the epiglottis is more anterior.

10. When air has inadvertently been pushed into the stomach, the stomach expands. The enlarged air-filled stomach prevents complete downward movement of the diaphragm and the lungs as well as presents an aspiration risk if the stomach refluxes into the airway.

Student Name: _____   Date: _____

Skill: Assembly of Laryngoscope and Blade
Equipment Needed:
Appropriate PPE
Laryngoscope Handle
Variety of Blade Types and Sizes
Spare Light Bulbs and Batteries

YES: _____   RE-TEACH: _____   RETURN: _____   INSTRUCTOR INITIALS _____

Step 1: The proximal end of the blade has a notched end that fits onto the handle securely.

YES: _____   RE-TEACH: _____   RETURN: _____   INSTRUCTOR INITIALS _____

Step 2: The notched end of the blade should be firmly attached to the handle with the blade in a closed position.

YES: _____   RE-TEACH: _____   RETURN: _____   INSTRUCTOR INITIALS _____

Step 3: Once properly attached, the blade can be extended and the light bulb at its distal end should turn on.

YES: _____   RE-TEACH: _____   RETURN: _____   INSTRUCTOR INITIALS _____

Step 4: The bulb should be quickly checked for security in position (be sure it is tightly screwed on) and bright quality of light. If the light is dim, the bulb may be poorly connected or the batteries may be low. It is the EMT's responsibility at the beginning of a shift to check the handles and blades to be sure they are functioning optimally.

YES: _____   RE-TEACH: _____   RETURN: _____   INSTRUCTOR INITIALS _____

Student Name: _____ Date: _____

Skill: Endotracheal Intubation
Equipment Needed: Gloves
Mask
Eye Protection
Suction Unit
Yankauer Catheters
Bag-Valve Mask Device
Laryngoscope Handle
Laryngoscope Blades
Endotracheal Tubes (Different Sizes)
Stylet
10 cc Syringe
Oropharyngeal Airway
Tape or Other Securing Device

YES: _____   RE-TEACH: _____   RETURN: _____   INSTRUCTOR INITIALS _____

Step 1: The EMT who will be intubating is above the head of the patient with the lit laryngoscope in his left hand and the prepared endotracheal tube and suction catheter within reach of his right hand.

YES: _____   RE-TEACH: _____   RETURN: _____   INSTRUCTOR INITIALS _____

Step 2: Ventilation must be discontinued. The intubating EMT then places the patient's head in a sniffing position (assuming no spinal injury) and uses his right hand to open the patient's mouth and remove the OPA and dentures (if present). An assisting provider should be applying gentle cricoid pressure.

YES: _____   RE-TEACH: _____   RETURN: _____   INSTRUCTOR INITIALS _____

Step 3: The laryngoscope blade is placed in the right side of the patient's mouth and slid gently into the pharynx.

YES: _____   RE-TEACH: _____   RETURN: _____   INSTRUCTOR INITIALS _____

Step 4: The blade is swept toward the patient's left, moving the tongue out of the visual field.

YES: _____   RE-TEACH: _____   RETURN: _____   INSTRUCTOR INITIALS _____

Step 5: The EMT then lifts the laryngoscope upward in order to move the patient's mandible out of the view. (Care should be taken not to allow the left wrist to bend and to cause pressure from the laryngoscope on the upper teeth. Unnecessary pressure on the upper teeth can result in broken teeth, which can then become airway foreign bodies and might also lead to an untoward cosmetic result.)

YES: _____   RE-TEACH: _____   RETURN: _____   INSTRUCTOR INITIALS _____

Step 6: This maneuver should lift the upper airway structures out of the way. The EMT should be able to visualize the vocal cords and trachea. It should be noted that the trachea is the most anterior hollow structure and the esophagus is the most posterior. Suction should be used to clear any obstructing liquids for better visualization.

YES: _____   RE-TEACH: _____   RETURN: _____   INSTRUCTOR INITIALS _____

Step 7: Once the triangular-shaped white-pink vocal cords have been visualized, the EMT picks up the preformed tube with his right hand and places the distal end through the cords. (It is very important to continue to visualize the tube as it passes through the cords and into the trachea to avoid inadvertent misplacement.)

YES: _____   RE-TEACH: _____   RETURN: _____   INSTRUCTOR INITIALS _____

Step 8: The tube is advanced until the distal cuff is just past the vocal cords (or until the heavy black line at the distal end of an uncuffed pediatric tube has passed the cords).

YES: _____   RE-TEACH: _____   RETURN: _____   INSTRUCTOR INITIALS _____

Step 9: The EMT then holds the tube in that position with his right hand while removing the laryngoscope from the patient's mouth with his life.

YES: _____   RE-TEACH: _____   RETURN: _____   INSTRUCTOR INITIALS _____

Step 10: The left hand then grasps the stylet and removes it from the endotracheal tube, being careful not to displace the tube in the process.

YES: _____   RE-TEACH: _____   RETURN: _____   INSTRUCTOR INITIALS _____

Step 11: While maintaining a constant grip on the tube itself, the EMT then picks up the syringe (it should still be attached to the pilot balloon at the proximal end of the tube) and instills 5 to 10 cc of air. (When the pilot balloon is full but still easily compressed, the right amount of air has been instilled and the distal cuff will be adequately inflated.)

YES: _____   RE-TEACH: _____   RETURN: _____   INSTRUCTOR INITIALS _____

Step 12: Once the cuff is inflated, the syringe is removed from the pilot balloon to prevent inadvertent withdrawal of air. The syringe should be kept at hand, however, in case there is a need to readjust the tube position.

YES: _____   RE-TEACH: _____   RETURN: _____   INSTRUCTOR INITIALS _____

Step 13: The placement of the tube is assessed. Once confirmed to be in the trachea, it is secured in place and the patient ventilated.

YES: _____   RE-TEACH: _____   RETURN: _____   INSTRUCTOR INITIALS _____

Student Name: _____   Date: _____

Skill: Endotracheal Suctioning
Equipment Needed:
Sterile Gloves
Mask
Goggles
Functioning Suction Unit and Tubing
Sterile Water
Various Sizes of Soft French Catheters

YES: _____   RE-TEACH: _____   RETURN: _____   INSTRUCTOR INITIALS _____

Step 1: After applying appropriate PPE, the EMT opens the package with the catheter and sterile gloves, taking care not to contaminate either.

YES: _____   RE-TEACH: _____   RETURN: _____   INSTRUCTOR INITIALS _____

Step 2: The suction unit is tested and the catheter attached to the suction tubing.

YES: _____   RE-TEACH: _____   RETURN: _____   INSTRUCTOR INITIALS _____

Step 3: The EMT applies the sterile gloves and picks up the sterile catheter in the right hand. The left hand will be used to disconnect the bag-valve device from the endotracheal tube.

YES: _____   RE-TEACH: _____   RETURN: _____   INSTRUCTOR INITIALS _____

Step 4: The EMT threads the suction catheter as far into the endotracheal tube as it can go or until the patient coughs.

YES: _____   RE-TEACH: _____   RETURN: _____   INSTRUCTOR INITIALS _____

Step 5: Suction is then applied as the catheter is slowly withdrawn.

YES: _____   RE-TEACH: _____   RETURN: _____   INSTRUCTOR INITIALS _____

Step 6: The EMT should keep the catheter in the right hand (which will remain the sterile hand) and use the left hand to reconnect the bag-valve device to the ET tube and ventilate the patient again for a minute.

YES: _____   RE-TEACH: _____   RETURN: _____   INSTRUCTOR INITIALS _____

Step 7: After the tube has been cleared, the catheter may then be used to suction the patient's oropharynx if needed prior to discarding it. A hard Yankaeur catheter may also be used at any point to suction the patient's oropharynx if needed.

YES: _____   RE-TEACH: _____   RETURN: _____   INSTRUCTOR INITIALS _____

Student Name: _____   Date: _____

Skill: Gastric Decompression
Equipment needed:
Gloves
Mask and Goggles
Orograstric tubes (assorted sizes 9–16 French)
60 cc Syringe
Water-Soluble Lubricant
Tape
Stethoscope
Suction Unit and Catheters

YES: _____   RE-TEACH: _____   RETURN: _____   INSTRUCTOR INITIALS _____

Step 1: After applying appropriate PPE, the EMT properly positions the patient. In the nonintubated, nontrauma patient, the head can be placed in a somewhat flexed position to allow for easier passage of the tube into the esophagus. Most of the patients that an EMT will perform gastric decompression on will have been intubated already and such head movement may jeopardize the position of the endotracheal tube. The head should be kept in a neutral position.

YES: _____   RE-TEACH: _____   RETURN: _____   INSTRUCTOR INITIALS _____

Step 2: The proper depth of the tube is measured from the mouth, around the ear, to a point below the xyphoid process.

YES: _____   RE-TEACH: _____   RETURN: _____   INSTRUCTOR INITIALS _____

Step 3: The distal end of the gastric tube is coated with a water-soluble lubricant prior to the initiation of the procedure.

YES: _____   RE-TEACH: _____   RETURN: _____   INSTRUCTOR INITIALS _____

Step 4: If the patient is intubated and the EMT will be performing orogastric tube placement, the endotracheal tube should be firmly held in place by one provider while another places the orogastric tube. The tube should be passed into the mouth and down toward the esophagus. The tube should pass easily. If any resistance is met, the tube should be withdrawn and the procedure begun again.

YES: _____   RE-TEACH: _____   RETURN: _____   INSTRUCTOR INITIALS _____

Step 5: The tube should be placed to the premeasured depth and then held there while its position is confirmed.

YES: _____   RE-TEACH: _____   RETURN: _____   INSTRUCTOR INITIALS _____

Step 6: The syringe can be placed on the end of the orogastric tube and stomach contents withdrawn, or the tube can be hooked directly to a suction unit to withdraw any contents. It is important to realize that the return of stomach contents alone does not confirm proper placement.

YES: _____   RE-TEACH: _____   RETURN: _____   INSTRUCTOR INITIALS _____

Step 7: Proper gastric placement is confirmed by placing the syringe filled with air on the end of the orogastric tube, and while listening over the epigastrium, rapidly instilling at least 20 cc of air. If the tube is properly placed in the stomach, the injected air will be heard over the epigastrium. If it is not, then the tube is not in the correct place and should be withdrawn and repositioned.

YES: _____   RE-TEACH: _____   RETURN: _____   INSTRUCTOR INITIALS _____

Step 8: Once the orogastric tube is confirmed to be in the stomach, it is hooked to suction and the stomach contents allowed to empty. When the tube no longer drains stomach contents, the suction may be discontinued and the tube left open to air with intermittent suction being applied.

YES: _____   RE-TEACH: _____   RETURN: _____   INSTRUCTOR INITIALS _____

CHAPTER 10

Shock: A State of Hypoperfusion

OBJECTIVES

Upon completion of this chapter, the reader should be able to:

1. Define perfusion and identify the significance of hypoperfusion.
2. Identify five specific etiologies of shock.
3. List the signs and symptoms of compensated shock.
4. Explain the importance of capillary refill in children.
5. Define decompensated shock.
6. Describe the appropriate initial evaluation of the patient in shock.
7. List appropriate steps in management of the patient with signs and sympto-ms of shock.
8. List the indications and contraindications for the use of MAST.
9. Describe the application of MAST.

GLOSSARY:

anaphylactic shock   A hypoperfused state resulting from a severe allergic reaction.

anaphylaxis   An exaggerated allergic reaction that can result in life-threatening airway, breathing, or circulatory compromise.

capillary refill time   The time it takes to see refill (evidenced by a return to normal color) of a capillary bed after blanching(loss of color in area of skin when pressed).

cardiac output   The amount of blood pumped out of the heart in one minute.

cardiogenic shock   A hypoperfused state resulting from inadequate cardiac pumping, usually due to multiple heart attacks.

compensated shock   A hypoperfused state that the body is compensating for by increasing heart rate, increasing respiratory rate, and shunting blood from certain organs.

decompensated shock   A hypoperfused state for which the body is no longer able to compensate and hypotension results.

evisceration   An injury resulting in abdominal organs being outside the abdomen, usually after penetrating abdominal trauma.

hemorrhagic shock   A hypoperfused state resulting from loss of blood.

hypoperfusion   Inadequate supply of oxygenated blood to a tissue or organ.

hypovolemia   A state of low fluid levels.

hypovolemic shock   A hypoperfused state resulting from low fluid levels.

irreversible shock   Hypoperfusion that has progressed to a point that survival is highly unlikely.

military anti-shock trousers (MAST)   A device that is inflated over the lower extremities and pelvis to attempt to increase blood flow to the core organs; also called Pneumatic Anti-Shock Garment (PASG).

neurogenic shock A hypoperfused state resulting from injury to the spinal cord and generalized vasodilation.

orthostatic vital signs   Heart rate and blood pressure measured in different positions, usually lying then standing.

perfusion   Supply of oxygenated blood to organs and tissues throughout the body.

pneumatic anti-shock garment (PASG)   Another name for military anti-shock trousers (MAST), a device that is inflated over the lower extremities and pelvis to attempt to increase blood flow to the core organs.

postural hypotension   A drop in blood pressure associated with a change in position, usually from lying to standing.

septic shock   A hypoperfused state resulting from overwhelming infection and generalized vasodilation.

shock A state in which the body is hypoperfused, resulting in inadequate oxygenation of cells, tissues, and organs.

stroke volume   The amount of blood the heart pumps out with each beat.

tilt test   The process of measuring orthostatic vital signs.

urticaria   A raised, red rash caused by localized dilation and leaking of blood vessels resulting in red, warm, swelling to the surface of the skin; also known as hives.

PREPARATORY

Materials: EMS Equipment: Sterile dressings, bandages, splints, pneumatic anti-shock garment, triangular bandage, stick or rod, air splints, gloves, eye protection, blanket.

Personnel: Primary Instructor: One EMTBasic instructor knowledgeable in bleeding and shock (hypoperfusion). Assistant Instructor: The instructor-to-student ratio should be 1:6 for psychomotor skill practice. Individuals used as assistant instructors should be knowledgeable in bleeding and shock.

Recommended Minimum Time to Complete: 2 hours

STUDENT OUTLINE

I. Chapter Overview
II. Cardiovascular Anatomy and Physiology
    A. Circulation
    B. Cardiac Output
    C. Perfusion
III. Hypoperfusion
    A. Causes of Hypoperfusion
        1. Fluid
            a) Hypovolemic Shock
        2. Container
            a) Anaphylactic Shock
            b) Septic Shock
            c) Neurogenic Shock
        3. Pump
            a) Cardiogenic Shock
IV. Physiologic Response to Shock
    A. Compensated Shock
        1. Pecking Order
        2. Signs and Symptoms
    B. Decompensated Shock
    C. Irreversible Shock
V. Assessment
    A. The Look Test
    B. Mental Status
    C. ABCs
    D. Vital Signs
        1. Orthostatic Vital Signs
VI. Management of Hypoperfusion
    A. Oxygen
    B. Control Bleeding
    C. Trendelenburg
    D. MAST
        1. Indications
        2. Contraindications
            a) Relative Contraindications
        3. MAST Application
        4. MAST Removal
    E. Reduce Heat Loss
    F. Transport
        1. Intercept
        2. Destination Issues
VII. Conclusion

LECTURE OUTLINE

I. Chapter Overview
    A. Cellular Demand
        1. Oxygen
        2. Glucose
    B. Adequate Supply
        1. Perfusion
    C. Inadequate Supply
        1. Hypoperfusion
    D. Prolonged Deprivation
        1. Shock States
            a) Cellular Death
            b) Organ Failure
            c) Death

II. Cardiovascular Anatomy and Physiology
    A. Circulation
        1. Systemic
            a) Vascular Tree
            (1) Arteries
            (2) Arterioles
            (3) Capillaries
            (4) Venules
            (5) Veins
    B. Cardiac Output
        1. Pumping Action
            a) Stroke Volume
            b) Heart Rate
    C. Perfusion
        1. Delivery of oxygen and nutrients
            to cells

III. Hypoperfusion
    A. Causes of Hypoperfusion
        1. Failure of Circulatory System
            a) Pump
            b) Pipes/Container
            c) Fluid
            (1) Red Blood Cells
        2. Fluid
            a) Blood Components
            (1) Red Blood Cells
                (a) Oxygen-carriers
                  (i) Hemoglobin
            (2) White Blood Cells
                (a) Infection-
                    fighters
            (3) Platelets
                (a) Clot-formers
            b) Hypovolemic Shock
            (1) Loss of Fluids
                (a) External Blood
                    Loss
                (b) External Fluid
                    Loss
                  (i) Diarrhea
                (a) Internal Blood
                    Loss
                (b) Internal Fluid
                    Loss
        3. Container
            a) Vascular Changes
            (1) Nervous Control
                (a) Dilation
                (b) Constriction
            b) Anaphylactic Shock
            (1) Stimulus
                (a) Allergen
                  (i) Bee Stings
            (2) Response
                (a) Vasodilation
                (b) Relative Hypovolemia
                (c) Hypoperfusion
            c) Septic Shock
            (1) Stimulus
                (a) Infection
                  (i) Pneumonia
            (2) Response
                (a) Vasodilation
                (b) Relative Hypovolemia
                (c) Hypoperfusion
            d) Neurogenic Shock
            (1) Loss of Nervous control
            (2) Response
                (a) Vasodilation
                (b) Relative Hypovolemia
                (c) Hypoperfusion
        4. Pump
            a) Cardiogenic Shock
            (1) Heart Failure
                (a) Heart Attack (Acute
                    Myocardial Infarction)
            (2) Loss of Cardiac Output
                (a) Hypoperfusion

IV. Physiologic Response to Shock
    A. Compensation
    B. Compensated Shock
        1. Alterations
            a) Heart Rate

b) Selective Capillary Bed Shut-
    down
  (1) Degree of Response
    (a) Varied Degrees
  (2) Shunting
    (a) Pecking Order
      (i) Fetus First
      (ii) Skin
      (iii) Large Muscles
      (iv) Gut
      (v) Heart/Lungs
      (vi) Brain
2. Signs and Symptoms
  a) Fetus First
    (1) Save the Baby, Save the
      Mother
  b) Skin
    (1) Pallor
    (2) Cool and Clammy
  c) Large Muscles
    i) Lethargy
  d) Gut
    (1) Nausea
  e) Heart/Lungs
    (1) Tachycardia
    (2) Tachypnea
  f) Brain
    (1) Altered Mental Status
C. Decompensated Shock
  1. Organ Failures
    a) Hallmark
      (1) Loss of Systolic Pressure
D. Irreversible Shock
  1. Multiple Organ System Failure
    (MOSF)
V. Assessment
  1. Methodical
  A. The Look Test
    1. Ill appearing
  B. Mental Status
    1. Level of Consciousness
      a) AVPU
  C. ABCs
    1. Priority
  D. Vital Signs
    1. Signs
      a) Tachypnea
      b) Tachycardia
      c) Hypotension
    2. Orthostatic Vital Signs aka Tilt
      Test

a) Precautions
  (1) Spinal Injury
  (2) Fainting
b) Standing and Sitting
  (1) 20/20 Rule
VI. Management of Hypoperfusion
  A. Oxygen
    1. First Priority
  B. Control Bleeding
    1. External Bleeding
  C. Trendelenburg
    1. Precautions
      a) Pelvic Fractures
      b) Fractured Extremities
    2. Elevate Legs
      a) 12 to 16 inches above heart
  D. MAST
    1. Action
      a) Compression of Lower Exter-
        mities and Abdomen
        (1) Autotransfusion
        (2) Increased Peripheral Resis-
          tance
    2. Indications
      a) Profound Hypotension
        (1) Systolic less than 50 mm
          Hg
        (2) Systolic less than 90 mm Hg
          with Pelvic Injury
      b) Follow Regional or State Pro-
        tocols
    3. Contraindications
      a) Absolute
        (1) Penetrating Trauma above
          the Diaphragm
        (2) Head Injury
        (3) Pulmonary Edema
          (a) Crackles (Rales)
      b) Relative Contraindications
        (1) Pregnancy
          (a) Do not inflate abdomi-
            nal section
        (2) Evisceration
          (a) Do not inflate abdomi-
            nal section
        (3) Impaled Object
          (a) Do not inflate affected
            limb section
    4. MAST Application
      a) Assessment
      b) Decision

CASE STUDY   INDUSTRIAL ACCIDENT

Jon was just completing his equipment check when his pager went off. "Medical emergency, building 12, man caught in machine, EMS has been notified, time 13:44."

Jon had just completed his first EMT course. The course had been part of his job training as plant security officer at the Greenwood Industrial Park. He was eager to show everybody what he had learned, so he grabbed his kit, jumped into the company pickup, and sped off.

Upon arrival, Jon was met by the plant supervisor, Paul, who led him to the patient. Jon found a young man seated on the floor next to a machine in which his arm seemed to be entangled. His co-workers were in the process of dismantling the machine in order to free his arm.

There was significant tissue damage to the man's upper arm. Then Jon noticed the large pool of blood on the floor next to the machine. Looking around, Jon also noted additional blood inside the machine.

The man cried out in pain as a piece of machinery shifted. Then he looked up to Jon and yelled, "My arm's caught!"

STOP AND THINK

1. Is this patient at risk of developing any life-threatening conditions?
2. What signs and symptoms would this patient predictably develop?
3. What treatment and transportation decisions are indicated?

ANSWERS TO STOP AND THINK

1. If the patient's bleeding continues unabated, he will become hypoperfused, leading to shock and eventually to death.

2. Initially the patient may complain of thirst and have pale, clammy skin. As the shock continues, his muscles, guts, and kidneys will shut down and shunt blood to the core organs. Eventually, if the bleeding continues, the patient's heart will beat faster (tachycardia) and the patient will breathe faster (tachypnea).

3. Entanglement of an extremity is a surgical emergency. Surgical emergencies are best treated in a trauma center. When this patient is disentangled from the machinery, he should be transported immediately, with lights and siren, to a trauma center.

CASE STUDY PNEUMONIA

Mrs. Gray was diagnosed with "pneumonia" after she was seen for a persistent cough. Her doctor prescribed a ten-day course of antibiotics and strict bed rest. On the third day after diagnosis, Mrs. Gray became increasingly lethargic. Her granddaughter, who was concerned about her change in condition, called the doctor's office.

She told the nurse that her grandmother was periodically running high fevers and was not eating well. She also related that her grandmother's pulse, at her wrist, was rapid and weak.

This morning, she told the nurse, her grandmother was very difficult to arouse and then wouldn't even take a sip of water. The nurse advised her to call an ambulance.

When the ambulance arrived, the granddaughter met them at the door. She told the EMTs, "My grandmother has pneumonia."

STOP AND THINK

1. Why is this patient exhibiting the signs and symptoms of shock?
2. What are other possible causes of hypoperfusion and what is the pathophysiology involved?

ANSWERS TO STOP AND THINK

1. While the patient is not bleeding externally, fluids are being lost internally. This loss of fluid creates hypovolemia and then hypoperfusion. The cause of the fluid loss is infection (septic shock).

2. It is not beyond reason to think that an elderly woman whose body is stressed by any infection could have had a heart attack (myocardial infarction), leading to pump failure and hypoperfusion. While an EMT is not expected to come to this conclusion, the point emphasizes the importance of closely monitoring the patient and transporting her to the emergency department.

ADDITIONAL CASE STUDY   BEE STING

While working in his garden, Jack is stung by a bee. Not thinking much of the insect bite, he continues to work. Shortly afterward, he starts to feel itchy and notices that his tongue feels fatter. Thinking he may have gotten some insecticide on himself, he decides to go into the house and shower. While undressing to shower he notices a rash is forming on his chest and his breathing is getting more labored. Not willing to take a chance, he decides to call 9–1-1. While waiting for EMS he starts to feel faint so he quickly sits down on the floor and immediately passes out.

STOP AND THINK

1. What are the symptoms of hypoperfusion and shock?
2. What is the reason (pathophysiology) for these symptoms?

ANSWERS TO STOP AND THINK

1. Loss of consciousness signals a medical emergency. In this case the loss of consciousness is due to hypoperfusion and shock. The first indication of hypoperfusion was the feeling of faintness.

2. The bee sting has caused Jack's body to have an abnormal reaction called anaphylaxis. The result is that all of Jack's blood vessels are enlarging, or dilating, so that not enough blood can fill them. The result is hypoperfusion and hypotension.

TEACHING STRATEGIES

1. Have the students draw an oxygen molecule. Then ask them to describe the path of the oxygen molecule from the environment to the cell, drawing each step. Have the student list under each step possible problems that could interfere with the body getting oxygen from the environment to the cell. When this drawing is complete, go back over the drawing and label the different types of shock.

2. Using a closed model of a hand-pump (the type used to siphon gas) and a bucket show how problems with the pump (pump the siphon weakly), problems with the fluids (empty the bucket), and problems with pipes (puncture the tubing to allow leakage) can impair circulation and lead to hypoperfusion.

3. As a contest, teams of students should use the trouser method, the wrapper method, and any other method they devise to apply MAST/PASG quickly. Time each team's efforts and announce the results. Then ask the students what injuries would not make the trouser method acceptable and what injuries would not make the wrapper method acceptable. The emphasis should be placed on when to apply MAST/PASG and not on how to apply the MAST/PASG.

FURTHER STUDY

Domeier, R. M., et al. (1997). Use of the pneumatic anti-shock garment (PASG). National Association of EMS Physicians. *Prehospital Emergency Care, 1*(1), 32–35.

O'Connor, R. E., & Domeier, R. M. (1997). An evaluation of the pneumatic anti-shock garment (PASG) in various clinical settings. *Prehospital Emergency Care, 1*(1), 36–44.

ANSWERS TO TEST YOUR KNOWLEDGE

1. Shock occurs when the body is unable to meet its metabolic demands. Specifically, the body is unable to perfuse organs and tissues with oxygen-laden blood (hypoperfusion).

2. Shock can be caused by external bleeding (hemorrhagic shock), internal fluid loss from infection (septic shock), or a relative fluid loss from vasodilation that can be due to loss of nervous control (neurogenic shock) or anaphylaxis (anaphylactic shock). Hypoperfusion and shock can also be caused by failure of the heart as a pump (cardiogenic shock).

3. The signs of shock include cool and clammy skin, muscular weakness, tachycardia, tachypnea, and hypotension. The symptoms of shock include thirst, weakness, agitation, nausea, dizziness, and lightheadedness.

4. The body's response to hypoperfusion is to selectively shut down organs in a predictable manner (called the pecking order). The first system to shut down is usually the skin (integumentary system), followed by the bones and muscles (musculoskeletal system), then the gut (gastrointestinal system), and finally the heart and lungs (cardiovascular and respiratory systems). If all these efforts fail, then the brain (central nervous system) suffers and the patient loses consciousness.

5. Decompensated shock is when the body's protective responses fail to maintain normal perfusion (hemostatis). The result is injury or death of organs and eventually the patient's death.

6. The initial evaluation of the patient in shock revolves around assessing and managing the ABCs of the initial assessment, then making a decision to rapidly transport the patient to an appropriate emergency facility.

7. Initial steps in treating the patient in shock include managing the airway, administering high-flow oxygen, assisting ventilation as needed, controlling external bleeding, treating hypoperfusion, and transporting immediately.

8. MAST is used for the patient with severe hypoperfusion, usually manifest with a blood pressure less than 50 mm Hg and a loss of consciousness.

9. MAST must not be used when there is penetrating trauma, such as a gunshot wound (GSW) above the diaphragm or signs of head injury with increased intracranial pressure. MAST must also not be used if the patient has pulmonary edema as evidenced by crackles in the lungs. These are cases of absolute contraindication. MAST must be used cautiously, if at all (cases of relative contraindication), whenever the patient is pregnant (inflate legs only), has an evisceration (inflate legs only), or has an impaled object (inflate unaffected portions only).

SKILLS

Skill 10–1 Orthostatic Vital Signs

Equipment Needed:
Gloves
Stethoscope
Blood Pressure Cuff
Watch with Second Hand
Assistant

Step 1: Obtain a full set of vital signs from the patient while she or he is lying down.

YES: _____   RE-TEACH: _____   RETURN: _____   INSTRUCTOR INITIALS _____

Step 2: Help the patient stand up, with an assistant behind the patient.

YES: _____   RE-TEACH: _____   RETURN: _____   INSTRUCTOR INITIALS _____

Step 3: Repeat vital signs.

YES: _____   RE-TEACH: _____   RETURN: _____   INSTRUCTOR INITIALS _____

Step 4: Compare vitals signs lying and standing.

YES: _____   RE-TEACH: _____   RETURN: _____   INSTRUCTOR INITIALS _____

Step 5: Treat for shock as indicated.

YES: _____   RE-TEACH: _____   RETURN: _____   INSTRUCTOR INITIALS _____

Step 6: Record or report significant changes.

YES: _____   RE-TEACH: _____   RETURN: _____   INSTRUCTOR INITIALS _____

Skill 10–2: Application of MAST

Equipment needed:
Gloves
MAST with Foot Pump Attachment
Stethoscope
Blood Pressure Cuff

Step 1: Perform initial assessment and take vital signs.
YES: _____   RE-TEACH: _____   RETURN: _____   INSTRUCTOR INITIALS _____

Step 2: Identify indications for MAST application: injured patient with severe hypotension (SBP < 50) or hypotension (SBP < 90) with associated pelvic instability WITH other signs of shock (less than two of the following: altered mental status, persistent tachycardia, cool and clammy skin, diaphoresis, thirst, or nausea).
YES: _____   RE-TEACH: _____   RETURN: _____   INSTRUCTOR INITIALS _____

Step 3: Assure lack of absolute contraindications (pulmonary edema, penetrating chest injury).
YES: _____   RE-TEACH: _____   RETURN: _____   INSTRUCTOR INITIALS _____

Step 4: Assess for relative contraindications (pregnancy, impaled object, evisceration).
YES: _____   RE-TEACH: _____   RETURN: _____   INSTRUCTOR INITIALS _____

Step 5: Apply trousers to patient's lower body. (Be sure not to allow trousers to cover ribcate.)
YES: _____   RE-TEACH: _____   RETURN: _____   INSTRUCTOR INITIALS _____

Step 6: Secure velcro fasteners.
YES: _____   RE-TEACH: _____   RETURN: _____   INSTRUCTOR INITIALS _____

Step 7: Attach air pump hoses and set to open position.
YES: _____   RE-TEACH: _____   RETURN: _____   INSTRUCTOR INITIALS _____

Step 8: Use foot pump to inflate trousers until gauge reaches 106 mm Hg or pop-offs release.
YES: _____   RE-TEACH: _____   RETURN: _____   INSTRUCTOR INITIALS _____

Step 9: Set air pump hoses to closed position.
YES: _____   RE-TEACH: _____   RETURN: _____   INSTRUCTOR INITIALS _____

Step 10: Reassess patient's ABCs and vital signs.
YES: _____   RE-TEACH: _____   RETURN: _____   INSTRUCTOR INITIALS _____

CHAPTER 11

Baseline Vital Signs and SAMPLE History

OBJECTIVES

Upon completion of this chapter, the reader should be able to:

1. Identify the vital signs.
2. Describe how to assess the quality and quantity of respiration.
3. Recognize a normal respiratory rate and quality.
4. Describe how to assess the quality and quantity of the pulse.
5. Recognize a normal pulse rate and quality.
6. Describe the methods used to assess blood pressure.
7. Define systolic pressure.
8. Define diastolic pressure.
9. Describe the methods to assess the pupils.
10. Identify normal and abnormal pupil size, shape, and reaction.
11. Describe the methods to assess the skin color, temperature, and condition.
12. Describe how to assess capillary refill in infants and children.
13. Identify normal and abnormal skin colors, temperatures, and conditions.
14. Identify normal and abnormal capillary refill in infants and children.
15. Discuss the use of pulse oximetry.
16. Describe how to measure oxygen saturation using a pulse oximeter.
17. Identify the components of the SAMPLE history.
18. Differentiate between a sign and a symptom.
19. State the importance of accurately reporting and recording the baseline vital signs.

GLOSSARY

accessory muscle use   The excessive use of the neck and chest muscles to assist in respiration.

anisocoria   Unequal pupils.

antecubital fossa   The anterior surface of the elbow, in the bend of the arm.

baseline vital signs   The first set of vital signs obtained, used as a baseline with which to compare subsequent sets.

diastolic   The lower number in the blood pressure; the pressure in the vessels when the heart is resting between contractions.

exhalation   Breathing out.

grunting   A noise made upon exhalation during periods of respiratory distress.

gurgling   Sound of liquid moving; if heard at the airway, indicates a need for suctioning.

inspiration   Breathing in.

jaundice   A yellow skin color.

pallor   Pale skin color.

PERRL   Acronym to report an eye exam: **P**upils **E**qual, **R**ound, and **R**eactive to **L**ight.

pulse oximeter   A tool that allows noninvasive measurement of the blood's oxygen saturation.

pupil   The black center of the eye.

SAMPLE   Acronym to remember the most important basic history questions: **S**igns and symptoms, **A**llergies, **M**edications, **P**ast medical history, **L**ast oral intake, **E**vents leading up to the incident/illness.

sign   Something the examiner can objectively see.

snoring   The sound made when a partial upper airway obstruction, such as from the tongue, exists in the supine patient.

sphygmomanometer   A device that is used to measure blood pressure; a blood pressure cuff.

stridor   A harsh inspiratory sound heard from a narrowed upper airway.

symptom   What a patient subjectively complains of.

systolic   The top number in a blood pressure; refers to the pressure in the vessels when the heart is contracting.

wheezing   A high-pitched expiratory sound heard when lower airway narrowing exists.

PREPARATORY

Materials: Exam gloves, stethoscope (dual and single head) (1:6), blood pressure cuffs (adult, infant, and child) (1:6), penlights (1:6).

Personnel: Primary Instructor: One EMT-Basic instructor knowledgeable in patient assessment. Assistant **Instructor:** The instructor-to-student ratio should be 1:6 for psychomotor skill practice. Individuals used as assistant instructors should be knowledgeable in assessing baseline vital signs and taking SAMPLE histories.

Recommended Minimum Time to Complete: 2 hours

STUDENT OUTLINE

I. Baseline Vital Signs
    A. Respiration
        1. Quantity
        2. Quality
        3. Labored Breathing
    B. Pulse
        1. Quantity
        2. Quality
    C. Blood Pressure
        1. Cuff Application
        2. Measurement by Auscultation
        3. Measurement by Palpation
    D. Skin
        1. Temperature and Moisture
        2. Color
        3. Capillary Refill in Children
    E. Pupils
        1. Size and Shape
        2. Reactivity
    F. Pulse Oximetry
II. Reassessment of Vital Signs
III. History-Taking
        1. Patient Rapport
        2. Proper Introduction of the Crew
        3. The EMT and Proper Etiquette
        4. Comforting Touch
    A. Sample History
        1. Signs and Symptoms
        2. Allergies
        3. Medications
        4. Past Medical/Surgical History
        5. Last Oral Intake
        6. Events Leading Up to Incident/Illness
IV. Conclusion

LECTURE OUTLINE

I. Chapter Overview
   A. Frequently Used Skills
      1. Vital Signs
         a) Respiratory Rate
         b) Heart Rate
         c) Blood Pressure
         d) Skin Temperature
      2. Pupil Check
      3. Pulse Oximetry
      4. Sample History

II. Baseline Vital Signs
      1. Completed After Initial Assessment
      2. Lifesaving Measures First
      3. Establishes Basis for Comparison
      4. Proficiency
      5. Practice Important
   A. Respiration
      1. Quantity
         a) Observation
            (1) Slow
            (2) Fast
         b) Measurement
            (1) Regular
               (a) 30 Seconds × 2
            (2) Irregular
               (a) Full Minute
      2. Quality
         a) Depth
            (1) Shallow
            (2) Moderate
            (3) Deep
         b) Regularity
         c) Quiet
      3. Labored Breathing
         a) Effort
            (1) Accessory Muscle Use
            (2) Intercostal Muscles
               (a) Neck or "Strap" Muscles
            (3) Nasal Flaring
               (a) Pediatrics
            (4) Noise
               (a) Stridor
               (b) Snoring
               (c) Wheezing
               (d) Grunting
                  (i) Pediatrics
   B. Pulse
      1. Defined

         a) Artery Next to Bone Near Surface
      2. Pulse Points
         a) Carotid
         b) Femoral
         c) Radial
            (1) Most Common
         d) Brachial
            (1) Pediatrics
      3. Quantity
         a) Measurement
            (1) Regular
               (a) 30 Seconds × 2
            (2) Irregular
               (a) Full Minute
      4. Quality
         a) Strength
            (1) Strong
            (2) Bounding
            (3) Thready
            (4) Weak
   C. Blood Pressure
      1. Tools
         a) Stethoscope
         b) Sphygmomanometer
      2. Values
         a) Systolic
            (1) Force of Contract
         b) Diastolic
            (1) Resting Pressure or Resistance
      3. Cuff Application
         a) Two-Thirds of Upper Arm
         b) Bare Upper Arm
      4. Measurement by Auscultation
         a) Palpate Brachial Pulse
         b) Antecubital Fossa
         c) Cuff Inflation
         d) Loss of Pulse + 20 mm Hg
         e) Gradual Deflation
         f) First Beat Heard
            (1) Systolic Pressure
         g) Last Beat Heard
         h) Diastolic Pressure
      5. Measurement by Palpation
         a) Palpation of Radial Pulse
         b) Inflation of Cuff
         c) Gradual Release of Pressure
         d) Pulse Felt

(1) Systolic Pressure Only

D. Skin
   1.Temperature and Moisture
      a) Condition
         (1) Warm and Dry
         (2) Hot to Touch
         (3) Cool and Clammy
   2. Color
      a) Assessment
         (1) Nailbeds
         (2) Oral Mucosa
         (3) Conjunctiva
   3. Quality
      a) Pink
         (1) Normal Perfusion
      b) Pale/Pallor/Gray
         (1) Hypoperfusion
      c) Blue
         (1) Poor Oxygenation
            (a) Cyanosis
               (i) Peripheral
                  (1) Poor Circulation
               (ii) Central
                  (1) Poor Oxygenation
      d) Red
         (1) Flushed
            (a) Carbon Monoxide Poisoning
            (b) Heat Exposure
            (c) Sunburn
      e) Yellow
         (1) Jaundice
            (a) Liver Disease
E. Capillary Refill in Children
   1. Reliability
      a) Children
         (1) Good
      b) Adults
         (1) Poor
            (a) Smoking
            (b) Medications
            (c) Age
   2. Technique
      a) Compress First Finger
      b) Release
   3. Value
      a) Return of Circulation in Less Than 2 Seconds
F. Pupils

1. Definitions
   a) Pupil
      (1) Black Center of Eye
   b) Iris
      (1) Colored Ring Around Pupil
         (a) Muscular Ring
            (i) Muscle Contraction
               (1) Constricted Pupil
            (ii) Muscle Relaxation
               (1) Dilated Pupil
2. Shape
   a) Normal
      (1) Round
   b) Abnormal
      (1) Surgery
3. Reactivity
   a) Response to Light
      (1) Bilateral
         (a) Consensual
      (2) Unilateral
         (a) Dilated
            (i) Anisocoria
4. Abbreviation
   a) PERRL
5. Implications of Abnormal Results
   a) Head Injury
   b) Eye Injury
G. Pulse Oximetry
   1. Machine
      a) Noninvasive
      b) Infrared Light Beam
         (1) Measures Absorption
            (a) Oxygenated versus Deoxygenated Blood
      c) Saturation Percentage
         (1) Normal
            (a) 96%–100%
         (2) Abnormal Low
            (a) Less Than 96%
         (3) Critically Low
            (a) Less Than 90%
   2. False Reading
      a) Carbon Monoxide Poisoning
      b) Nail Polish
      c) Blood Pressure Measurement
H. Reassessment of Vital Signs
   1. Standards
      a) Stable
         (1) Every 15 Minutes

b) Minimum Standard
   (2) Two Sets of Recordings
c) Unstable
   (3) Every 5 Minutes
d) After Medication Administration

III. History-Taking
   A. Barriers To History-Taking
      1. Anxiety
      2. Cultural Taboos
      3. Familial Interference
      4. Physical Condition
   B. Patient Rapport
      1. Cultural Considerations
   C. Proper Introduction of the Crew
      1. Self-Introduction
        a) Title
        b) Name
      2. Patient Introduction
        a) First Name Familiarity
          (1) Unprofessional
        b) Respectful
          (1) Title
          (1) Last Name
            (a) Exception
              (i) Invitation
              (ii) Pediatrics
                (1) First Name
      3. Comforting Touch
        a) Cultural Considerations
          (1) Taboos

IV. SAMPLE History
   A. Signs and Symptoms
      1. Symptoms
        a) Patient's Perception
      2. Signs
        a) Visible Physical Indicators
   B. Allergies

      1. Medications
      2. Vital Health Information
   C. Medications
      1. Prescription
        a) Name
          (1) Careful Spelling
        b) Dose
          (1) Label
        c) Frequency
          (1) Compliance
        d) Over-the-Counter
   D. Past Medical/Surgical History
      1. Disease Categories
        a) Stroke
        b) Seizure
        c) Hypertension
        d) Heart Attack
        e) Asthma
        f) Emphysema
        g) Diabetes
        h) Cancer
      2. Personal Physician
        a) Name
        b) Practice
      3. Sources of Information
        a) Patient
        b) Medic-Alert
        c) Family
        d) Personal Belongings
          (1) Law Enforcement
             Officer
   E. Last Oral Intake
      1. Vomiting and Aspiration
      2. Surgical Risk
   F. Events Leading Up to Incident/Illness
      1. Trigger
      2. Mechanism of Injury
IV. Conclusion

TEACHING STRATEGIES

1. Ask the students to interview a friend or family member with a medical condition. Have them report the SAMPLE history and vital signs.

2. Arrange for the students to visit the local hospital's emergency department. Have the students assigned to the triage desk assist the nurse with SAMPLE history and vital signs.

3. Arrange for the students to visit a local nursing home. Have them assigned to specific patients. The students should obtain a SAMPLE history and vital signs on those patients and report them to the charge nurse.

FURTHER STUDY

DeLaune, S., & Ladner, P. (1998). *Fundamentals of nursing: Standards and practice*. Albany, NY: Delmar Thompson Learning.
Lindh, W., et al. (1998). *Comprehensive medical assisting*. Albany, NY: Delmar-Thompson Learning.
Estes, M. E. (1998). *Health assessment and physical examination*. Albany, NY: Delmar Publishers.

ANSWERS TO TEST YOUR KNOWLEDGE

1. The vital signs are temperature, pulse, respiration, and blood pressure. Pulse oximetry has been referred to as the fifth vital sign.

2. The quality of respiration is a subjective assessment as the EMT observes the patient's breathing, looking for labored breathing, and as she or he describes the breathing. The quantity of respiration is a function of counting the breaths per minute.

3. The normal respiratory rate of an adult is 12 to 20 breaths per minute. Pediatric respiratory rates are slightly faster. Pediatric respiratory rates should be compared to a chart of normal respiratory rates for children. A child's respiratory rate is not normally slower than an adult's.

4. The quality of the pulse is a subjective assessment as the EMT feels the pulse, looking for strength and regularity. The quantity of the pulse is a function of counting the number of beats per minute.

5. The normal pulse rate of an adult is 70 to 100 beats per minute. The normal pulse rate of a child is faster. Pediatric pulse rates should be compared to a chart of normal pulse rates for children. A child's pulse rate is not normally slower than an adult's.

6. The more traditional method of obtaining a blood pressure reading is with the aid of a stethoscope and listening for the systolic and diastolic pressure. In some special limited cases a systolic blood pressure can be felt using a blood pressure cuff only and obtaining a radial pulse.

7. The systolic pressure is the pressure created by the contraction of the heart.

8. The diastolic pressure is the pressure within the blood vessels between beats, when the heart is at rest, and can be thought of as the resistance that the heart will have to beat against.

9. The pupils are assessed by shading the eyes from room light, then using a penlight directed at each pupil and observing the constriction of the iris and the size of the pupil.

10. A patient's pupils are normally midline, brisk to react, and consensual. Some EMTs will note that the pupils were equal, round, and reactive to light (PERRL). Abnormal pupils are unequal (anisorcia) or sluggish to react.

11. The skin temperature is best assessed by pressing the flesh on the back of one's hand on the patient's forehead. The skin color is observed by looking at the conjunctiva, the mucosa, or the nailbeds.

12. To test the capillary refill in a child, the EMT would compress the nailbed of the first finger and release it. The nailbed would initially be pale, then return to its normal color within 2 seconds if it is normal and the capillary bed is perfused.

13. Several atypical skin conditions include cyanosis (a sign of hypoxia), jaundice (a sign of liver disease), and flushed (a sign of heat exposure, carbon monoxide poisoning, or sunburn).

14. The normal capillary refill time for a child is less than 2 seconds. Capillary refill times greater than 2 seconds are abnormal.

15. Pulse oximetry is a useful adjunct to the EMT's assessment of the patient's respiratory status. It helps the EMT determine if oxygen administration is sufficient or if the patient needs assistance with ventilation.

16. The probe of the pulse oximeter is placed on the first finger and the machine is turned on. Once the machine has an adequate sample, as indicated by the flashing light or graph, the EMT can take a reading.

17. The components of the SAMPLE history are S = Signs and Symptoms, A = Allergies, M = Medications, P = Past medical history, L = Last meal, and E = Events preceding.

18. A sign is an indicator that the EMT observes whereas a symptom is a condition that the patient senses and can describe.

19. Serial vital signs, obtained after the initial baseline vital signs, help the EMT determine if the patient is improving or deteriorating as a result of treatment.

Student Name: _____ Date: _____

Skill: Measurement of Respiration
Equipment Needed:
Personal Protective Equipment (minimally gloves)
Watch/clock with Second Hand

YES: _____   RE-TEACH: _____   RETURN: _____   INSTRUCTOR INITIALS _____

Step 1: Apply any appropriate personal protective equipment.

YES: _____   RE-TEACH: _____   RETURN: _____   INSTRUCTOR INITIALS _____

Step 2: Observe patient's chest or abdomen for rise and fall with respiration, noting any irregular patterns, noises, or effort.

YES: _____   RE-TEACH: _____   RETURN: _____   INSTRUCTOR INITIALS _____

Step 3: Note whether the respiration is shallow or particularly labored.

YES: _____   RE-TEACH: _____   RETURN: _____   INSTRUCTOR INITIALS _____

Step 4: Count the number of complete breaths taken (one inspiration and one exhalation count as ONE breath) over a 30-second period.

YES: _____   RE-TEACH: _____   RETURN: _____   INSTRUCTOR INITIALS _____

Step 5: Multiply this number by 2 to obtain breaths per minute.

YES: _____   RE-TEACH: _____   RETURN: _____   INSTRUCTOR INITIALS _____

Step 6: Record the respiratory rate and quality.

YES: _____   RE-TEACH: _____   RETURN: _____   INSTRUCTOR INITIALS _____

Student Name: _____   Date: _____

Skill: Measurement of Pulse
Equipment needed:
Personal Protective Equipment (minimally gloves)
Watch/clock with Second Hand

YES: _____   RE-TEACH: _____   RETURN: _____   INSTRUCTOR INITIALS _____

Step 1: Apply appropriate personal protective equipment.
YES: _____   RE-TEACH: _____   RETURN: _____   INSTRUCTOR INITIALS _____

Step 2: Find radial pulse at thumb side of wrist and note the quality and regularity of the pulse.
YES: _____   RE-TEACH: _____   RETURN: _____   INSTRUCTOR INITIALS _____

Step 3: Count the number of pulse beats felt over a 30-second period.
YES: _____   RE-TEACH: _____   RETURN: _____   INSTRUCTOR INITIALS _____

Step 4: Multiply this number by 2 to obtain beats per minute.
YES: _____   RE-TEACH: _____   RETURN: _____   INSTRUCTOR INITIALS _____

Step 5: Record the pulse rate, quality, and regularity.
YES: _____   RE-TEACH: _____   RETURN: _____   INSTRUCTOR INITIALS _____

Student Name: _____   Date: _____

Skill: Measurement of Blood Pressure by Auscultation
Equipment needed:
Personal Protective Equipment (minimally gloves)
Stethoscope
Proper Size Blood Pressure Cuff
YES: _____   RE-TEACH: _____   RETURN: _____   INSTRUCTOR INITIALS _____

Step 1: Apply appropriate personal protective equipment.
YES: _____   RE-TEACH: _____   RETURN: _____   INSTRUCTOR INITIALS _____

Step 2: Place the blood pressure cuff around the patient's upper arm snugly.
YES: _____   RE-TEACH: _____   RETURN: _____   INSTRUCTOR INITIALS _____

Step 3: Find the brachial pulse.
YES: _____   RE-TEACH: _____   RETURN: _____   INSTRUCTOR INITIALS _____

Step 4: Close the valve on the cuff.
YES: _____   RE-TEACH: _____   RETURN: _____   INSTRUCTOR INITIALS _____

Step 5: Inflate the cuff until the brachial pulse is no longer felt, then 20 points higher.
YES: _____   RE-TEACH: _____   RETURN: _____   INSTRUCTOR INITIALS _____

Step 6: Place the stethoscope on the brachial pulse and in your ears.
YES: _____   RE-TEACH: _____   RETURN: _____   INSTRUCTOR INITIALS _____

Step 7: Slowly deflate the blood pressure cuff using the valve next to the bulb.
YES: _____   RE-TEACH: _____   RETURN: _____   INSTRUCTOR INITIALS _____

Step 8: Note the systolic and the diastolic pressures.
YES: _____   RE-TEACH: _____   RETURN: _____   INSTRUCTOR INITIALS _____

Step 9: Allow complete deflation of cuff.
YES: _____   RE-TEACH: _____   RETURN: _____   INSTRUCTOR INITIALS _____

Step 10: Record blood pressure.
YES: _____   RE-TEACH: _____   RETURN: _____   INSTRUCTOR INITIALS _____

Student Name: _____   Date: _____

Skill: Measurement of Blood Pressure by Palpation
Equipment needed:
Personal Protective Equipment (minimally gloves)
Proper Size Blood Pressure Cuff

YES: _____   RE-TEACH: _____   RETURN: _____   INSTRUCTOR INITIALS _____

Step 1: Apply appropriate personal protective equipment.

YES: _____   RE-TEACH: _____   RETURN: _____   INSTRUCTOR INITIALS _____

Step 2: Place the blood pressure cuff around the patient's upper arm snugly.

YES: _____   RE-TEACH: _____   RETURN: _____   INSTRUCTOR INITIALS _____

Step 3: Find the radial pulse.

YES: _____   RE-TEACH: _____   RETURN: _____   INSTRUCTOR INITIALS _____

Step 4: Close the valve on the cuff.

YES: _____   RE-TEACH: _____   RETURN: _____   INSTRUCTOR INITIALS _____

Step 5: Inflate the cuff until the radial pulse is no longer felt, then 20 points higher.

YES: _____   RE-TEACH: _____   RETURN: _____   INSTRUCTOR INITIALS _____

Step 6: Slowly deflate the blood pressure cuff using the valve next to the bulb.

YES: _____   RE-TEACH: _____   RETURN: _____   INSTRUCTOR INITIALS _____

Step 7: Note the pressure on the valve at the time that you feel the return of the radial pulse.

YES: _____   RE-TEACH: _____   RETURN: _____   INSTRUCTOR INITIALS _____

Step 8: Allow complete deflation of cuff.

YES: _____   RE-TEACH: _____   RETURN: _____   INSTRUCTOR INITIALS _____

Step 9: Record blood pressure.

YES: _____   RE-TEACH: _____   RETURN: _____   INSTRUCTOR INITIALS _____

Student Name: _____   Date: _____

Skill: Pulse Oximetry
Equipment needed:
Appropriate Personal Protective Equipment
Pulse Oximeter with Indicator Light
Nail Polish Remover
YES: _____   RE-TEACH: _____   RETURN: _____   INSTRUCTOR INITIALS _____

Step 1: Apply appropriate personal protective equipment.
YES: _____   RE-TEACH: _____   RETURN: _____   INSTRUCTOR INITIALS _____

Step 2: Assess the patient and apply oxygen as thought appropriate.
YES: _____   RE-TEACH: _____   RETURN: _____   INSTRUCTOR INITIALS _____

Step 3: Turn on pulse oximeter.
YES: _____   RE-TEACH: _____   RETURN: _____   INSTRUCTOR INITIALS _____

Step 4: Place probe on patient's finger
(if nail polish is present, you must remove polish first).
YES: _____   RE-TEACH: _____   RETURN: _____   INSTRUCTOR INITIALS _____

Step 5: Note indicator light assuring adequate sampling.
YES: _____   RE-TEACH: _____   RETURN: _____   INSTRUCTOR INITIALS _____

Step 6: Note reading as "percent saturated" and document it.
YES: _____   RE-TEACH: _____   RETURN: _____   INSTRUCTOR INITIALS _____

Step 7: Turn device off and store in safe location.
YES: _____   RE-TEACH: _____   RETURN: _____   INSTRUCTOR INITIALS _____

CHAPTER 12

Lifting and Moving Patients

OBJECTIVES

Upon completion of this chapter, the reader should be able to:

1. Discuss proper back care.
2. Define body mechanics as it pertains to the tasks of an EMT.
3. Discuss the guidelines and safety precautions that need to be followed when lifting a patient.
4. State the guidelines for reaching and their application.
5. Describe the guidelines and safety precautions for carrying patients and/or equipment.
6. State the guidelines for pushing and pulling.
7. Discuss the general considerations of moving patients.
8. State several situations that may require the use of an emergency move.
9. Describe and demonstrate four emergency drags.
10. Describe and demonstrate six emergency carries.
11. Describe and demonstrate two lifts used for routine transportation.
12. Describe the utilization the following patient carrying devices:
    a. Orthopedic or scoop stretcher
    b. Stairchair
    c. Basket stretcher
    d. Flexible stretcher
    e. Portable stretcher (litter)
    f. Wheeled stretcher
13. Describe correct and safe carrying procedures on stairs.
14. Describe correct and safe carrying procedures for stretchers.
15. Describe proper patient packaging.
16. Describe correct and safe transferring procedures.

GLOSSARY

arm drag   A patient movement technique in which the EMT grasps the wrists of the patient, pulls the arms to the patient's chest, and drags the patient by the arms.

back strap carry   A carrying technique whereby the EMT steps in front of a standing patient and, using the patient's arms, hoists the patient onto his back with the patient's feet dragging.

basket stretcher   A type of stretcher, such as the Stokes basket, that allows complete immobilization of the patient and protection during a move over rough terrain.

bedroll   The linen on the stretcher to cover the patient.

blanket drag A technique used to move patients by placing them on a blanket to drag them across the ground.

body mechanics The proper or most efficient way to perform physical activities that are safe, are energy-conserving, and help prevent the physical strains that may cause injury.

carry transfer A means of moving a patient from one stretcher to another by lifting and carrying the patient.

caterpillar pass A means of replacing tired rescuers with fresh ones in carrying a patient on a stretcher without actually putting the patient down.

chair carry The use of a standard kitchen chair to move a patient.

clothing drag The technique of pulling a patient to safety using the clothing he or she is wearing.

cradle carry An emergency means of moving a patient involving lifting the patient up and cradling him or her in the arms for a rapid move from the dangerous environment.

cravat A simple cotton triangular bandage useful in many circumstances.

diamond stretcher carry A technique in which four EMTs carry a patient on a stretcher, one at either end and one on each side.

direct carry Lifting a patient and carrying her or him a short distance directly to the stretcher.

direct lift A technique that allows three EMTs to lift a patient from the ground without using assistive devices.

drawsheet Either a regular sheet folded over in half or a sturdy linen of equal length used to move a patient from a bed to a stretcher, or vice versa.

drawsheet transfer Use of a drawsheet to move a patient from one stretcher to another.

emergency drag A technique used by a single EMT to move a patient quickly in an emergency.

emergency move The technique that an EMT uses to quickly remove a patient from danger.

end-to-end stretcher carry The use of one EMT on either end of a stretcher to carry it.

extremity lift A lifting technique whereby one EMT stands behind a seated patient and grasps her or him under the shoulders, while a second EMT grasps the patient under the knees and they lift and carry her or him.

firefighter's carry A technique that involves lifting a supine patient up onto the EMT's shoulder to quickly move the patient from a dangerous environment.

firefighter's drag A carrying technique that involves the patient's arms being around the EMT's neck and the EMT crawling on hands and knees dragging the patient underneath him or her.

flexible stretcher A lightweight plastic stretcher that may be rolled up when not in use; it is commonly used in confined space and cave rescue.

four corners carry A patient conveyance technique in which four or more EMTs carry a stretcher over a distance.

litter A stretcher or other means of patient conveyance that does not have wheels and must be carried.

orthopedic stretcher A stretcher that splits in half and can be placed under the patient one half at a time; also known as the scoop stretcher.

power grip A technique of lifting with the palms up to provide a better grip.

power lift A technique used to lift a heavy object, such as a patient on a backboard, from the ground; also called a squat lift.

Reeves(R) stretcher A commercially available long, flat litter with handles on all corners that can be wrapped around the patient and allows for easy movement of the nonspinal-injured patient.

rescuer assist The use of one EMT on one side of a walking patient for assistance with walking.

scoop stretcher A stretcher that splits in half and can be placed under the patient one half at a time; also known as the orthopedic stretcher.

seat carry A technique of carrying a conscious patient that utilizes two EMTs who join arms and allow the patient to sit on their arms as if they formed a seat.

squat lift A technique used to lift a heavy object, such as a patient on a backboard, from the ground; also called the power lift.

stairchair A specially designed chair that has handles on the back and on the front that a patient may be secured into and then carried down a flight of stairs by two EMTs.

sling A loop of webbing used to help even the load when carrying a litter or basket; also known as a stringer.

Stokes basket A type of basket stretcher that allows complete immobilization and protection of the patient during moves over rough terrain.

stringer Another name for a sling.

transfer board A smooth, flat device that is used when transferring a patient from one stretcher to another to reduce friction and the work involved in the transfer; also called a slide board.

PREPARATORY

Material: EMS Equipment: Wheeled stretcher, stairchair, scoop stretcher, flexible stretcher, ambulance, long and short backboards, bed.

Personnel: Primary Instructor: One EMT-Basic instructor knowledgeable in this area. Assistant Instructor: The instructor-to-student ratio should be 1:6 for psychomotor skills practice. Individuals used as assistant instructors should be knowledgeable about lifting and moving patients.

Recommended Time to Complete: 3 hours

STUDENT OUTLINE

1) Back Injuries
   a) Anatomy Review
      i) Back Care
   b) Know Your Limitations
      i) Is There Enough Help?
   c) What Is the "Right Stuff"?
      i) Safety First
2) Body Mechanics
   a) Reaching
   b) Lifting
   c) Power Lift
   d) The Power Grip
   e) Carrying
   f) Pushing and Pulling
3) Planning a Move
   a) Emergency Moves
   b) Emergency Drags
      i) The Clothing Drag
      ii) The Arm Drag
      iii) The Blanket Drag
      iv) The Firefighter's Drag
   c) Emergency Carries
      i) The Rescuer Assist
      ii) The Pack Strap Carry
      iii) The Cradle Carry
      iv) The Firefighter's Carry
      v) The Seat Carry
      vi) The Chair Carry
   d) Nonurgent Moves
   e) Command and Coordination
      i) The Extremity Lift
      ii) The Direct Lift
      iii) Scoop Stretcher
      iv) Stairchairs
   f) The Stair Carry
   g) Off-Road Stretchers
      i) The Basket Stretcher
      ii) The Flexible Stretcher
   h) Off-Road Carries
      1) The End-to-End Carry
      2) The Diamond Stretcher Carry
      3) The Four Corners Carry
         a) The Use of Slings
      4) Passing over Obstacles
4) Packaging the Patient
   a) Positioning
   b) Strapping
   c) Transfer to the Ambulance
   d) Loading the Ambulance
   e) Transfer to Hospital Bed
      i) The Carry Transfer
      ii) The Drawsheet transfer
      iii) The Use of a Transfer Board

LECTURE OUTLINE

1) Back Injuries
    a) Anatomy Review
        (1) Lumbar
            (a) Weight-bearing
            (b) Injury-prone
        (2) Vertebrae
            (a) Support
                (i) Muscles
                (ii) Ligaments
            (b) Cushion
                (i) Intervertebral discs
                (ii) Back Care
        (1) strong muscles
            (a) regular exercise program
                (i) weight training
                (ii) tai chi
        (2) preparation for lifting
            (a) warm-up
    b) Know your limitations
        i) Critical Questions
            (1) Is there enough help?
            (2) Is the right equipment being used?
        ii) Is There Enough Help?
            (1) Functional job description
                (a) each EMT lifts 125 pounds
        iii) What is the "Right Stuff"?
            (1) adjunctive equipment
                (a) weight/strength
                (b) ease of function—carrying
        iv) Safety First
            (1) orthopedic back braces
                (a) Caution—proper use
            (2) proper footwear
                (a) nonskid soles
                (b) ankle protection
2) Body Mechanics
    a) efficient lifting
        (1) injury prevention
        (2) energy-conserving
    b) Reaching
        i) never lean backwards
        ii) never twist lower back
        iii) keep back straight
        iv) keep elbows close to body
            (1) no more than 12 inches reach

        v) bend at the knees
    c) Lifting
        i) back straight
        ii) load close to center of gravity
        iii) use of strong leg muscles
    d) Power Lift
        i) stand close to object
            (1) about 6 inches
            (2) feet under object if possible
                (a) feet flat
            (3) squat to object
    e) The Power Grip
        i) palms up
        ii) elbows locked out
    f) Carrying
        i) shoulder slings
            (1) slip load off shoulder
        ii) balanced load
            (1) one each shoulder
    g) Pushing and Pulling
        i) Push rather than pull
        ii) push at waits level
        iii) elbows close to body
        iv) use axillary device to extend reach
            (1) rope, for example
3) Planning a Move
    i) preplanning
        (1) prevents injuries
    ii) elements of preplan
        (1) survey the scene
        (2) determine urgency of carry
        (3) determine resources
            (a) personnel
            (b) equipment
        (4) communicate the plan
            (a) typical standard approaches
                (i) person at head calls the start of the move
                (ii) EMT is usually on patient's left side
                (iii) strongest person at the head
    b) Emergency Moves
        i) risk-benefit analysis
            (1) reality of danger
            (2) potential for further injury
        ii) first priority
            (1) EMT safety

c) Emergency Drags
    (1) performed alone
  ii) The Clothing Drag
    (1) grab collar of clothing
    (2) walk backwards
  iii) The Arm Drag
    (1) grasp wrists
      (a) cross-chest carry
    (2) conscious patient
      (a) head and neck injuries
  iv) The Blanket Drag
    (1) blanket or similar object
    (2) patient log-rolled onto blanket
    (3) blanket pulled
  v) The Firefighter's Drag
    (1) forward-facing drag
      (a) permits danger ahead to be seen
    (2) cravat
      (a) secure hands
      (b) protects patient from falling debris
d) Emergency Carries
    (1) lift and carry of patient
    (2) limitations
      (a) EMT strength
      (b) patient size
      (c) distance to cover
  ii) The Rescuer Assist
    (1) partially ambulatory
  iii) The Pack Strap Carry
    (1) semiconscious to unconscious
    (2) physically demanding
  iv) The Cradle Carry
    (1) small adults and children
    (1) physically demanding
  v) The Firefighter's Carry
    (1) classic carry
    (2) assistant can help with lift to back
    (3) physically demanding
  vi) The Seat Carry
    (1) two EMTs needed
    (2) hands interlaced to form seat
  vii) The Chair Carry
    (1) use of readily available adjunct
      (a) straightback chair
e) Nonurgent Moves
  i) time is not as import ant
  ii) patient safety is more important
    (1) prevention of further injury
f) Command Coordination

    (1) clear communication
    (2) improved efficiency
    (3) lowered risk of injury
  ii) The Extremity Lift
    (1) two EMTs
    (2) cross-chest wrist carry
  iii) The Direct Lift
    (1) two or three EMTs
    (2) cradle lift
    (3) cross-arms support
  iv) Scoop Stretcher
    (1) clam-shell device
    (2) useful in tight spaces
  v) Stairchairs
    (1) collapsible chair-like device
    (2) small spaces
      (a) stairwells
      (b) narrow hallways
g) The Stair Carry
  i) third EMT
    (1) bracing back of first
    (2) calling out steps
h) Off-Road Stretchers
    (1) special off-road operations
      (a) farmer in field
      (b) hunter in woods
      (c) hiker on trail
  ii) The Basket Stretcher
    (1) carrying device
      (a) rigid
      (b) rugged
      (c) designed for rope rescue
  iii) The Flexible Stretcher
    (1) materials
      (a) plastic
        (i) SKED(R)
      (b) Canvas
        (i) Reeves(R)
        (ii) Litters
  i) Off-Road Carries
      (a) Utility
        (i) long carry
        (ii) uneven ground
    (2) The End-to-End Carry
      (a) two EMTs
      (b) short distance
      (c) all facing forward
        (i) fall prevention
    (3) The Diamond Stretcher Carry
      (a) four EMTs
      (b) short distance
      (c) assisting civilians

(4) The Four Corners Carry
    (a) multiple EMS
    (b) long distance
        (i) back country rescue
    (c) team carry
    (d) The Use of Slings
        (i) reduces fatigue
            1. reduces back injury
        (ii) load-sharing
        (iii) balance
(5) Passing over Obstacles
    (a) catepillar pass
        (i) human bucket brigade
        (ii) EMT static, basket
            moves

4) Packaging the Patient
  i) many names
    (1) gurney
    (2) trundle
    (3) stretcher
    (4) cot
  ii) qualities
    (1) portable
    (1) wheeled
  b) Positioning
    i) high-Fowlers
    ii) modified Trendelenburg
  c) Strapping
    i) points of fixation
      (1) shoulder girdle
      (2) pelvic girdle
    ii) crash-worthy
      (1) three-point harnesses
    iii) comfort
      (1) padding

    (a) buckles
    (b) objects
        (i) oxygen bottles
d) Transfer to the Ambulance
  i) lowest position
e) Loading the Ambulance
  i) lifting principles
    (1) power lift
      (a) bend knees
      (b) lift with back
    (2) power grip
      (a) leather gloves
f) Transfer to Hospital Bed
  (1) travel
    (a) feet first typical
  (2) completion of patient care
  ii) The Carry Transfer
    (1) device-assisted
      (a) backboard
      (b) flexible stretcher
    (2) manual carry
  iii) The Drawsheet Transfer
    (1) sling carry
      (a) strength of material
    (2) The Use of a Transfer Board
      (a) plastic device
        (i) sliding board
5) Conclusion
  a) Lifting common
    i) Function of every EMS call
  b) injuries common
    i) lost providers
  c) safety first
    i) EMT safety

TEACHING STRATEGIES

1. Take the class to a three-story home and provide them with a variety of lifting and carrying situations. Include some emergency moves as well as a large number of routine moves. Have each situation conclude with the loading of the patient into the ambulance.

2. Contact the local search and rescue team and ask them to come and do a presentation of backwoods rescue techniques, including cross-country carry. Have the students assist with a quarter-mile carry so that they can understand how labor-intensive a cross-country carry is.

FURTHER STUDY

Hegner, B. R., & Caldwell, E. (1995) . *Nursing assistant: A nursing process approach* (4th ed.) . Albany, NY: Delmar-Thompson Learning.

U.S. Fire Administration and Federal Emergency Management Agency (1994) *EMS safety: Techniques and applications* (Publication FA-144) . Emmitsburg, MD: USFA Publications.

CASE STUDY   FIRE-RESCUE

The smoke was choking, and the pace was maddeningly slow as firefighter-EMT Santulli crawled along on all fours. He had been detailed to the rescue company to cover a sick call-out. The first alarm this morning was a fire in an abandoned house.

"The house fire was probably the work of arsonists," he thought as he did the room-by-room search.

Suddenly, he felt something move. Yes, something, or someone had grabbed his leg. He yelled out, "Someone's in here!"

Turning, he saw an elderly man who appeared to be coughing in fits and then collapsed to the ground. Santulli thought, "Maybe he was trying to crawl out and got lost. It's easy to understand how someone could get lost in all this thick black smoke."

Firefighter-EMT Deso joined him at the patient's side. Yelling at the top of his lungs, through his mask, he told Santulli that the ambulance was at the backdoor "standing by."

STOP AND THINK

1. What about this situation makes it urgent that the firefighter-EMT move the patient?

2. Are there any risks with moving the patient?

3. Is the move justified in light of those risks?

4. What method could the firefighter use to move the patient if he is ambulatory? If the patient is injured but conscious?

5. How could the EMT move the unconscious patient to a safe area? What can the EMT do if there is another EMT available?

ANSWERS TO STOP AND THINK

1. The heavy smoke and the presence of fire make it imperative that this patient be rescued immediately.

2. This elderly patient may have sustained injuries that prevented him from escaping. Movement may further injure the patient.

3. The situation described is potentially life-threatening, and life comes before limb.

4. If the patient is ambulatory, the FF-EMT could help the patient using an emergency assist or an emergency drag.

5. The FF-EMT would use an emergency carry if the patient was unconscious. If another FF-EMT was available, a seat carry or chair carry may be useful.

CASE STUDY   A FALL AT HOME

The scene is a house call for a medical emergency. An elderly patient, who has fallen, called EMS. Paramedics from the fire department are already on-scene.

As A. J. steps out of the ambulance, he looks up at the three-story house. Located in an older section of the city, the house is in the old Victorian style, including narrow halls and even narrower stairs.

Once A. J. reaches the top of the stairs, he is greeted by the fire lieutenant. Lieutenant Groat explains that the patient had slipped on a throw rug, fallen, and appears to have broken her hip. The patient's vital signs are stable. A routine transfer is needed to a local hospital for further evaluation and possible surgical repair of the hip.

The only problem is that she fell in the bathroom between the toilet and the bathtub. There is plenty of help available. Her condition is not urgent at this time, so the EMT discusses the method of removal with the paramedic.

STOP AND THINK

1. What methods could the EMT use to move the patient in this case?

2. Suppose the patient had fallen in the dining room. Would that location change the method used?

3. What method would be used if the patient's problem was shortness of breath instead of a probable hip injury?

ANSWERS TO STOP AND THINK

1. The patient movement will be dictated by physical conditions. If there is room in the hallway, a log-axis drag may be in order. If there is not room, either a three-person lift or an orthopedic stretcher may be appropriate.

2. If a larger area was available to work in, the EMT can choose a variety of moving devices, including a Reeves® stretcher or a long backboard.

3. If the patient is short of breath, it is unlikely that he would tolerate lying flat (orthopnea) . The patient would therefore have to moved onto a stairchair or carried down the stairs in a cradle carry to the ambulance gurney.

CASE STUDY   A HUNTING ACCIDENT

The day was perfect for hunting. The leaves were down, the sky was clear, the sun was warm, and the wind was calm. Everything was perfect, or so Tom through as he climbed into the old tree stand for a look around. He knew he wasn't supposed to climb up anything he hadn't set up himself, but he just wanted a quick look.

Now, here he was lying on the ground, at the foot of the tree, with an arrow impaled in his thigh. Thank goodness for cellular phones.

One quick call and a lengthy description of where he was and help was on the way. He estimated that he was about 4 miles north of Beaver Dam Road.

He started to wonder, "How are they going to get me out of here?"

STOP AND THINK

1. What method would be used to carry this hunter out of the woods?

2. What method would be used if the trail were narrow?

3. What would the team do if a fallen tree obstructed their pathway?

ANSWERS TO STOP AND THINK

1. The hunter would likely be carried out on either a Stokes basket or similar device using a four-person carry.

2. If the trail is narrow, the basket would be carried using the diamond configuration. If the trail is too narrow for this approach, an end-to-end carry with frequent breaks would be necessary.

3. When coming across an obstruction in the pathway, the team would have to perform a caterpillar pass over the obstacle before continuing.

ANSWERS TO TEST YOUR KNOWLEDGE

1. Backcare is an attitude that an EMT takes to exercise, to lift properly, and to protect her or his back from injury.

2. An EMT should always keep his back straight, keep the weight over his center of gravity, and lift with his legs, not his back or arms.

3. An EMT should always check to be sure the ground is level and that her feet are flat. Then she should practice good backcare.

4. Never twist or overextend to reach something. Heavy objects being reached for should be within 12 inches of the body.

5. An EMT should never lift more than 125 pounds without assistance. An EMT should always use proper lifting techniques.

6. An EMT must also be careful of the amount being carried. The assistance of other EMTs or the use of assistive carrying devices should be considered.

7. When possible, an object should be pushed rather than pulled. Pushing from waist height reduces injuries. Use of straps, ropes, and other devices helps lengthen an EMT's reach.

8. The type of lift and carry is determined by the danger on-scene, the urgency or priority of the medical emergency, and personnel and equipment that is available.

9. An emergency move should be considered whenever there is a greater risk of injury from the dangers present than from moving the patient.

10. The four emergency drags are the clothing drag, the arm drag, the blanket drag, and the firefighter's drag.

11. The six emergency carries are the rescuer assist, the pack strap carry, the cradle carry, the firefighter's carry, the seat carry, and the chair carry.

12. The EMT could move the patient from the ground to the stretcher using the extremity lift or the cradle carry.

13. The orthopedic or scoop stretcher is used in narrow spaces. Split in half, each half is placed alongside the patient and then the stretcher is reassembled. The stairchair is used in narrow spaces, like hallways and stairwells, to carry patients. It is brought in and reassembled and the patient placed in the chair to be carried. The basket stretcher is an off-road rescue device. The patient is simply lifted into the basket and then secured. The flexible stretcher is designed to be carried into a scene, where it is unrolled or unraveled; the patient is then placed inside the litter for transportation. The portable stretcher (litter) is the original means of conveyance for the sick and injured. It is carried end-to-end. The modern wheeled stretcher is found in every ambulance. While each operates slightly differently, all provide the ability to sit the patient upright or to elevate the patient's feet.

14. A spotter or "backer" should be used to help brace the EMT. This backer is responsible for calling out steps as well as obstacles.

15. Depending on the number of EMTs available, the stretcher can be carried end-to-end, or diamond, or at all four corners.

16. The patient is bundled in a blanket, then secured to the stretcher with seatbelts at the shoulders and hips.

17. The patient may be physically lifted from the ambulance stretcher to the hospital gurney by either a direct lift and carry, or by using a drawsheet or a slide board.

SKILL CHECKLISTS

Student Name: _____   Date: _____

Skill 12–1/Proper Lifting Techniques

Equipment Assembled:
1. Appropriate Personal Protective Equipment
2. Appropriate Back Support
3. Proper Footwear
4. Adequate Number of Trained Assistants

Step 1: The EMT positions his feet about shoulder length apart, facing forward.

Step 2: The EMT then lowers his body by bending at the knees, one knee down, keeping the back straight.

Step 3: Grasping the object with both hands, palms upward (power grip) , the EMT lifts evenly and smoothly.

Step 4: With arms locked out straight, the EMT stands fully upright.

Student Name: _____   Date: _____

Skill 12–2/Clothing Drag

Equipment Assembled:
1. Appropriate Personal Protective Equipment

Step 1: The EMT grasps the patient's clothing at the collar, while cradling the patient's head on her forearms.

Step 2: Crouching down, with back straight, the EMT walks backward.

Student Name: _____   Date: _____

Skill 12–3/Arm Drag

Equipment Assembled:
1. Appropriate Personal Protective Equipment

Step 1: Kneeling down, the EMT slides his arms under the patient's arms, grasping the wrists across the chest.

Step 2: Standing up, the EMT walks backward.

Student Name: _____ Date: _____

Skill 12–4/Blanket Drag

Equipment Assembled:
1. Appropriate Personal Protective Equipment
2. Blanket, Tarp, Drape, or Similar Covering

Step 1: Place the blanket along the long axis of the body, leaving about a foot of material at the head.

Step 2: Log-roll the patient onto the blanket, pulling the blanket from underneath the patient.

Step 3: Wrap the patient with the blanket, protecting the patient.

Step 4: Roll up the excess material at the head and grasp the roll.

Student Name: _____ Date: _____

Skill 12–5/Firefighter's Drag

Equipment Assembled:
1. Appropriate Personal Protective Equipment
2. Triangular Bandage

Step 1: Using the triangular bandage, folded into a cravat, the EMT secures the patient's wrists together.

Step 2: While on all fours, the EMT drapes the tied hands over her shoulders and drags the patient underneath her.

Student Name: _____ Date: _____

Skill 12–6/The Rescuer Assist

Equipment Assembled:
1. Appropriate Personal Protective Equipment

Step 1: The EMT crouches to the patient's level, and swings one arm over his shoulders.

Step 2: With one hand grasping the patient's beltline, and another grasping the patient's other wrist, the EMT stands and assists the patient with walking.

Student Name: _____ Date: _____

Skill 12–7/The Pack Strap Carry

Equipment Assembled:
1. Appropriate Personal Protective Equipment

Step 1: Kneeling in front of the seated patient, grasp the patient's wrists and pivot on the heels, draping the patient's arms over the shoulders.

Step 2: Stand and hoist the patient onto the shoulders and off his feet.

Student Name: _____   Date: _____

Skill 12–8/The Cradle Carry

Equipment Assembled:
1. Appropriate Personal Protective Equipment

Step 1: The EMT first kneels next to the supine patient, placing one hand under the shoulders and the other hand under the knees.

Step 2: The EMT then stands, keeping the patient's body close to hers.
(Tying the hands together with a cravat helps with some of the work of carrying.)

Student Name: _____   Date: _____

Skill 12–9/The Firefighter's Carry

Equipment Assembled:
1. Appropriate Personal Protective Equipment

Step 1: The EMT starts by standing toe to toe with the supine patient. Crouching down, he grabs the patient's wrists and proceeds to roll the patient to a seated position.

Step 2: Without stopping, the EMT then pulls the patient as nearly erect as possible.

Step 3: Quickly crouching again, the EMT places his shoulder into the patient's abdomen, while simultaneously standing.

Step 4: The EMT then puts one arm through the patient's legs and grasps the patient's hand lying across his chest, effectively locking the patient over his shoulders.
(Another EMT may help hoist the patient up onto the shoulders of the EMT. The second EMT waits until the patient is up and over the first EMT's shoulders then, grasping the patient's knee, helps hoist the patient.)

Student Name: _____   Date: _____

Skill 12–10/The Seat Carry

Equipment Assembled:
1. Appropriate Personal Protective Equipment

Step 1: The two EMTs kneel on opposite knees, and clasp arms. Each EMT should grasp the other EMT at the elbow.

Step 2: With one pair of arms low and one pair high, the patient sits back into the seat that has been created. The EMTs then stand together, at the same time.

Student Name: _____   Date: _____

Skill 12–11/The Chair Carry

Equipment Assembled:
1. Appropriate Personal Protective Equipment

2. Hardback Chair

Step 1: The patient is assisted to a sitting position in the chair.

Step 2: One EMT kneels in front of the chair, facing forward, and between the patient's legs. He reaches back and grasps the legs of the chair.

Step 3: The second EMT, at the back of the chair, grasps the uprights of the chair, and leans the chair backwards.

Step 4: Simultaneously, the two EMTs lift the patient up and proceed to walk forward together.

Student Name: _____   Date: _____

Skill 12–12/The Extremity Lift

Equipment Assembled:
1. Appropriate Personal Protective Equipment

Step 1: The first EMT kneels behind the patient and helps the patient up to a sitting position. The patient can be rested against the EMT's knee for a moment.

Step 2: The EMT then reaches under the patient's arms and grasps the patient's wrists, pulling them against the patient's chest tightly.

Step 3: The second EMT crouches between the patient's knees. Reaching down on each side, the EMT grasps under the patient's knees.
(In some cases it may be more convenient to crouch beside the patient's knees and hook arms under the patient's knees.)

Step 4: Simultaneously, the two EMTs stand with the patient and walk forward together.

Student Name: _____ Date: _____

Skill 12–13/The Direct Lift

Equipment Assembled:
1. Appropriate Personal Protective Equipment

Step 1: All of the EMTs stand on one side of the supine patient then kneel, on the same knee, beside the patient.

Step 2: The first EMT places one arm under the patient's head and neck and the other arm under the shoulders. The second EMT places her arms under the patient's lower back and buttocks.

Step 3: Simultaneously, the two EMTs hoist the patient to their knees. If the patient is being transferred to a stretcher on the other side of the patient, they need only drop the one knee to move forward and over the stretcher.

Step 4: If the patient is to be carried any distance, the EMTs should roll the patient against their chests and then walk forward together.

Student Name: _____ Date: _____

Skill 12–14/The Scoop Stretcher

Equipment Assembled:
1. Appropriate Personal Protective Equipment

2. Orthopedic Stretcher

Step 1: The scoop stretcher is split in half and the two halves adjusted to the patient's height.

Step 2: The patient is then log-rolled to one side and the scoop stretcher half placed along the patient's axis. This is repeated with the other side and the two ends are secured.

Student Name: _____ Date: _____

Skill 12–15/End-to-End Stretcher Carry

Equipment Assembled:
1. Appropriate Personal Protective Equipment

2. Stretcher or Litter

Step 1: Each EMT takes a position at each end of the litter. Both EMTs should be facing in the direction of travel. Kneeling down, each EMT grasps the nearest handhold.

Step 2: Simultaneously, the EMTs stand together. If the patient is to be carried any distance, the EMTs walk forward together.

Student Name: _____ Date: _____

Skill 12–16/The Diamond Stretcher Carry

Equipment Assembled:
1. Appropriate Personal Protective Equipment
2. Stretcher or Litter

Step 1: An EMT takes a place at each side of the stretcher and one on each end. All EMTs should be facing in the direction of travel. Kneeling down, each EMT grasps the nearest handhold.

Step 2: Simultaneously, the EMTs stand together. If the patient is to be carried any distance, the EMTs walk forward together.
(Whenever a patient is carried on a stretcher over rough ground, the EMT in charge should choose a diamond carry.)

Student Name: _____ Date: _____

Skill 12–17/The Four Corners Stretcher Carry

Equipment Assembled:
1. Appropriate Personal Protective Equipment
2. Stretcher or Litter

Step 1: An EMT takes a place at each corner of the stretcher. All EMTs should be facing in the direction of travel. Kneeling down, each EMT grasps a corner of the stretcher.

Step 2: Simultaneously, the EMTs stand together. If the patient is to be carried any distance, the EMTs walk forward together.

Student Name: _____ Date: _____

Skill 12–18/Use of a Stringer

Equipment Assembled:
1. Appropriate Personal Protective Equipment
2. Loop of One Webbing, Approximately 6 Feet Long

Step 1: The EMT places the webbing under the bar, or handhold, and loops it back through itself, in effect creating a half-hitch.

Step 2: The EMT then kneels next to the stretcher and slips the loop of webbing over his shoulder, being sure that the webbing knot was not on the shoulder.

Step 3: Then the EMT slips his opposite hand inside the loop. It may be necessary to shorten the length of the loop by tying a knot in the webbing.

Step 4: Once standing, the EMT adjusts the loop over his shoulders. One hand should be carrying the stretcher and the other hand should be exerting downward force on the loop, in effect, balancing the load.

Student Name: _____ Date: _____

Skill 12–19/The Caterpillar Pass

Equipment Assembled:
1. Appropriate Personal Protective Equipment
2. Stretcher or Litter

Step 1: Coming to the obstacle, all EMTs stop and turn toward each other.

Step 2: Two EMTs go around or over the obstacle and take a position across from the litter. The front of the litter is then handed to them across the object.

Step 3: As the litter is passed forward, the two EMTs in the rear move forward to take position beyond the obstacle. All EMTs remain standing with feet firmly planted as the litter is passed.

Step 4: Once the litter is clear of the obstacle, all EMTs turn and face forward. The EMTs may then move forward together as a unit.

Student Name: _____ Date: _____

Skill 12–20/The Bedroll

Equipment Assembled:
1. Appropriate Personal Protective Equipment
2. Stretcher, Blanket, Sheet, Pillow, Pillowcase

Step 1: The first EMT would center the blanket on the stretcher, then the sheet on top of that.

Step 2: The first and second EMTs grasp half of the linen and fold it in half, creating a collar. Repeat with the other side.

Step 3: To open the bedroll, the EMTs simply grasp the collars and folded edges.

Step 4: With the patient lying supine, the EMTs can fold the upper edge over the patient's head, then secure the edge with the lower edge. The pillow should then be placed behind the head, outside the linen.

Student Name: _____   Date: _____

Skill 12–21/The Carry Transfer

Equipment Assembled:
1. Appropriate Personal Protective Equipment
2. Two stretchers, gurneys

Step 1: The first stretcher is placed with the patient's head at the foot of the other stretcher at a 90 degree angle.

Step 2: The two EMTs stand on the side of patient. The first EMT places one arm under the patient's head and neck and the other arm under the shoulders. The second EMT places her arms under the patient's lower back and buttocks.

Step 3: Simultaneously, the two EMTs hoist the patient to their chests. Shuffling sideways, the two EMTs move the patient to the awaiting stretcher.

Step 4: The patient is gently laid onto the awaiting stretcher. The EMT should be sure that all stretcher brakes are engaged before moving the patient.

Student Name: _____   Date: _____

Skill 12–22/Drawsheet Transfer

Equipment Assembled:
1. Appropriate Personal Protective Equipment
2. Two Stretchers, Drawsheet, or Bed Linen

Step 1: The two stretchers are placed side by side. The EMT should be sure that the stretcher brakes are engaged before moving the patient. Any siderails present will have to be lowered.

Step 2: Two EMTs are on the open side of both stretchers. Rolling the edge of the drawsheet or bed linen into a collar, the EMTs grab a firm purchase. (It is a good practice to have the two teams of EMTs pull vigorously against each other to test the strength of the sheet.)

Step 3: Simultaneously, the four EMTs slide the patient from one stretcher to the other in one fluid motion.

Step 4: Once the patient is on the new stretcher, the siderails should be replaced.

CHAPTER 13

Scene Size-Up

OBJECTIVES

Upon completion of this chapter, the reader should be able to:

1. List important safety regulations that pertain to EMS.
2. Describe a "standard approach" to an EMS call.
3. List the scene information that may be obtained from the prearrival instructions.
4. Discuss the importance of staging as a protective behavior.
5. Describe what is meant by the term *scene size-up*.
6. List risk factors at residential EMS calls.
7. List the elements of a global survey.
8. List risk factors at the scene of a motor vehicle collision.
9. Describe how the EMT can manage those risks.
10. Describe how to protect the public's safety.
11. Describe what to look for during a damage survey.
12. Demonstrate the minimum actions required to stabilize an automobile.

GLOSSARY

crumple zone   Automobile fenders designed to absorb energy while compacting.

dangerous instrument   Anything capable of producing death or serious bodily harm when used in certain circumstances.

deadly weapon   Any device that, by its nature, is intended to produce death.

environmental assessment   An EMT's visual overview of an entire scene while identifying potential hazards.

global assessment   The EMT's general feeling about the entire scene; should involve thoughts of safety and need for additional rescuers.

high index of suspicion   Based on the noted mechanism of injury, the feeling that there is a high likelihood of injury.

initial report   The first radio report of scene conditions by the first emergency responder; includes hazards, number of patients, and requests for additional resources.

loaded bumper   A front or rear bumper that, when compressed and locked, is able to suddenly and unexpectedly spring forward.

mechanism of injury The way an injury happened.

Occupational Safety and Health Administration (OSHA) The federal organization that regulates safety requirements for businesses.

perimeter An imaginary boundary that divides safe areas from dangerous areas.

risk factor Predictable hazard that is encountered on certain scenes.

safety corridor A zone of protection, created by a barrier, that permits the EMT to work safely.

size-up A rapid determination of the situation, including hazards at the scene of an emergency.

staging Designating a specific area for emergency vehicles and providers entering a scene.

step blocks Prefabricated cribbing designed for use in rapidly stabilizing a vehicle.

triage A method of sorting patients according to the severity of their injury or illness.

PREPARATORY

Materials: None.

Personnel: Primary Instructor: One EMT-Basic instructor, knowledgeable in scene management.

Assistant Instructor: The instructor-to-student ratio should be 1:6 for psychomotor skill practice. Individuals used as assistant instructors should be knowledgeable about scene size-up.

Recommended Minimum Time to Complete: 0.5 hour.

STUDENT OUTLINE

I. Introduction
    A. History of Safety in EMS
II. Standard Approach
    A. Tip from the Field
    B. Dispatch Information
        1. Prearrival Instructions
    C. Personal Protective Equipment
    D. Staging
    E. Scene Size-Up
        1. Why Do a Scene Size-Up?
        2. Scene Size-Up—the View from the Windshield
    F. Hazard Identification
        1. Risk Factors
            a) High Index of Suspicion
            b) Information Overload
        2. Risk Factors at a House Call
        3. Risk Factors at a Motor Vehicle Collision
            a) Downed Power Lines
    G. Risk Management
        1. Risk Management at a Motor Vehicle Collision
            a) Vehicle Placement
            b) Warning Lights
            c) Road Flares
    H. Public Safety
    I. Damage Survey
    J. Number of Patients
    K. First Contact
        1. Vehicle Stabilization
    L. Global Assessment
III. Conclusion

LECTURE OUTLINE

I. Introduction
  A. Continuum
    1. Personal Well-Being
    2. Healthy Lifestyles
    3. Scene Safety
  B. History of Safety in EMS
    1. Dangerous Occupation
      a) Routine Job Function
        (1) Infectious Disease
        (2) Personal Injury
    2. Growing Attention
      a) Litigation
      b) Costs of Care
        (1) Rehabilitation
    3. Federal Report
      a) America Burning
    4. Changing Paradigm
      a) Then—"It's the Job"
      b) Now—"Safety First"
        (1) Private
          (a) National Fire Protective
            Association
              (i) Recommenda-
                tions
              (ii) Safety Standards
        (2) Public Pressure
          (a) Occupational Health
            and Safety Adminstra-
            tion
              (i) Regulations
                (1) Force of
                  Law
                (2) Fines
        (3) Landmark Regulations
          (a) Bloodborne Patho-
            gens
              (i) 1910.1030
          (b) Confined Space
              (i) 1910.10.146
          (c) Respiratory Protec-
            tion
              (i) 1910.134
          (d) Hazardous Materials
              (i) 1910.120
      c) Safety Officer
        (1) Command Staff
          (a) Surveillance
          (b) Management
II. Standard Approach

  A. Elements
    1. Assessment
    2. Hazard Control
  B. Dispatch Information
      a) First Source of Information
        (1) Nature of Call
          (a) Medical
          (b) Trauma
        (2) Additional Resources
          (a) Heavy Rescue
          (b) Law Enforcement
        (3) Hazards En Route
          (a) Other emergency vehi-
            cles
    1. Prearrival Instructions
      a) Heads Up
        (1) On-Scene Conditions
      b) Computer Aided Dispatch
        (CAD)
        (1) Weather Conditions
        (2) Call History
  C. Personal Protective Equipment
    1. Barrier Devices
      a) Nature of Call
        (1) Trauma
          (a) Turnout Gear
        (2) Medical
          (a) Complaint-specific
          (b) Gloves
              (i) Minimum protec-
                tion
                (1) Latex Aller-
                  gies
  D. Staging
    1. Functions
      a) Out of Harm's Way
        (1) Fire and Explosions
        (2) Gunfire
      b) Assessment Time
        (1) Hazardous Conditions
  E. Scene Size-Up
    1. Elements
      a) Environmental Assessment
        (1) Hazards
      b) Initial Report
        (1) Request for Resources
    2. Why Do a Scene Size-Up?
      a) Ensures
        (1) Organized Approach

(2) Attention to Detail
(3) Prevents Hasty Entrance
(a) Personal Injury
3. Scene Size-Up—The View from the Windshield
a) Method
(1) Stop, Look, and Listen
(2) Use of Binoculars
F. Hazard Identification
1. Broadbased Assessment
a) Safety is everyone's job
2. Risk Factors
a) High Index of Suspicion
(1) Scene-Specific
(a) Medical versus Trauma
b) Information Overload
(1) Scene Size-up as a skill
(a) Mentor
(b) Sutton's Law
(i) Anticipation of Hazard
3. Risk Factors at a House Call
a) Animals
(1) Number One Hazard
(a) Dogs
b) Environmental Hazards
(1) Poor Lighting
(2) Broken Stairs
c) Weapons
(1) Deadly Weapons
(2) Dangerous Instruments
4. Risk Factors at a Motor Vehicle Collision
a) Environmental Hazards
(1) Spilled Fluids
(a) Gasoline
(b) Antifreeze
(i) Trip Hazard
(2) Hazardous Materials
(a) Vapors and Fumes
(3) Downed Power Lines
(a) Hot Spots
(b) Switching
(i) Power Grids
G. Risk Management
1. Hazard Mitigation
a) Identification
b) Management
2. Risk Management at a Motor Vehicle Collision
a) Traffic Number One Hazard

(1) Vehicle Placement
(a) Safety Corridor
(b) Distance
(i) Speed of Traffic
(1) Faster = farther
(ii) Vehicles in Traffic
(1) Bigger = farther
(c) Warning Lights
(i) Rear-facing Yellow Lights
(ii) Farthest Vehicle Only
(d) Direction of Exit
(i) Toward Destination Hospital
(2) Road Flares
(a) Advantages
(i) Portable
(ii) Highly Visible
(b) Disadvantage
(i) Dangerous
(1) Severe Burns
(c) Personal Protective Equipment Recommended
(i) Gloves
(1) Firefighter
(2) Leather
(ii) Eye Protection
(1) Goggles
(2) Helmet Shields
(d) Position
(i) Distribution
(1) Farthest Point First
(2) Pattern
(a) Top of the Curve
(b) Hilltop
H. Public Safety
1. Perimeter
a) Law Enforcement Officer
I. Damage Survey
1. Bumpers
a) Loaded
b) Damage
(1) Low Speed

2. Crumple Zones
   a) Damage
     (1) Higher Speed
3. Windshields
   a) Damage
     (1) Highest Speed
       (a) Stars or Spiders
4. Airbags
   a) Deployed
     (1) Steering Wheel under the bag
       (a) Bent = Abdominal Injuries

J. Number of Patients
  1. Multiple Causality
   a) Incident Management System
     (1) Triage

K. First Contact
  1. Inspect Seatbelts
   a) Locked up
   b) Frayed
  2. Vehicle Stabilization
   a) Unstable = unsafe
     (1) Immediate Actions
       (a) Vehicle Out of Gear

       (b) Turn Car Off
         (i) Keys from Ignition
           (a) Keys to Floorboard
       (c) Emergency Brake Engaged
     (1) Cribbing
       (a) Rolling
         (i) Wheel Chocks
       (b) Off Wheels
         (i) Step Blocks

L. Global Assessment
  1. Elements
   a) Mechanism of Injury or Nature of Illness
   b) Number of Patients
  2. Initial Report
   a) Additional Resources
     (1) Interdisciplinary

III. Conclusion
  A. Critical Questions
   1. Am I safe?
   2. Is my team safe?
   3. What is the nature of the call?
   4. How many patients do I have?
   5. What resources will I need?

TEACHING STRATEGIES

1. Scene size-up is best taught by having students perform repeated scenarios. For example, one scenario should be a stable motor vehicle collision, the next scenario an unstable motor vehicle.

2. EMTs can become complacent about responding to a house call. Consider having the students respond to a house with an unlighted doorway, then let shots ring out from a starter's pistol.

FURTHER STUDY

Dernocoeur, K. B. (1996). *Streetsense: Communication, safety, and control* (3rd ed.). St. Louis: Mosby.

Krebs, D., et al. (1990). *When violence erupts: A survival guide for emergency responders.* St. Louis: Mosby.

Leisner, K. (1989). Managing the pre-violent patient. *Emergency Medical Services, 18*(7), 18–20, 23, 26, 28–29.

Rice, M. M., & Moore, G. Management of the violent patient, therapeutic and legal considerations. *Emergency Medical Clinics of North America.*

Richards, E. (1995). *Knife and gun club: Scenes from an emergency room.* St. Louis: Mosby.

CASE STUDY   ACCIDENT ON THE INTERSTATE

"Ambulance 24, motor vehicle collision on Interstate 66 at mile post marker 124, unknown injuries, time out 16:20." After pouring out their lukewarm coffee, Joe and Kenny fasten their seatbelts and turn on the emergency lights.

As typical, the situation is an unknown collision. The 9-1-1 caller was probably on a cell phone and cannot be reached again. Looking ahead, they can see that traffic is backed up for about half a mile. Joe carefully turns the ambulance onto the shoulder of the roadway and slowly proceeds toward the scene.

STOP AND THINK

1. What are the risk factors on the scene of a motor vehicle collision?
2. If this had been a house call, would the risk factors be different?
3. How does an EMT routinely approach every scene?
4. How do you prepare for the hazards involved in a motor vehicle collision?
5. What type of additional resources would be needed to handle those hazards?

ANSWERS TO STOP AND THINK

1. The risk factors can be broadly categorized into situational and environmental risk factors. The location of the motor vehicle collision creates unique hazards. A motor vehicle collision on the interstate has the speed of passing motor vehicles as an inherent risk factor whereas a motor vehicle collision on a city street may present risk factors from the assembled crowd.

Once the EMT is on-scene, environmental conditions, such as rain, snow, slopes, and fallen leaves, may present additional risk factors.

2. House calls present unique risk factors. These risk factors can be broadly categorized into structural risk factors and occupancy. A dog barking at the door certainly presents a significant risk factor. Unrepaired stairs and railings, as well as unlit doorways, are examples of a few structural risk factors.

3. The EMT approaches *every* scene with a stop, look, and listen attitude. A moment spent surveying the scene may prevent unnecessary injuries later.

4. First, an EMT should stage his vehicle and prepare himself for the scene ahead. This includes using personal protective equipment that is appropriate to the situation. For example, an EMT would wear turnout gear on the scene of a heavy rescue.

5. Other emergency services offer protection from specific hazards. For example, law enforcement officers will help protect the EMT from sniper fire, while firefighters would help protect the EMT from fires and explosions. The list of potential resources on the scene of an emergency is almost endless and specific to each situation.

ANSWERS TO TEST YOUR KNOWLEDGE

1. The key regulatory agency for EMS is the Occupational Health and Safety Administration (OSHA). Other regulatory agencies exist at both the state and local levels. Each EMT should be aware of these agencies and their regulatory authority.

2. All EMTs approach an emergency scene with the same "heads up" attitude. Standard approach includes staging a safe distance from the scene and taking a "stop, look, and listen" posture before entering the scene.

3. The initial dispatch usually includes information about the location, the type of call, the presence of any known hazards, and if other emergency services agencies are responding.

4. Staging at the scene of an emergency call gives the EMT time to assess the scene for hazards while at a safe distance.

5. The two major categories of risk factors at a house call are related to occupancy and structural integrity. The two major categories of risk factors on a trauma scene are related to the situation and the environment.

6. Each risk factor represents a potential hazard that the EMT must address. For example, gunfire may indicate that there is criminal activity and in most cases the EMT must call for law enforcement officers to first secure the scene. The students should list local emergency services that are available to the EMT.

7. It is the central tenet of EMS that the EMT's safety comes first. This principle has been upheld in the court of law and should be at the forefront of every EMT's mind. Along with personal safety, the EMT should consider the entire team's safety as well.

8. The most common method of protecting the public is by excluding the public from the immediate area. By establishing an enforceable perimeter, the EMT is protecting the public. In some cases, it is necessary to evacuate the public from the immediate area to protect them.

9. Minimally, an EMT should ensure that every motor vehicle is turned off, in gear, and the keys removed from the ignition. Furthermore, the EMT should engage the emergency brake as an extra precaution.

10. The global survey includes the assessment of the nature of the call, medical or trauma, and an assessment of any scene hazards as well as the number of patients and any additional resources that may be needed on-scene.

Student Name: _____   Date: _____

Skill 13–1/Lighting a Road Flare

Equipment:
1. Road Flare
2. Helmet with Eye Shield
3. Gloves
4. Turnout Coat

Step 1: The EMT first puts on eye protection and gloves, minimally. The EMT should wear a turnout coat as well.

Step 2: The EMT removes the striker from the end of the flare.

Step 3: The EMT briskly strikes the striker against the flare's igniter while aiming it away from her body.

Step 4: The EMT keeps the lit flare away from her body and places it on the ground.

Student Name: _____   Date: _____

Skill 13–2/Vehicle Stabilization

Equipment:
1. Flashlight
2. Turnout Gear

Step 1. The first EMT circles the car starting from the driver's side. The EMT advises the patient to sit still for a minute. The EMT checks for vehicle damage.

Step 2: The second EMT circles the car from the opposite side. The EMT checks for hazards above and underneath the car.

Step 3: After the second EMT calls "all clear," the first EMT enters the passenger side and takes stabilization of the patient's head.

Step 4: The first EMT reaches in and checks to see that the car is in PARK.

Step 5: The EMT confirms the car is turned OFF.
The EMT checks for electric locks windows and seats first.

Step 6: The EMT confirms that the car's emergency brake is engaged.

CHAPTER 14

Initial Assessment

OBJECTIVES

Upon completion of this chapter, the reader should be able to:

1. Summarize the reasons for forming a general impression of the patient.
2. Discuss methods of assessing mental status.
3. Differentiate among assessing the mental status in the adult, child, and infant patient.
4. Discuss methods of assessing the airway in the adult, child, and infant patient.
5. Describe methods used for determining whether a patient is breathing.
6. State the care that should be provided to the adult, child, and infant patient with adequate breathing.
7. State the care that should be provided to the adult, child, and infant patient without adequate breathing.
8. Differentiate between a patient with adequate breathing and one with inadequate breathing.
9. Distinguish among methods of assessing breathing in the adult, child, and infant patient.
10. Compare the methods of providing airway care to the adult, child, and infant patient.
11. Differentiate among obtaining a pulse in an adult, child, and infant patient.
12. Discuss the need for assessing the patient for external bleeding.
13. Describe normal and abnormal findings when assessing skin color, temperature, and condition.
14. Describe normal and abnormal findings when assessing capillary refill in the infant and child patient.
15. Explain the reason for prioritizing a patient for care and transport.

GLOSSARY

ABCs The techniques involved in assessing the airway, breathing, and circulation.

alert Term used to describe the mental status of a patient who is awake and interacting with his or her environment.

AVPU Acronym used to remember the classifications of mental status: **A**lert, **V**oice, **P**ain and **U**nresponsive.

crepitus The feeling of air under the skin (feels like Rice Crispies® popping under the fingertips).

flail chest segment Two or more ribs broken in two or more places, resulting in a free-floating segment of ribcage.

general impression The initial feeling, based on observation, of how seriously ill or injured a patient is.

initial assessment   The first assessment done on every patient to address life-threatening problems.

paradoxical motion   The movement of a flail chest segment in a direction opposite to that of the rest of the chest wall.

responsive to painful stimuli   Term used to describe the mental status of a patient who is aroused only by painful stimuli.

responsive to voice   Term used to describe the mental status of a patient who is aroused by verbal stimuli but is not spontaneously awake and interactive.

sternal rub   Technique used to assess a patient's response to a painful stimuli; with this technique the knuckles are rubbed against the patient's sternum.

sucking chest wound   A wound on the chest through which air can enter the pleural space, making a sucking sound.

unresponsive   Term used to describe the mental status of a patient who cannot be aroused by verbal or even painful stimuli.

PREPARATORY

Materials: EMS Equipment: Exam Gloves, Airway Management Equipment.

Personnel: Primary Instructor: One EMT-Basic instructor knowledgeable in patient assessment.

Assistant Instructor: The instructor-to-student ratio should be 1:6 for psychomotor skill practice. Individuals used as assistant instructors should be knowledgeable about patient assessment.

Recommended Minimum Time to Complete: 1 hour

STUDENT OUTLINE

I. Chapter Overview

II. The Initial Assessment

    A. Steps of the Initial Assessment

        1. General Appearance

        2. Mental Status

            a) Alert

            b) Responsive to Voice

            c) Responsive to Pain

            d) Unresponsive

        3. Airway

        4. Breathing

            a) Look

            b) Listen

            c) Feel

        5. Circulation

            a) Assess for a Pulse

            b) Assess for Bleeding

            c) Circulatory Support

III. Determine Priority

    A. Load and Go

    B. Stay and Play

IV. Conclusion

LECTURE OUTLINE

I. Chapter Overview
II. The Initial Assessment
    A. Steps of the Initial Assessment
        1. General Appearance
        2. Mental Status
            a) Alert
            b) Responsive to Voice
            c) Responsive to Pain
            d) Unresponsive
        3. Airway
        4. Breathing

            a) Look
            b) Listen
            c) Feel
        5. Circulation
            a) Assess for a Pulse
            b) Assess for Bleeding
            c) Circulatory Support
III. Determine Priority
    A. Load and Go
    B. Stay and Play
IV. Conclusion

TEACHING STRATEGIES

1. Using various photographs of patients taken in the emergency department, with their permission, ask the students to form a general impression of each patient's state of health.

2. Using the first case study and the additional case study, compare and contrast the condition of the two patients. Ask the students which patient is in grave risk of permanent injury or even death.

3. Giving the students a list of seriously ill and not so seriously ill or injured patients, ask them to determine the patients' priority for transport.

FURTHER STUDY

Dalton, A. L., Limmer, D., Mistovich, J. J., & Werman, H. A. (1999). *Advanced medical life support.* Upper Saddle River, NJ: Brady/Prentice Hall.

CASE STUDY   CHEST PAIN

After a scene size-up proves not to show any danger to his crew, Will enters the patient's living room and observes a man seated in a chair. The patient is an older man, in his seventies, who looks pale and sweaty. He is leaning back in the chair with both hands rubbing his chest, complaining of a "heavy" sort of chest pain and slight difficulty in breathing.

STOP AND THINK

1. What is your general impression of this patient?
2. Does he seem to be acutely ill?
3. Are any immediate treatments indicated?

ANSWERS TO STOP AND THINK

1. This patient appears "ill" as is apparent from his pale skin and his actions.

2. The fact that the patient is still seated indicates that his blood pressure has not fallen dangerously low. However, the hands rubbing his chest suggests that he is having a cardiac event and is therefore a high-priority patient.

3. This patient should receive oxygen immediately while the EMT completes his history and physical.

ADDITIONAL CASE STUDY

A quick survey of the scene and Maggie determines that the scene is safe and proceeds toward the first wreck. The patient was extricated by helpful bystanders and is lying face-up on the roadway. The face of the seventeen-year-old is covered in blood from a scalp wound. The whites of his eyes are a stark contrast to the rest of his face. Looking up at Maggie, the young man asks, "Am I going to do die?"

STOP AND THINK

1. What is your general impression of this patient?
2. Does he seem to be acutely ill?
3. Are any immediate treatments indicated?

ANSWERS TO STOP AND THINK

1. The scene of carnage described would suggest that the patient was involved in a high-energy motor vehicle collision. The serious mechanism of injury plus the patient's physical appearance would suggest that this patient may have significant injuries.

2. The fact that the patient remains lying on the ground, and is not up walking around the scene surveying the damage, may indicate that he is seriously injured. On the positive side, the patient is speaking, suggesting an open airway, and is able to form and express coherent thoughts. These facts indicate that the patient's blood pressure must be adequate enough to sustain the brain.

3. After assuring the patient's airway and breathing are adequate, including administering oxygen, the EMT should assess and treat the patient's scalp laceration to control the bleeding.

ANSWERS TO TEST YOUR KNOWLEDGE

1. The general impression an EMT forms typically helps the EMT decide the pace of assessment and treatment. From the EMT's first impression, she decides whether the patient is "sick" or "not sick." Experience helps the EMT develop a finer sense of which patients are sick and need immediate attention.

2. The levels of consciousness can first be broken into conscious and unconscious. The level of consciousness can be further subdivided into alert and oriented or confused and disoriented. The unconscious patient can be either responsive to pain, by moaning or uttering undistinguishable words, or be unresponsive to pain.

3. At first the EMT determines whether the patient is conscious or not. If the patient is conscious, the EMT would proceed with questioning the patient to determine level of consciousness. If the patient is unconscious, the EMT would start with calling out loudly to the patient, followed by shaking then painful stimuli, typically a sternal rub. The patient's response to these noxious stimuli would be noted.

4. Initially a conscious patient's airway could be thought to be open if the patient can speak. However, experienced EMTs know they must look into a patient's airway as well. The unconscious patient's airway must be manually opened, cleared of secretions and debris, and then secured with a device such as an oral airway.

5. A blocked airway must be cleared. The EMT would clear the airway using the standard approach advocated by the American Heart Association and the American Red Cross.

6. The patient's breathing is assessed by looking at the effort of breathing as well as counting respirations. Then the EMT should listen to the patient's lungs for extraordinary sounds. Finally, the EMT should palpate the patient's chest wall for deformity or point tenderness as well as crepitus.

7. If breathing is inadequate, the EMT must ventilate the patient. If the oxygenation is inadequate, the EMT must oxygenate the patient using an oxygen mask.

8. The fundamental question of circulation is: Is the patient bleeding to death on the outside or bleeding to death on the inside? Gross external bleeding should be readily apparent and needs immediate treatment. Internal bleeding is not so apparent and therefore the EMT must look for external signs of internal bleeding.

9. External bleeding is typically controlled with direct pressure and elevation of the injury. While measures, such a heat preservation and leg elevation, can help support the circulation, it takes surgery to definitively control the bleeding.

10. A high-priority patient has either a life- or limb-threatening injury that requires immediate medical attention. A low-priority patient has a significant injury or illness that requires medical attention that cannot wait for an office visit.

Skill 14.1 Initial Assessment

Student Name: _____   Date: _____

Purpose: To obtain a baseline examination for assessment and comparison as well as detection and treatment of life-threatening injuries.

Standard Precautions:
Icon— Handwashing— Gloves

Equipment:
Stethoscope
Scissors

1. The EMT surveys the scene for safety hazards as well as any potential mechanism of injury. Needed personal protective equipment would be donned.

YES: _____   RE-TEACH: _____   RETURN: _____   INSTRUCTOR INITIALS _____

2. The EMT forms a general impression of the scene, deciding, for example, whether it is trauma or medical.

YES: _____   RE-TEACH: _____   RETURN: _____   INSTRUCTOR INITIALS _____

3. The EMT next determines mental status on the AVPU scale. If the scene is trauma, another EMT immediately take head stabilization first.

YES: _____   RE-TEACH: _____   RETURN: _____   INSTRUCTOR INITIALS _____

4. The EMT assesses and manages the airway, as needed.

YES: _____   RE-TEACH: _____   RETURN: _____   INSTRUCTOR INITIALS _____

5. Next, the EMT assesses and manages breathing.

YES: _____   RE-TEACH: _____   RETURN: _____   INSTRUCTOR INITIALS _____

6. Finally the EMT assesses and manages circulation.
If the patient is high-priority, transportation should be initiated immediately.

YES: _____   RE-TEACH: _____   RETURN: _____   INSTRUCTOR INITIALS _____

CHAPTER 15

Focused History and Physical Examination of the Trauma Patient

OBJECTIVES

Upon completion of this chapter, the reader should be able to:

1. State the main objectives of a rapid trauma assessment.
2. Give examples of patients who should, and should not, have a rapid trauma assessment.
3. Describe the importance of the patient-physician relationship to the practice of EMS and its impact on the performance of a focused history and physical examination.
4. Discuss the reasons an EMT should consider mechanism of injury.
5. List the mechanisms of injury that would cause an EMT to have a high index of suspicion that significant injuries exist.

6. Describe the advantages that an advanced life support provider can bring to the injured patient.
7. List the steps in the assessment of a trauma patient with a significant mechanism of injury.
8. Describe each of the components of DCAP-BTLS.
9. Describe the rapid trauma assessment by body regions.
10. Describe the importance of obtaining a baseline set of vital signs and a SAMPLE history.

GLOSSARY

abrasion   A superficial scrape to the skin.
burn   An injury caused by significant heat applied to the skin.
contusion   Bruising of tissue caused by blunt force.
DCAP-BTLS   Abbreviation for assessment of signs of serious underlying injuries: **D**eformity, **C**ontusion, **A**brasion, **P**uncture, **B**urns, **T**enderness, **L**aceration, **S**welling.
deformity   Misshapen or not in the usual position.

focused trauma assessment An assessment that is focused on the patient's complaint or injury.

guarding Muscular tension created by a patient to protect an underlying injury.

jugular venous distention(JVD) Bulging veins on the side of the neck.

laceration A nonsurgical tear in skin and tissue.

puncture A hole in skin created by an object.

rapid trauma assessment A quickly performed head-to-toe examination of a seriously injured trauma patient to discover hidden or suspected injuries.

swelling An increase in soft tissue size due to inflammation.

tenderness referring to an area that is sensitive or painful upon palpation.

PREPARATORY

Materials: EMS Equipment: Exam gloves, stethoscope (dual and single head)(1:6), blood pressure cuffs (adult, child, and infant)(1:6), penlight (1:6).

Personnel: Primary Instructor: One EMT-Basic instructor, knowledgeable in patient assessment. Assistant **Instructor:** The instructor-to-student ratio should be 1:6 for psychomotor skill practice. Individuals used as assistant instructors should be knowledgeable in assessing the history and physical exam of the trauma patient.

Recommended Minimum Time to Complete: 4 hours

STUDENT OUTLINE

I. Overview

II. Determination of Trauma

III. Focused History and Physical Assessment

    A. General Principles of Physical Examination

    B. Reconsider the Mechanism of Injury

        1. Basic Assumptions

        2. ALS Backup

IV. The Rapid Trauma Assessment

    A. Physical Signs of Injury

        1. Deformity

        2. Contusion

        3. Abrasion

        4. Puncture

        5. Burn

        6. Tenderness

        7. Laceration

        8. Swelling

    B. Steps of the Rapid Trauma Assessment

        1. Head and Neck

        2. Chest

        3. Abdomen

        4. The Extremities

        5. Back and Buttocks

        6. Baseline Vital Signs and SAMPLE History

V. Focused Trauma Assessment

VI. Conclusion

LECTURE OUTLINE

I. Chapter Overview
    A. Initial Assessment First
    B. History and Physical of Trauma Patient
II. Determination of Trauma
    A. Mechanism of Injury (MOI)
        1. Inapparent MOI
            a) Assume Trauma
III. Focused History and Physical Assessment
        1. Physical Examination
            a) Significant MOI
                (1) Rapid Trauma Assessment
            b) Minor MOI
                (1) Focused Trauma Assessment
    A. General Principles of Physical Examination
        1. Medical Examination
            a) Patient-Physician Privilege
        2. Courtesy
            a) Privacy
            b) Introductions
            c) Explanations
            d) Eye Contact
            e) Honesty
    B. Reconsider the Mechanism of Injury
        1. List of Serious Mechanisms of Injury
            a) Falls
            b) Motor Vehicle Collisions
        2. Basic Assumptions
            a) All trauma potentially involves the spine
        3. ALS Backup
            a) Airway control
IV. The Rapid Trauma Assessment
        1. All patients with significant mechanism of injury
    A. Physical Signs of Injury
        1. Deformity
            a) Irregular body shape
                (1) Indicates trauma to underlying structures, including bones
        2. Contusion
            a) Bleeding under the skin
                (1) Indicates significant force to cause internal bleeding

        3. Abrasion
            a) Scraped skin with capillary bleeding
                (1) Indicates application of force to an area
        4. Puncture
            a) Hole in the skin
                (1) Indicates application of force to a focus point
        5. Burn
            a) Destruction of skin as a result of friction or heat
        6. Tenderness
            a) Indicates injury of underlying tissues
        7. Laceration
            a) Indicates a force great enough to tear the skin
        8. Swelling
            a) Accumlation of blood or body fluids under the skin
                (1) Internal bleeding or injury
    B. Steps of the Rapid Trauma Assessment
            a) Systematic approach to physical examination
        1. Head and Neck
            a) Scalp
                (1) Skull Fractures
                    (a) Lacerations
                    (b) Tenderness
            b) Facial Bones
                (1) Eye Injuries
                (2) Jaw Injury
                    (a) Airway Control
            c) Neck
                (1) Jugular Venous Distention (JVD)
                    (a) Chest Injury
        2. Chest
            a) Look
                (1) DCAP-BTLS
            b) Listen
                (1) Crackles
                    (a) Contusion to Lungs
                (1) Absence
                    (a) Punctured Lung
            c) Feel

(1) Deformity
    (a) Broken Ribs
(2) Uneven (Paradoxical) Motion
    (a) Several Broken Ribs
(3) Crepitus
    (a) Broken Ribs
3. Abdomen
  a) Palpation
    (1) Guarding
      (a) Internal Injury
  a) Pain
    (1) Broken Pelvis
4. Extremities
  a) Broken Bones
    (1) Laceration of Nerves and Blood Vessels
      (a) Pulses, Movement, and Sensation (PMS)

5. Back and Buttocks
  a) Hidden Injury
  b) In-Line Stabilization of Spine
6. Baseline Vital Signs and SAMPLE History
  a) Vital Signs
    (1) Foundation for later assessments
  b) SAMPLE History
    (1) Pre-operative Checklist
V. Focused Trauma Assessment
  A. Restricted
    1. Affected Area Only
  B. Baseline Vital Signs and SAMPLE History
VI. Conclusion
  A. Rapid Trauma Assessment versus Focused Trauma Assessment
    1. Function of Mechanism of Injury

TEACHING STRATEGIES

1. Using a series of pictures of trauma, ask the students to decide whether they would perform a rapid trauma assessment or a focused trauma assessment. Video clips and photographs of "sports bloopers" are sources rich with examples of trauma.

2. Jugular venous distention (JVD) is a difficult concept for students to visualize. Ask the students to pair up and have one student placed in a modified Trendelenburg position. The jugular veins should be prominent as they run from the proximal clavicle to the angle of the jaw.

3. Similarly, crepitus is a difficult concept for students to understand. Place a 4 × 4 inch sheet of small bubble-wrap under the skin of a CPR manikin and ask the students to first listen then feel for the crepitus.

FURTHER STUDY

Prehospital Trauma Life Support Committee of National Association of EMTs and the American College of Surgeons/Committee on Trauma (1999). *Basic and advanced prehospital trauma life support* (4th ed.) Philadelphia: Mosby.

CASE STUDY   HIGH-SPEED ROLLOVER

"Ambulance one, high-speed crash, possible rollover on Cornish Hill."

"Ambulance one en route."

Upon arrival, the ambulance pulls ahead of the crash scene. A teenager can be seen lying on the side of the road, covered with a blanket. Sue, the EMT in charge, prepares to care for the patient, while Carrie carefully goes down the hill to check out the car in the ravine.

Walking completely around the car, Carrie observes the driver's-side front fender damage. Then she notices that although the car is now on four wheels, the roof is caved in.

Carrie then peers into the driver's-side window. The windshield is intact, and a deflated airbag is hanging from the steering wheel. She lifts the airbag off the steering wheel and observes that the steering wheel is bent. Continuing, she tugs on the seat belt and notes that it unrolls easily.

Returning to the ambulance, Carrie finds that Sue has completed her initial assessment. The patient's only complaint is sore wrists.

STOP AND THINK

1. Does this patient need a rapid trauma assessment?

2. What observations should make an EMT have a higher index of suspicion that there may be serious hidden injury?

3. Does this change the patient's priority?

ANSWERS TO STOP AND THINK

1. Based on the high-energy involved in a motor vehicle collision the patient should have a rapid trauma assessment performed.

2. Both the roll-over of the vehicle as well as the crushed roof would lead the EMT to suspect multiple impacts with the interior of the vehicle and possible serious injury as a result.

3. Based on the mechanism of injury, this patient would be a high-priority patient.

CASE STUDY   ANKLE INJURY

The radio crackled. "Officer Sherman, go to the lower-level food court escalator for a woman who may have fallen." The mall had trained its security officers as EMTs about 6 months before. This was Officer Sherman's first call as an EMT.

When Officer Sherman arrived he did a quick scene size-up. There was one patient sitting on the floor at the foot of the escalator. Officer Sherman quickly donned a pair of gloves and reached under the rail to turn off the escalator.

A woman in her twenties was sitting cross-legged on the floor. Officer Sherman directed another officer to perform manual stabilization of her neck while he asked the woman what had happened. As she was speaking Officer Sherman did a quick initial assessment. He noted that she was awake and alert, her airway was patent, and she was breathing a little fast but not too fast. He further noted that she had no obvious bleeding and her pulse was a little rapid.

"Where do you hurt, ma'am?" Officer Sherman asked. She replied that she had been distracted for "just a minute" and had tripped at the bottom of the stairs when getting off; now her right ankle hurt.

STOP AND THINK

1. What potential does this mechanism of injury have?
2. What sort of assessment does the patient need?
3. What priority does this type of injury create?

ANSWERS TO STOP AND THINK

1. The potential for injury from this mechanism of injury is proportionate to the height of the fall. If the patient had fallen from the top of the escalator to the bottom she could have been seriously injured. Fortunately, the patient fell at the bottom of the escalator and, without the added complication of entrapment, had sustained only a minor trauma.

2. After completing the initial assessment, the EMT should proceed to a focused trauma examination while obtaining a SAMPLE history and baseline vital signs.

3. Barring any new information obtained after the assessment it, would be safe to assume that the patient has a minor injury and would be low-priority.

ADDITIONAL CASE STUDY

The sickening sound of breaking bones was muffled by the umpire as he cried out "Safe!" Jared had beat the pitch but right now his mind was focused on the excruciating pain coming from his left ankle. Seeing the deformity, the umpire motioned to the EMT sitting in the dugout to come over and assess the patient.

As he grabbed his bag and ran out to home-plate, Jonathan watched Jared grab his ankle, which was dangling at an odd angle, and start to roll around on the ground.

STOP AND THINK

1. Does this patient need a rapid trauma assessment?
2. What observations should make an EMT have a higher index of suspicion that there may be serious hidden injury?
3. Does this change the patient's priority?

ANSWERS TO TEST YOUR KNOWLEDGE

1. The objective of the rapid trauma assessment is to discover serious and potentially life-threatening injuries.

2. Any patient who may have sustained injury as a result of a significant mechanism of injury, such as a high fall or motor vehicle collision.

3. A show of respect for the patient's privacy indicates that the EMT values the patient-physician relationship.

4. Any patient who may have sustained injury as a result of one of the significant mechanisms of injury listed in Table 15–2.

5. After the scene size-up, the EMT would immediately stabilize the cervical spine and proceed with the initial assessment, paying close attention to the ABCs. Once the initial assessment has been completed, the EMT could elect to package the patient for transport, and complete a rapid trauma assessment while inbound to the hospital, or complete a rapid trauma assessment while on-scene. The EMT would follow the rapid trauma assessment with a baseline vital signs and a SAMPLE history of the patient.

6. DCAP-BTLS stands for deformity, contusion, abrasion, puncture, burns, tenderness, laceration, swelling.

7. The EMT should look for clear fluid from the ears or nose, jugular venous distention of the neck, crepitus of the chest wall, guarding of the abdomen, instability of the hips, loss of peripheral pulses in the extremities, and undiscovered injuries of the back.

8. The first, or baseline, set of vital signs forms the foundation for the future assessment of the patient's clinical condition (for example, improving or deteriorating).

Skill 15.1 Focused Trauma Assessment

Student Name: _____ Date: _____

Purpose: To assess for other non-life threatening injuries of the major trauma patient.

Standard Precautions:

Icon— Handwashing— Gloves

Equipment:
Penlight
Stethoscope, Cervical Collars
Blood Pressure Cuff
Scissors

Procedural Steps:

Step 1: After completing an appropriate scene size-up and initial assessment, the EMT performs a rapid trauma assessment of the trauma patient with a significant mechanism of injury. Manual head stabilization is maintained for the duration of the rapid trauma assessment.

YES: _____   RE-TEACH: _____   RETURN: _____   INSTRUCTOR INITIALS _____

Step 2: The EMT should consider a request for ALS backup and determine the transport priority. Transport is begun.

YES: _____   RE-TEACH: _____   RETURN: _____   INSTRUCTOR INITIALS _____

Step 3: The EMT next assesses the head by careful inspection and palpation for signs of injury. Deformities, contusions, abrasions, punctures/penetrations, burns, tenderness, lacerations, or swelling should be noted. Moving in a methodical fashion, the EMT next inspects and palpates the neck.

YES: _____   RE-TEACH: _____   RETURN: _____   INSTRUCTOR INITIALS _____

Step 4: The EMT next looks, listens, and feels the chest to assess for presence of any signs of injury. Breath sounds are carefully assessed at the apices and bases. Presence and equality of air movement are noted.

YES: _____   RE-TEACH: _____   RETURN: _____   INSTRUCTOR INITIALS _____

Step 5: The abdominal assessment includes looking and feeling for any signs of injury. The pelvis is visually inspected, then gently compressed downward and inward in order to find any signs of injury.

YES: _____   RE-TEACH: _____   RETURN: _____   INSTRUCTOR INITIALS _____

Step 6: After rolling the patient to the side using a log-roll technique, and continuing to maintain spinal immobilization, the EMT inspects and palpates the back and buttocks to find signs of injury.

YES: _____   RE-TEACH: _____   RETURN: _____   INSTRUCTOR INITIALS _____

Step 7: After completing the rapid trauma assessment, a complete baseline set of vital signs must be taken.

YES: _____   RE-TEACH: _____   RETURN: _____   INSTRUCTOR INITIALS _____

Step 8: A SAMPLE history is then elicited.

YES: _____   RE-TEACH: _____   RETURN: _____   INSTRUCTOR INITIALS _____

Skill 15:12 Focused Trauma Assessment

Student Name: _____ Date: _____

Purpose: To obtain a baseline physical examination for assessment and comparison of the minor trauma patient.

Standard Precautions:

Icon— Handwashing— Gloves— Goggles— Gown

Equipment:
Stethoscope
Blood Pressure Cuff
Assortment of Cervical Collars

Step 1: The EMT considers the mechanism of injury. Depending on the mechanism of injury, the EMT decides whether to perform a rapid trauma assessment or a focused physical examination.

YES: _____ RE-TEACH: _____ RETURN: _____ INSTRUCTOR INITIALS _____

Step 2: The EMT next determines the chief complaint.

YES: _____ RE-TEACH: _____ RETURN: _____ INSTRUCTOR INITIALS _____

Step 3: The EMT performs a focused examination specific to the injury.

YES: _____ RE-TEACH: _____ RETURN: _____ INSTRUCTOR INITIALS _____

Step 4: The EMT then obtains baseline vital signs.

YES: _____ RE-TEACH: _____ RETURN: _____ INSTRUCTOR INITIALS _____

Step 5: The EMT completes the assessment with a SAMPLE history.

YES: _____ RE-TEACH: _____ RETURN: _____ INSTRUCTOR INITIALS _____

CHAPTER 16

Detailed Physical Examination

OBJECTIVES

Upon completion of this chapter, the reader should be able to:

1. List the patients who require a detailed physical examination.
2. Describe the primary objective of the detailed physical examination.
3. Describe how the detailed physical examination is both similar to and different from the rapid trauma assessment.
4. List the points of examination for the following areas of the body: head, neck, chest, abdomen, pelvis, extremities, and back.

GLOSSARY

Battle's sign   Bruising behind the ears on the mastoid process; indicates a fracture of the skull.
cerebrospinal fluid (CSF)   The nutrient-rich fluid that bathes and protects the spinal cord and brain.
halo test   Observing for a ring of CSF around blood spilled from the ears or nose in a head-injured patient.
hyphema   A collection of blood in the anterior part of the eye.
raccoon's eyes   Bruising around the eyes that may be indicative of a skull fracture.

PREPARATORY

Materials: EMS Equipment: Exam gloves, stethoscope (dual and single head) (1:6), blood pressure cuffs (adult, child, and infant) (1:6), penlight (1:6).
Personnel: Primary Instructor: One EMT-Basic instructor with knowledge in patient assessment.
Assistant Instructor: The instructor-to-student ratio should be 1:6 for psychomotor skill practice. Individuals used as assistant instructors should be knowledgeable in conducting a detailed physical exam.
Recommended Minimum Time to Complete: 1 hour

STUDENT OUTLINE

I. Chapter Overview

II. Detailed Physical Examination

    A. Steps in the Detailed Physical Examination

        1. Head

        2. Ears

        3. Eyes

        4. Face

        5. Nose

        6. Mouth

        7. Neck

        8. Chest

        9. Abdomen

        10. Extremities

        11. Vital Signs Revisited

III. Conclusion

LECTURE OUTLINE

I. Chapter Overview
    A. Patient-Specific
    B. Injury-Specific
II. Detailed Physical Examination
    A. Objective
        1. Life-threatening Injuries
        2. Treated En Route
    B. Order of Assessment
        1. Initial Assessment First
        2. Rapid Trauma Assessment
        3. Detailed Physical Examination
            a) Change in Status
                (1) Upgrade Response
                (2) Divert Trauma Center
                (3) Intercept Advanced Life Support
    C. Steps in the Detailed Physical Examination
        1. Details
            a) Head-to-Toe Examination
            b) Preempted by Lifesaving Treatments
            c) Restricted
                (1) Major Trauma
                (2) Major Illness
        2. Head
            a) Inspection (Look)
                (1) Penlight
            b) Palpate (Feel)
                (1) DCAP-BTLS
        3. Ears
            a) Inspection (Look)
                (1) Clear Fluid
                      (a) Cerebrospinal Fluid (CSF)
                (2) Blood
                (3) Bruising
                      (a) Mastoid Process
                          i) Battle's Sign
        4. Eyes
            a) Inspection (Look)
                (1) Penlight
                (2) Bilateral Comparison
                      (a) PERRL
                (3) Blood
                      (a) Hyphema
                (4) Bruising
                      (a) Raccoon's Eyes
        5. Face
            a) Palpation (Feel)
                (1) Bony Prominences
                      (a) Orbital Rims
                      (b) Cheeks
                      (c) Jaw
        6. Nose
            a) Inspection (Look)
                (1) Clear Fluid
                      (a) Cerebrospinal Fluid (CSF)
                (2) Blood
        7. Mouth
            a) Inspection (Look)
                (1) Blood
                      (a) Control
                          (i) Local Pressure
                (2) Broken Teeth
                (3) Dentures
                      (a) Secured
            b) Palpate (Feel)
                (1) Broken Incisors
        8. Neck
            a) Inspection (Look)
                (1) DCAP-BTLS
            b) Palpate (Feel)
                (1) Trachea
                      (a) Suprasternal Notch
                          (i) Midline
        9. Chest
            a) Inspection (Look)
                (1) Gross Inspection
                      (a) Effort
                      (b) Pain
            b) Ausculate (Listen)
                (1) Crackles
                (2) Rubs
            c) Palpate (Feel)
                (1) Point Tenderness
                (2) Crepitus
      10. Abdomen
            a) Inspection (Look)
                (1) Gross Inspection
                      (a) DCAP-BTLS
                      (b) Incontinence
            b) Listen
                (1) Patient Complaints
            c) Feel
                (1) Tenderness
                (2) Guarding

TEACHING STRATEGIES

1. Have the students follow a patient who was delivered from the field to a local hospital emergency department. Ask the students to compare and contrast the physical examination findings.

2. Have the students visit a patient who was admitted to the intensive care unit following a motor vehicle collision. Have the students research the mechanism of injury, then create a list of suspected injuries. Afterward have the students take the list of suspected injuries with them to the intensive care unit and compare their findings with the patient's actual findings.

CASE STUDY   SILO ACCIDENT

The high-angle rescue team had successfully lowered the patient from the pinnacle of the silo to the ground using a basket. The patient, a sixteen-year-old male, had climbed the conveyer to fix a jam when it suddenly lurched forward, throwing the youth some 20 feet to the grain pile below.

The initial assessment was unremarkable, and the rapid trauma assessment uncovered only some minor contusions on his arms and legs. Because of the height of the fall and the length of time that it took to rescue him, the EMTs decided to transport him to the regional trauma center. The youth was quickly assessed and packaged for immediate transportation to the hospital.

STOP AND THINK

1. On the basis of the mechanism of injury, what injuries should be suspected?
2. What, if any, further signs of injury would the detailed physical examination uncover?
3. On the basis of the limited information provided, what conditions could develop en route that would necessitate either an ALS intercept or a change in the patient's transportation priority?

ANSWERS TO STOP AND THINK

1. The typical pattern of injuries seen in a fall of greater than three times the patient's height has been loosely called the "Don Juan" syndrome. Starting at the feet, the patient may experience bilateral heel fractures, then possible knee injuries. If the patient's legs were straight when he struck the grain pile, the force should flow the long bones and create bilateral hip injuries. Next, the line of force would follow the curvature of the spine, causing spinal column compression at the lumbar and cervical curves. The patient would then either fall forward or backward, possibly injuring either his scapulas or his outstretched arms.

2. Slow venous and capillary bleeding within the tissues will typically take upwards of 30 minutes to manifest. Therefore, the EMT performing a detailed physical examination may uncover contusions and abrasions.

3. With continued internal bleeding, as may or may not be manifested by contusions, etc., the patient could experience hypoperfusion of vital organs. The EMT must diligently monitor the patient's vital signs as well as repeatedly assess for DCAP-BTLS.

FURTHER STUDY

Prehospital Trauma Life Support Committee of the National Association of EMTs and the American College of Surgeons/Committee on Trauma (1999). *Basic and advanced prehospital trauma life support* (4th ed.). Philadelphia: Mosby.

ANSWERS TO TEST YOUR KNOWLEDGE

1. Any patient with either a prolonged transportation time or any high-priority trauma patient, human resources permitting.

2. The primary objective of the detailed physical examination is to uncover any undiscovered injuries as well as any new signs that may be developing.

3. The detailed physical examination inspects the same areas as the rapid trauma examination but in more detail and with attention given to even minor injury.

4. Beyond DCAP-BTLS, the EMT should assess the ears and nose for clear cerebrospinal fluid (CSF) leaking as well as the development of Battle's signs and/or raccoon's eyes. The EMT should further check the neck for the presence of jugular venous distention (JVD) as well as tracheal deviation. Turning to the chest, the EMT should assess for diminished breath sounds, which may indicate a developing pneumothorax. The abdomen should be closely examined for the presence of contusions as well as rebound tenderness or guarding. Ending with the extremities, the EMT should repeatedly monitor all of the limbs for pulse, movement, and sensation (PMS).

5. The following is a definition of each physical finding:

halo sign A ring of red and a clear center created by cerebrospinal fluid.

Battle's sign A contusion found behind the ear that may indicate a skull fracture.

consensual light reflex A pupillary response by one eye when a light is shone in the other eye.

crepitus The crackling sound of air under the skin heard when the lung has been punctured.

pallor A lighter or paler color of skin seen with hypoperfusion of the skin.

paralysis The inability to move an extremity; due to either central spinal cord injury or, if unilateral, a long bone fracture.

paraesthesia A loss of sensation for the same reasons there is a loss of movement.

pulselessness A loss of pulses in an extremity; usually due to an interruption of a blood vessel because of a long bone fracture.

Skill 16–1 Detailed Physical Examination

Student Name: _____ Date: _____

Purpose: To obtain a more thorough physical examination of injuries to a trauma patient; usually performed en route to the hospital.

Standard Precautions:

Icon — Handwashing — Gloves — Goggles — Gown

Equipment:
Penlight
Stethoscope
Blood Pressure Cuff
Scissors

Step 1: The EMT starts at the top of the head and assesses the scalp and the face for DCAP-BTLS.

YES: _____   RE-TEACH: _____   RETURN: _____   INSTRUCTOR INITIALS _____

Step 2: Next, he assesses the ears, nose, and throat, noting any bleeding or drainage of fluids as well as jugular venous distention or displacement of the trachea.

YES: _____   RE-TEACH: _____   RETURN: _____   INSTRUCTOR INITIALS _____

Step 3: The EMT proceeds to look, listen, and feel the chest wall for injury, including crepitus and paradoxical motion.

YES: _____   RE-TEACH: _____   RETURN: _____   INSTRUCTOR INITIALS _____

Step 4: Turning next to the abdomen and the pelvis, the EMT assesses for DCAP-BTLS. Assessment of the pelvis should include gentle pressure inward on the hips to check for a hip fracture.

YES: _____   RE-TEACH: _____   RETURN: _____   INSTRUCTOR INITIALS _____

Step 5: The extremities are assessed for pulses, movement, and sensation as well as DCAP-BTLS.

YES: _____   RE-TEACH: _____   RETURN: _____   INSTRUCTOR INITIALS _____

Step 6: After checking as much of the posterior as possible, the EMT obtains another set of vital signs.

YES: _____   RE-TEACH: _____   RETURN: _____   INSTRUCTOR INITIALS _____

CHAPTER 17

Focused History and Physical Examination of the Medical Patient

OBJECTIVES

Upon completion of this chapter, the reader should be able to:

1. Describe the different priorities when assessing a medical versus a trauma patient.
2. List the steps followed when assessing a responsive medical patient.
3. Identify the importance of eliciting any past medical history from the medical patient.
4. List the steps followed when assessing an unresponsive medical patient.

5. Identify the importance of eliciting information regarding the present illness and any past medical history from the family of an unresponsive medical patient.
6. Differentiate between the assessment that is performed for a patient who is unresponsive or has an altered mental status and other medical patients requiring assessment.

GLOSSARY

chief complaint The patient's main problem and reason for calling.
focused physical examination A physical exam focused on the medical patient's chief complaint.
medic-alert bracelets Jewelry that may be worn that relates important medical information.
ongoing assessment The continuing observation of the patient throughout contact.
OPQRST An abbreviation used to prompt questions related to a patient's complaint: **O**nset; **P**rovocation; **Q**uality; **R**adiation; **S**everity; **T**ime.
rapid physical examination A quick head-to-toe exam done on a patient who is unable to provide a history owing to a decreased level of consciousness.
vial of life A small plastic tube with a piece of paper inside that contains the patient's name, address, and essential medical information.

PREPARATORY

Materials: EMS Equipment: Exam gloves, stethoscope (dual and single head)(1:6), blood pressure cuffs (adult, child, and infant)(1:6), penlight (1:6).

Personnel: Primary Instructor: One EMT-Basic instructor, knowledgeable in patient assessment. **Assistant Instructor:** The instructor-to-student ratio should be 1:6 for psychomotor skill practice. Individuals used as assistant instructors should be knowledgeable in obtaining the history and conducting a physical exam for medical patients.

Recommended Minimum Time to Complete: 2 hours

STUDENT OUTLINE

I. Chapter Overview
II. Assessment of the Medical Patient
    A. History
    B. Physical Examination
III. The Responsive Medical Patient
    A. History of the Present Illness
        1. Chief Complaint
        2. OPQRST
    B. SAMPLE History
    C. Focused Physical Examination
    D. Baseline Vital Signs
    E. Treatment and Transport
        1. On-Line Medical Control
        2. Consider ALS
    F. Ongoing Assessment
IV. The Unresponsive Medical Patient
    A. Rapid Physical Examination
        1. Head and Neck
        2. Chest
        3. Abdomen and Pelvis
        4. Extremities
        5. Back and Buttocks
    B. Vital Signs
    C. History
    D. Treatment and Transport
        1. Medical Control/ALS
    E. Ongoing Assessment
V. During Transport
VI. Conclusion

LECTURE OUTLINE

I. Chapter Overview
    A. Illness-Oriented
II. Assessment of the Medical Patient
    A. History
        1. Direct Source
            a) SAMPLE History
        2. Indirect Source
            a) Vial of Life
    B. Physical Examination
        1. Focused Physical Examination
            a) Organ-Specific
III. The Responsive Medical Patient
    A. History of the Present Illness
        1. Chief Complaint
        2. OPQRST
    B. SAMPLE History
    C. Focused Physical Examination
        1. Organ-Specific
            a) Chest Pain
                (1) Chest
    D. Baseline Vital Signs
        1. Complete Set
    E. Treatment and Transport
        1. Complaint-Specific
        2. On-Line Medical Control
            a) Assist Patient with Medications
        3. Consider ALS
            a) Loss of Consciousness
            b) Chest Pain
            c) Shortness of Breath
            d) Abdominal Pain
    F. Ongoing Assessment
IV. The Unresponsive Medical Patient
    A. Rapid Physical Examination
            a) DCAP-BTLS

        1. Head and Neck
            a) Consider Trauma
            b) Pupils
            c) Jugular Venous Distention
        2. Chest
            a) Accessory Muscle Use
        3. Abdomen and Pelvis
            a) Palpate
                (1) Point Tenderness
                (2) Guarding
                (3) Masses
                    (a) Pulstile
        4. Extremities
            a) Edema
                (1) Pedal
            b) PMS
            c) Medic-alert Bracelet
        5. Back and Buttocks
            a) Injury
            b) Breath Sounds
    B. Vital Signs
        1. Complete Set
    C. History
        1. SAMPLE
            a) Family
            b) Bystanders
    D. Treatment and Transport
            a) Life-Threatening Illness
        1. Medical Control/ALS
    E. Ongoing Assessment
V. During Transport
    A. Contact Destination Hospital
VI. Conclusion
    A. Medical versus Trauma
        1. History is the Key

TEACHING STRATEGIES

    1. Have the EMT students pair off and obtain a medical history from one another, emphasizing the SAMPLE format as well as a complete past medical history.

    2. Have the EMT students spend a shift in the emergency department gathering histories from the patients.

    3. Have the EMT students spend an afternoon in a nursing home obtaining medical histories from the residents. Ask the EMT students to then report, both written and verbal, to the class.

CASE STUDY   PALPITATIONS AND DIZZINESS

Crystal and Jeremy responded to a call for a woman having chest pain. Upon arrival, they were greeted by a young girl who directed them into the living room, where they found the girl's mother seated in a chair, with one hand clutched to her chest. She was holding herself upright and was awake but seemed very uncomfortable.

Jeremy approached the woman and introduced himself and his partner as EMTs with the local ambulance service. He asked the woman what the problem was. She responded easily and told him that she was feeling palpitations and chest pain and felt too dizzy to stand up. The woman's respirations did not appear to be labored and seemed to be a normal rate. Jeremy felt her radial pulse and noted it to be quite rapid and weak.

STOP AND THINK

1. What is the general impression of this patient? Is this trauma or medical?
2. What treatments are indicated immediately?
3. What are the priorities for further management?

ANSWERS TO STOP AND THINK

1. In the absence of mechanism of injury, the EMT would suspect that the patient had a medical complaint. However, the EMT should question the patient to ensure that the pain is not the result of an earlier trauma. Chest pain, regardless of origin, is serious and should be treated accordingly.

2. The first treatment, after placing the patient in a comfortable position, is to administer oxygen.

3. Apparently this patient's complaint is cardiac in origin. The first priority would be to administer oxygen to the patient. If the patient has nitroglycerine, the EMT might consider assisting the patient with administration of the nitroglycerine, assuming her blood pressure is sufficient. Having completed these few tasks, the EMT should prepare the patient for rapid transportation to the hospital while requesting an ALS intercept.

CASE STUDY   UNRESPONSIVE MALE

Ann Marie and Pedro arrived on-scene and approached their patient. The call was for an unresponsive male in his sixties. Ann Marie began to perform an initial assessment while Pedro asked the family what had happened.

Apparently, while watching television the patient had suddenly complained of a severe headache and then passed out. The family had not been able to wake him. Ann Marie found the man unresponsive with snoring respirations, requiring her to manually open his airway. He had a strong but slow radial pulse and no evidence of external hemorrhage.

STOP AND THINK

1. What's your general impression of this patient?
2. What treatments are immediately indicated?
3. What's the priority of this patient?
4. What further assessment should be done?

ANSWERS TO STOP AND THINK

1. The fact that the patient suddenly became unconscious after complaining of a severe headache makes him a high-priority patient.

2. In order of treatment, the airway should be opened, assessed, suctioned for secretions, and secured with an oral airway. After completing the reminder of the initial assessment, including oxygen administration, this patient should be rapidly transported to the hospital.

3. This patient is high-priority based on his unconsciousness.

4. The EMT should attempt to ascertain if the patient is a known diabetic to eliminate low blood sugar (hypoglycemia) as the cause of the unconsciousness.

ANSWERS TO TEST YOUR KNOWLEDGE

1. The history is the key to understanding a medical patient's illness, whereas the mechanism of injury is the guide to understanding the injuries of a trauma patient. Therefore, a complete and accurate history is important to the medical patient's care.

2. After completing the initial assessment, the EMT would proceed with a SAMPLE history, then a physical examination including a baseline set of vital signs.

3. Frequently patients are not experiencing a new illness but an acute exacerbation of a previous illness. The patient's past medical history can shed a great deal of light on the patient's present condition.

4. After completing an initial assessment and a rapid physical examination, the EMT should obtain a baseline set of vital signs. While preparing the patient for transport, the EMT should attempt to obtain any history of the present illness that he or she can from family and bystanders.

5. As many medical emergencies are a flare-up of a preexisting condition, the past medical history may shed light on the patient's present condition. Furthermore, if the patient is taking any medications, these medications may interfere with the emergency medications being administered.

6. The examination of the medical patient still depends heavily upon any medical history that can be provided by bystanders or family. Unfortunately, the scant history that is typically available forces the EMT to depend on the results of the physical examination more heavily than otherwise would be the case.

Skill 17.1/Focused Medical Assessment—Responsive Patient

Student Name: _____   Date: _____

Purpose: To obtain a baseline examination of the responsive medical patient.

Standard Precautions:
Icon — Handwashing—Gloves

Equipment:
Penlight
Stethoscope
Blood Pressure Cuff
Scissors

Step 1: The EMT obtains a chief complaint and a history of the present illness, using the OPQRST format when appropriate.

YES: _____   RE-TEACH: _____   RETURN: _____   INSTRUCTOR INITIALS _____

Step 2: After obtaining the history of the present illness, the EMT takes the patient's SAMPLE history.

YES: _____   RE-TEACH: _____   RETURN: _____   INSTRUCTOR INITIALS _____

Step 3: On the basis of the patient's chief complaint, the EMT performs a focused physical examination of the affected area. After the physical examination, the EMT obtains a baseline set of vital signs.

YES: _____   RE-TEACH: _____   RETURN: _____   INSTRUCTOR INITIALS _____

Step 4: It may be necessary for the EMT to assist the patient with medications, or transport the patient to the hospital. An ongoing assessment should be continued en route to the hospital.

YES: _____   RE-TEACH: _____   RETURN: _____   INSTRUCTOR INITIALS _____

Skill 17.2 Rapid Medical Examination—Unresponsive Patient

Student Name: _____   Date: _____

Purpose: To obtain a baseline examination of the unresponsive medical patient.

Standard Precautions:
Icon — Handwashing—Gloves

Equipment:
Penlight
Stethoscope
Blood Pressure Cuff
Scissors

Step 1: The EMT quickly performs an initial assessment.

YES: _____   RE-TEACH: _____   RETURN: _____   INSTRUCTOR INITIALS _____

Step 2: The EMT proceeds to a rapid physical examination of the patient.

YES: _____   RE-TEACH: _____   RETURN: _____   INSTRUCTOR INITIALS _____

Step 3: As soon as is practical, a baseline set of vital signs is obtained.

YES: _____   RE-TEACH: _____   RETURN: _____   INSTRUCTOR INITIALS _____

Step 4: Bystanders or family members should be questioned about the patient's illness and past medical history.

YES: _____   RE-TEACH: _____   RETURN: _____   INSTRUCTOR INITIALS _____

Step 5: The EMT transports the patient as soon as possible.

YES: _____   RE-TEACH: _____   RETURN: _____   INSTRUCTOR INITIALS _____

Step 6: En route to the hospital, the EMT contacts medical control and considers meeting with ALS.

YES: _____   RE-TEACH: _____   RETURN: _____   INSTRUCTOR INITIALS _____

CHAPTER 18

The Ongoing Assessment

OBJECTIVES

Upon completion of this chapter, the reader should be able to:

1. List the purpose of performing an ongoing assessment.
2. Describe the ongoing assessment in detail.
3. Give several examples of changes to be monitored.
4. Define the term *trend*.
5. List the frequency of reassessment for different types of patients.

GLOSSARY

ongoing assessment   The continuing assessment the EMT performs during the entire time of patient contact in order to note any changes in condition.

trend   Identification of a pattern over a period of time.

PREPARATORY

Materials: EMS Equipment: Exam gloves, stethoscope (dual and single head) (1:6), blood pressure cuffs (adult, child, and infant) (1:6), penlight.

Personnel: Primary Instructor: One EMT-Basic instructor with knowledge in patient assessment. Assistant Instructor: The instructor-to-student ratio should be 1:6 for psychomotor skill practice. Individuals used as assistant instructors should be knowledgeable in the aspects of the ongoing assessment.

Recommended Minimum Time to Complete: 1 hour

STUDENT OUTLINE

I. Chapter Overview

II. Ongoing Assessment

    A. Purpose

    B. Components of the Ongoing Assessment

        1. The Initial Assessment Repeated

            a) Mental Status

            b) Airway

            c) Breathing

            d) Circulation

            e) Reevaluate Patient Priority

            f) Destination

        2. Reassess Vital Signs

        3. Repeat History

        4. Repeat Physical Examination

            a) Focused

            b) Detailed

        5. Check ABCs and Interventions

        6. Note Changes

    C. How Often?

III. Conclusion

LECTURE OUTLINE

I. Chapter Overview
    A. Continuous Observation
        1. Changes in Condition
            a) Upgrade on Need
II. Ongoing Assessment
    A. Purpose
        1. Repeat Assessments
            a) Changes in Status
                (1) Improvements
            b) Trends
    B. Components of the Ongoing Assessment
        1. The Initial Assessment Repeated
            a) Mental Status
                (1) Changes Gradual
                (2) Effects Dramatic
            b) Airway
                (1) Fatigue Factor
            c) Breathing
                (1) Clinical Changes
                    (a) Improvement in Symptoms
                    (b) Deterioration
                        (i) Ventilation versus Oxygenation
            d) Circulation
                (1) Reassess Bandages
                    (a) Bleed-Through
                    (b) Tourniquet Effect
            e) Reevaluate Patient Priority
                (1) Sum of Assessment
            f) Destination
                (1) Appropriate
        2. Reassess Vital Signs
            a) Complete
                (1) Trends
        3. Repeat History
            a) Accuracy
            b) Completeness
                (1) Stress Impact
        4. Repeat Physical Examination
            a) Focused
            b) Detailed
        5. Check ABCs and Interventions
        6. Note Changes
        7. How Often?
            a) Function of Priority
                (1) High Priority
                    (a) Every 5 to 10 minutes
                (2) Low Priority
                    (a) Every 15 minutes
III. Conclusion
    A. Trends are Key
        1. Subtle Changes Noted
        2. Action Taken

TEACHING STRATEGIES

1. The importance of serial examinations can be driven home by having a mock patient with "subtle" changes. Have a model assessed by the students. During the next break, moulage the mock patient with some reddened areas. Then have the students reassess the patient. At the end of class, make the contusions obvious and add point tenderness and guarding to the assessment findings.

ANSWERS TO TEST YOUR KNOWLEDGE

1. The purpose of the ongoing assessment is to note any changes in the patient's condition from the initial baseline.

2. Changes in mental status due to increasing intracranial pressure can be very subtle. Attention to details, such as span of concentration, is important.

3. The reevaluation of the airway is performed as usual with emphasis on ensuring that mechanical adjuncts are functioning properly.

4. The reevaluation of breathing includes a reference to the initial assessment findings. The EMT should also verify that the oxygen delivery system is functioning properly, checking the volume in the oxygen tank to ensure continuous flow.

5. The EMT should check all bandages to ensure that they have not (1) bled through, (2) loosened, or (3) become so constricting that they are acting like a tourniquet. A repeat set of vital signs are also in order.

6. An EMT would "trend" a pulse, for example, to note changes in the pulse rates that represent a pattern.

7. A low-priority patient should be reassessed every 10 to 15 minutes.

8. High-priority patients are reassessed frequently—as often as every 5 minutes. The patient in cardiac arrest may be reassessed for pulses every minute.

9. The EMT should call for an ALS intercept whenever the patient's trends indicate that she or he is deteriorating.

10. Minimally, every patient should be assessed on-scene, en route, and upon arrival.

11. Every patient, regardless of status, should receive a minimum of two sets of vital signs. This includes patients who are refusing medical attention.

12. An EMT should change destination hospitals whenever the patient's condition, or trends in the patient's condition, indicate the necessity of immediate intervention that the EMT cannot provide.

Skill 18–1 Ongoing Assessment

Student Name: _____   Date: _____

Purpose: To continue to monitor the patient for assessment and comparison to baseline examinations.

Personal Protective Equipment: _____

Icon— Handwashing—Gloves

Equipment:
Penlight
Stethoscope
Blood Pressure Cuff

Step: 1: While en route to the hospital, the EMT repeats the initial assessment, reassessing the patient's mental status using the AVPU scale and monitoring the airway.

YES: _____   RE-TEACH: _____   RETURN: _____   INSTRUCTOR INITIALS _____

Step: 2: The patient's breathing must be reassessed for rate and quality, and lung sounds must be monitored.

YES: _____   RE-TEACH: _____   RETURN: _____   INSTRUCTOR INITIALS _____

Step: 3: The EMT reassesses the patient's circulatory status, including skin temperature, and notes any additional bleeding.

YES: _____   RE-TEACH: _____   RETURN: _____   INSTRUCTOR INITIALS _____

Step: 4: After mentally reviewing the patient's priorities, the EMT reassesses vital signs and repeats a physical examination as needed.

YES: _____   RE-TEACH: _____   RETURN: _____   INSTRUCTOR INITIALS _____

Step: 5: The EMT rechecks the interventions, such as oxygen tank pressures.

YES: _____   RE-TEACH: _____   RETURN: _____   INSTRUCTOR INITIALS _____

CHAPTER 19

Radio

OBJECTIVES

Upon completion of this chapter, the reader should be able to:

1. Discuss the role of the communications specialist.
2. Diagram a typical radio system.
3. Describe the role of the Federal Communications Commission.
4. Describe how modern technology has advanced communications.
5. Describe basic radio procedure when initiating and terminating a radio call.
6. List the elements of an alert report.
7. List the elements of a medical consultation report.
8. List the correct radio procedures used throughout the course of an emergency call.

GLOSSARY

base station The main radio transmitter used in a system, frequently located at the base of operations.

call sign An identifying name or number that is assigned to a particular radio or person.

channel guard A device that prevents extraneous interference from radio transmissions from outside the base station; also called a private line.

communications center A central dispatch point.

communications specialist (COMSPEC) A specially trained radio operator.

duplex A radio that allows the EMT to both speak and listen at the same time, like a telephone.

echo technique A technique that involves repeating what was originally said to confirm it and avoid mistakes.

Federal Communications Commission (FCC) The federal agency that regulates radio communications.

hailing The frequency the channel uses to call a particular agency or hospital.

Med channel A frequency that is frequently used by paramedics and EMTs to speak to base hospital physicians.

mobile radio A radio unit that is mounted inside a vehicle.

multiplex A multiple-channel radio that allows for complex data such as EKGs and spoken messages to be transmitted simultaneously.

portable radio A small handheld radio unit that typically has 1–5 watt power output.

radio head The main section of a mobile radio, often located in the driver's compartment of the vehicle.

repeater A radio receiver/transmitter that picks up the signal from a mobile unit and increases or boosts the signal to the base station receiver.

scanner   An electronic device that may be used to listen to various radio frequencies.

simplex   A type of radio that can only receive or transmit at one time; allows only one-way communication.

stand-by   Radio terminology meaning "hold on a minute."

tactical channel   A designated channel for special operations that permits efficient scene coordination.

telemetry   Sending an EKG rhythm strip to the base hospital for physician interpretation.

trunked line   A truncated frequency made possible by the use of computers; used to prioritize messages.

two-way radio   A wireless electronic device that permits the transmission of messages to distant radio receivers as well as receipt of signals from those distant radios.

UHF   Ultrahigh frequency.

VHF   Very-high frequency.

PREPARATORY

Materials: EMS Equipment: None.

Personnel: Primary Instructor: One EMT-Basic instructor knowledgeable in this area. Assistant Instructor: The instructor-to-student ratio should be 1:6 for psychomotor skill practice. Individuals used as assistant instructors should be knowledgeable in communications.

Recommended Minimum Time to Complete: 0.25 hour

STUDENT OUTLINE

I. Overview
II. Communication Systems
    A. Communication Specialist
    B. Radio Systems
        1. Mobile Radios
        2. Portable Radios
    C. Radio Array
    D. Radio Frequencies
        1. Federal Communications Commission
    E. Radio Channels
    F. Computers and Radios
    G. Telephones
        1. Cellular Phones
        2. Digital Technology
III. Basic Radio Operation
    A. Radio Procedures
        1. Standard Nomenclature
IV. Hospital Communication
    A. Alert Report
    B. Medical Consultation Report
        1. Accepting a Medical Order
V. Other Radio Communications
VI. Conclusion

LECTURE OUTLINE

I. Overview
   A. Early Beginnings
      1. Hot Lines
II. Communication Systems
   A. Communication Specialist
      1. Former Role
         a) Dispatcher
      2. Modern
         a) Telephone Interrogation
            (1) First First Responder
         b) Triage
         c) Radio Dispatch
            (1) Computer-Aided Dispatch
         d) Logistics Coordination
         e) Resource Networking
         f) Prearrival Instruction
   B. Radio Systems
      1. Base Station
         a) Two-Way Communications
         b) Wireless
      2. Mobile Radios
         a) Radio Control Head
            (1) Frequency/Channel Selection
         b) Radio Repeater
            (1) Retransmit over distance
      3. Portable Radios
         a) Handheld
            (1) Safety
               (a) Downgrade Response
            (2) Resource Requests
   C. Radio Array
      1. Simplex
         a) One-way transmission/ reception
            (1) Walkie-talkies
      2. Duplex
         a) Two-way transmission/ reception
            (1) Telephony
      3. Multiplex
         a) Telemetry plus Voice
            (1) Electrocardiogram
   D. Radio Frequencies
      1. Amplitude Modulation (AM)
      2. Frequency Modulation (FM)

         a) Very-High Frequency (VHF)
         b) Ultra-High Frequency (UHF)
      3. Federal Communications Commission
         a) Allocate Radio Frequencies
            (1) Medical Channels
         b) Issue Call Signs
         c) Moniter Radio Communications
            (1) Profanity
   E. Radio Channels
      1. Tactical Channels
   F. Computers and Radios
      1. Trunking
         a) Computer Controlled-Radio Frequency Selection
         b) 800 megaHertz
   G. Telephones
      1. Cellular Phones
         a) Advantage
            (1) Portability
         b) Disadvantage
            (1) Loss of Location Identification
      2. Digital Technology
         a) Fax Technology
            (1) Digital Electrocardiogram
III. Basic Radio Operation
   A. Elements
      1. Thoughtful Consideration
      2. Concise
         a) Useless Utterances
   B. Radio Procedures
      1. Radio Courtesy
         a) You First, Then Me
         b) No Profanity
      2. Standard Nomenclature
         a) Plain English
         b) Spell Out Numbers
            (1) One-Five instead of Fifteen
      3. Breaks in Communications
         a) Emergency Traffic
      4. Clear Frequency
IV. Hospital Communication
   A. Alert Report
      1. Unit Identifier
      2. Level of Provider

TEACHING STRATEGIES

1. Provide the students with several prepared scenarios, all of which are disorganized. Ask them to glean from the scenarios the important information and organize it into a coherent report. Using family channel radios, or a similar device, ask the students to give a radio report.

2. If the system utilizes a medical control center or hospital, the students should be encouraged to observe during a shift to hear radio reports.

3. Record radio transmissions of actual calls to medical control and ask the students to critique them. Ask the students to assume the role of medical control. Ask them if sufficient information was provided to make an intelligent decision.

4. Cut up a radio log, indicating all the radio transmissions for a call, and have the EMT students place the transmissions in order.

CASE STUDY   CAR OFF THE ROAD

In the middle of the night, in a desolate spot, a car slides off the wet pavement and into a tree. The driver is unconscious. The horn blares while steam rises from the hood. Driving home, a local volunteer EMT comes upon the scene.

STOP AND THINK

1. What various means of telecommunications could this EMT take advantage of to alert the EMS system?
2. What are the advantages of each telecommunications system?
3. What is meant by "standard radio procedure"?

ANSWERS TO STOP AND THINK

1. Depending on available telecommunications technology, the EMT could either radio the call in to the communications center using a portable or mobile radio or use a cellular phone to call 9-1-1. Alternatively, he could drive to the closest public telephone and make a 9-1-1 call.

2. Mobile and portable radios have the advantage of direct communication but are expensive. The cellular telephone is portable and easily accessible but, with current technology, does not provide the 9-1-1 communications specialist the location of the call.

3. Standard radio procedure refers to the common hailing and communications process agreed to by all radio users.

CASE STUDY   ALERT REPORT

"One, two, three, four, five, bag, one." All hands are occupied trying to revive this patient, a forty-five-year-old male who is in cardiac arrest. Jack is trying to help where he can, not really sure what to do because this is his first cardiac arrest experience. The crew chief looks up and says, "Jack, use the radio to call this one into the hospital."

STOP AND THINK

1. What are the fundamental elements of a radio report?
2. Does the hospital need to know the complete history and physical findings?
3. What specific information does the hospital need to know?

ANSWERS TO STOP AND THINK

1. The fundamental elements of a radio report are a unit identifier, the patient's demographic information (age, sex, weight), the patient's chief complaint, and a brief history followed by the physical examination findings as well as the vital signs. The report should end with a short explanation of treatments performed as well as an estimated time of arrival (ETA).

2. To conserve valuable radio time as well as allow the hospital time to prepare for the impending arrival of the patient, the EMT should only emphasize important, or pertinent, findings.

3. Minimally, the hospital will need the patient's chief complaint, vital signs, and an ETA.

CASE STUDY   CONSULTATION REPORT

Classic signs of a heart attack. Substernal chest pain radiating into the left arm. The patient took his nitroglycerin tablet without relief. He called EMS. Now he is asking the EMT if he should take another tablet. His blood pressure is borderline low. The EMT decides to call the base hospital for more directions, using a cellular telephone.

STOP AND THINK

1. When is it appropriate to request to speak to medical control?
2. What essential elements should be included in this report?
3. How does an EMT "accept" a medical control order?

ANSWERS TO STOP AND THINK

1. The EMT should never hesitate to call medical control any time there are questions about performing a skill and especially when administering a medication. Another time it is appropriate to contact medical control is when orders are to be anticipated—for example, after a prolonged entrapment and extrication.

2. The medical control physician is going to need as much information as is available to make an informed decision. The EMT is literally the eyes and hands of the physician in the field and therefore must be as descriptive as possible.

3. The usual method of accepting a medical control order is called the "echo technique." The echo technique requires no less than three communications before the order is accepted.

FURTHER STUDY

Clawson, J. (1997). The DNA of dispatch. *Journal of Emergency Medical Services, 22*(5), 55–57.

Hanneken, S. (1997). The most important piece of EMS equipment? The radio!. *Journal of Emergency Medical Services, 22*(5), 50.

MacKay, M. (1997) Bandwidths, rrequencies, and megahertz. *Journal of Emergency Medical Services, 22*(5), 42–49.

ANSWERS TO TEST YOUR KNOWLEDGE

1. The modern communication specialist is a triage officer, a dispatcher, and an emergency system manager whose role includes logistics coordination and resource networking.

2. A typical radio system has as its components a base station, one or more mobile radios, and frequently several portable radios. The modern radio system is also linked to computers for logistics coordination as well as computer-aided dispatch.

3. The Federal Communications Commission allocates radio frequencies and generally monitors radio frequencies for proper use.

4. The use of computers has provided the communication specialist instant information about the caller as well as the ability to retrieve preplans for certain locations, past call history at that location, and other important information.

5. Typical radio procedures require that a unit/radio coming on the air use the radio's designated identifier. Similarly, many systems require that radios "sign off" the air by indicating their designated identifier and stating "clear."

6. An alert report typically consists of the identifier, the patient's demographic data, a brief history of the present illness, any relevant past medical history, vital signs, pertinent physical findings, treatments in progress, and an estimated time of arrival.

7. The consultation report includes all the elements of an alert report, frequently with more detail, and ends with a request for advice or instruction from the medical control physician.

8. Calls typically start with the "alert" and dispatch information. Once the responding unit acknowledges and is en route to the call, more information from other responding emergency services units may be accepted. All emergency services units report when they are arriving. Once the EMT is at the patient's side it may be necessary to call for more resources and/or medical control. After the patient is packaged and transported to the hospital, the EMT will contact the destination hospital with an alert report. Finally, the ambulance will call in arrival as well as "back in service."

CHAPTER 20

Report

OBJECTIVES

Upon completion of this chapter, the reader should be able to:

1. Describe the importance of a verbal report.
2. Describe the three "rights" of effective interpersonal communications.
3. Describe the barriers to effective interpersonal communications.
4. Describe some techniques EMTs use to overcome these barriers.

GLOSSARY

confidentiality   Privacy; maintaining confidentiality means ensuring that medical information is provided only to the patient's health care providers.

repetitive persistence   Repeating a message several times until it is evident that the point has been taken.

verbal report   A spoken account of the patient encounter given to the accepting health care provider.

PREPARATORY

Materials: EMS Equipment: None.

Personnel: Primary Instructor: One EMT-Basic instructor knowledgeable in this area. Assistant Instructor: The instructor-to-student ratio should be 1:6 for psychomotor skill practice. Individuals used as assistant instructors should be knowledgeable in communications.

Recommended Minimum Time to Complete: 0.25 hour

STUDENT OUTLINE

I. Chapter Overview
II. The Verbal Report
    A. Right Person
    B. Right Place
    C. Right Time
II. Interpersonal Communications
    A. Communication Barriers
IV. Conclusion

LECTURE OUTLINE

I. Chapter Overview
    A. Transfer of Care
        1. Exchange of Observations
            a) Medical Handoff
        2. Turned Over To (TOT)
            a) Abandonment
II. The Verbal Report
        1. Bedside Report
    A. Right Person
        1. Primary Patient Care Provider
    B. Right Place
        1. Bedside
            a) Confidentiality
    C. Right Time

        1. Urgency versus Necessity
III. Interpersonal Communications
    A. Speech
    B. Body Language
        1. Facial Expressions
        2. Tone of Voice
    C. Communication Barriers
        1. Failure of Focus
            a) Repetitive Persistence
IV. Conclusion
    A. Purpose
        1. Urgent Communications
        2. Continuation of Care

TEACHING STRATEGIES

1. Distribute completed prehospital care reports to the students, then ask them to stand and "give report" to another EMT student or group of EMTs.

2. Ask the students to research the cultural history of the community, then visit historical cultural sites within the community.

CASE STUDY   TRANSFER OF CARE

The patient was a middle-aged African-American male with a history of hypertension. His wife called 9-1-1 when he started to complain of chest pain.

The patient appeared to be having a heart attack. Drew wasn't sure. The wife kept interrupting and the room started to get noisy. Feeling a little uncomfortable, Drew directed his partner to package the patient immediately. The patient insisted on going to Center Hospital, all the way across town and out of the district.

At the hospital, still unsure of the entire history, Drew rolled the patient into what could be called chaos. He got a room assignment over the radio, and he just wanted to give report.

The patient was starting to look grayer and was now grossly diaphoretic (perspiring). He grabbed the first orderly who went by. The orderly shook him off and told him he was busy.

Drew was starting to feel a little panic-stricken himself. He knew the patient was sick and nobody seemed to want to listen. He grabbed the next nurse who went by him.

STOP AND THINK

1. What communication barriers has this EMT encountered?
2. What are the essential elements of the bedside report?
3. Is it necessary for an EMT to provide a bedside report? What are the possible consequences if he or she does not?

ANSWERS TO STOP AND THINK

    1. The first communication barrier was the cultural differences this EMT encountered. Cultural differences can lead to as many difficulties as a language barrier. Next he encountered a situational barrier.

    2. The bedside report should minimally contain the same information as the alert report.

    3. The bedside report constitutes the transfer of care from the EMT to the hospital's emergency department. Failure to properly transfer, or turn over care, to another health care provider of equal or greater standing could lead to charges of patient abandonment.

FURTHER STUDY

Anderson, C. (1999). Patient care documentation. *Emergency Medical Services, 28*(3), 59–61.

Krafsur, J., & Nagorka, F. (2000). Prehospital rounds: Documentation in a two-tiered system. *Emergency Medical Services, 29*(3), 106–108.

TEST YOUR KNOWLEDGE

1. Describe the importance of a verbal report.
2. Describe the three rights of effective communications.
3. Describe the barriers to effective communications.
4. Describe some techniques EMTs use to overcome these barriers.

ANSWERS TO TEST YOUR KNOWLEDGE

1. The verbal report is often the first opportunity that the bedside health care provider has to obtain specific information about the patient's condition and, more important, to ask the EMT direct questions. The verbal report represents the continuation of care.

2. The three "rights" of effective interpersonal communication include the right person, at the right place, at the right time.

3. Language barriers, competing activities, and ineffective delivery are some of the barriers to effective communication.

4. To overcome these barriers to effective communication, the EMT must first ensure that she or he has the right person, at the right time and in the right place. Assuming this, the EMT needs to weigh the importance of the report over the activity at hand. If the patient's report is critically important, the EMT can practice repetitive persistence until the message is effectively conveyed.

CHAPTER 21

Record

OBJECTIVES

Upon completion of this chapter, the reader should be able to:

1. Describe the importance of an EMT's documentation.
2. List the standard elements of every EMT patient care report (PCR).
3. Describe how the PCR fits into the patient's medical record.
4. List four functions of the PCR.
5. Describe a minimum data set.
6. Differentiate between open and closed charting methods.
7. List the elements of the acroymn SOAP.
8. List the elements of the acroymn CHEATED.
9. Describe the importance of standardized abbreviations.
10. List the principles of good documentation.
11. Describe how to correct an error in the record.
12. Describe how to make an addition to the record.
13. List several reasons for writing a special incident report.
14. Describe the special documentation an EMT uses at a multiple-casualty incident.
15. Describe the critical elements that must be included in every patient refusal.
16. List people who would make good witnesses on a patient refusal form.

GLOSSARY

affidavit   Written testimony by a person.

CHEATED   An acronym to help recall the outline of a completely documented patient record: **C**hief **C**omplaint, **H**istory, **E**xam, **A**ssessment, **T**reatment, **E**valuation, **D**isposition.

mandated reporter   An individual who comes into contact with certain situations and is required by law to report these situations to the proper authorities; for example, child abuse.

minimum data set   The specific pieces of information that are required on a patient care report.

objective Information obtained by the EMT through direct observation or assessment.

patient care report (PCR)   The document on which an EMT records the evidence of the patient encounter.

patient refusal form   A specific form a patient must sign if he or she refuses to allow care or transport.

sentinel PCR   A report that requires special review by the medical director or a risk management group.

special incident report   A specific document upon which the EMT would write the details of a defined special incident, such as equipment failure.

subjective Information the patient or family members tell the EMT.

triage tag A special document that is used in multiple-casualty incidents to indicate the priority of each patient.

PREPARATORY

Materials: EMS Equipment: None.

Personnel: Primary Instructor: One EMT-Basic instructor knowledgeable in this area. Assistant Instructor: The instructor-to-student ratio should be 1:6 for psychomotor skill practice. Individuals used as assistant instructors should be knowledgeable in communications.

Recommended Minimum Time to Complete: 0.5 hour

1) Chapter Overview
2) The Record
    a) Functions of the Record
        i) Quality Improvement
        ii) Research
        iii) Administrative Purposes
        iv) Legal Document
    b) Minimum Data Sets
    c) Format for Documentation
        i) SOAP Charting Method
            (1) Subjective
            (2) Objective
            (3) Assessment
            (4) Plan
        ii) CHEATED Charting Method
            (a) Chief Complaint
            (b) History
            (c) Examination
            (d) Assessment
            (e) Treatment
            (f) Evaluation
            (g) Disposition
3) Principles of Documentation
    a) Documentation Standards
        i) Errors and Corrections
        ii) Legibility
4) Special Incident Reports
    a) Injury to EMT
    b) Infectious Disease Exposure
    c) Equipment Failure
5) The EMT as a Good Citizen
6) Multiple-Casualty Incident
7) Patient Refusal Documentation
8) Conclusion

LECTURE OUTLINE

1) Chapter Overview
   a) Patient Care Record
      i) Medical Documentation
      ii) Legal Documentation
2) The Record
      i) Problem-Oriented Medical Record-Keeping
   b) Functions of the Record
      i) Quality Improvement
         (1) Protocol Compliance
         (2) Peer Review Process
            (a) Sentinel Records
      ii) Research
         (1) Retrospective
      iii) Administrative Purposes
         (1) Contractual Obligations
            (a) Response Times
         (2) Revenue Recovery
      iv) Legal Document
         (1) Court Record
   c) Minimum Data Sets
      i) Demographics
      ii) Elements of History and Physical
   d) Format for Documentation
      i) Standard Report Format
      ii) SOAP Charting Method
         (1) Subjective
            (a) Information Expressed aka Symptoms
               (i) Family
               (ii) Bystanders
         (2) Objective
            (a) Information Assessed aka Signs
               (i) Vital Signs
         (3) Assessment
            (a) Decision-Making
         (4) Plan
            (a) Treatments
               (i) Protocol-Driven
      iii) CHEATED Charting Method
   (a) Chief Complaint
      (i) Patient's Own Words
   (b) History
      (i) Medical
         (1) Nature of Illness
         (2) History of Present Illness
         (3) Past Medical History
      (ii) Trauma
         (1) Mechanism of Injury

         (2) SAMPLE
   (c) Examination
      (i) Initial Assessment
      (ii) Detailed or Focused Physical Examination
   (d) Assessment
      (i) Protocol-Driven
   (e) Treatment
      (i) Care Rendered
   (f) Evaluation
      (i) Effectiveness of Care Rendered
   (g) Disposition
      (i) Turned Over To (TOT)
3) Principles of Documentation
   a) Legal Imperative
      i) Documentation of Good Care
   b) Documentation Standard
      i) Abbreviations
         (1) Standardization
      ii) Errors and Corrections
         (1) Cross-out
         (2) White-out
      iii) Legibility
         (1) Readability
            (a) Medical Document First
4) Special Incident Reports
   a) Circumstantial
      i) Evidence
   b) Examples
      i) Injury to EMT
      ii) Infectious Disease Exposure
      iii) Equipment Failure
5) The EMT as a Good Citizen
   a) Referring Criminal Activity
   b) Mandated Reporters
      i) Child Abuse
      ii) Elder Abuse
      iii) Domestic Violence
   c) Affidavit
      i) Sworn Testimony
6) Multiple-Casualty Incident
   a) Abbreviated Medical Documentation
      i) Triage Tags
7) Patient Refusal Documentation
   a) Refusal of Medical Attention versus Against Medical Advice
      i) Standards
         (1) Age of Majority
         (2) Capable of Understanding
8) Conclusion

TEACHING STRATEGIES

1. Have several students reenact a call. Then ask the rest of the students to complete a PCR detailing the call.

2. Have the students watch an episode of "Emergency." Take a specific episode and ask the students to complete a PCR for that call.

3. Consider asking a local attorney, familiar with malpractice, or the local hospital's risk manager to come to class and discuss documentation standards.

4. Provide the students with a mock scenario of a multiple-casualty incident. Ask them to complete a triage tag.

CASE STUDY   WRITING A REPORT

Mrs. Rocky lived in the third-floor apartment above the barbershop. Every few days she would call EMS for one complaint or another. Today she called because her back hurt; her "sciatica" was acting up, and she had a terrible headache.

Her past medical history included a heart attack in 1994, congestive heart failure, a "touch" of emphysema, and a thirty-year history of smoking two packs of cigarettes a day.

The EMT completed a focused history and physical exam based on her complaints. Her physical examination revealed she had jugular venous distention, audible wheezes, and abdominal tenderness, and her legs were swollen from the ankles to the knees.

After turning Mrs. Rocky over to the emergency department nurse, the EMT sat down to write the Patient Care Record.

ADDITIONAL CASE STUDY

A crowd had assembled around the "unknown, man down." The man appeared disheveled. Witnesses at the scene said he fell down and started to convulse. One bystander was heard to say, "just another bum. These people shouldn't be allowed on the street." What caught EMT Kuhne's eye was the fact that the man was dressed in a three-piece suit. No one seemed to know who he was, only that he had stumbled out the alley and then collapsed.

Officer Salerno pushed through the crowd and handed her the patient's driver license. "I'll call the house and see if I can get any information for you," he called out as he turned away.

While her partner accomplished manual head stabilization, Kuhne went through the initial assessment of the patient. There were no immediately life-threatening injuries. She went on to complete a rapid trauma assessment. Starting at the head, she noted a minor cut at the back of the head, perhaps from a fall or a blow to the head. She also discovered a Medic-alert(TM) tag that stated the patient was a known epileptic. Log-rolling the patient onto the backboard, she immobilized the patient. Although there were no life-threatening injuries, the fact that the patient was still confused left her uneasy. If this had been a simple seizure, the patient should become more alert. In fact, he was not, so she decided he was high-priority.

STOP AND THINK

1. What essential elements should be included in the patient care report?
2. What format could be used to organize the information?
3. What are some important documentation standards?

ANSWERS TO STOP AND THINK

1. The patient care report should minimally include the patient's demographic information, a brief history of the present illness, the patient's pertinent past medical history, and the physical examination findings, including vital signs. The PCR should also detail the treatments provided to the patient and the patient's response to those treatments.

2. Accepted formats include the SOAP format and the CHEATED format.

3. All documentation should be written legibly, in black pen, at the time of the call by the EMT in charge of patient care. The patient's chief complaint should be written in her or his own words (if possible) and the source of historical information noted. All treatments, as well as vital signs, should be noted in terms of time and effect. Finally, the patient's disposition should be noted.

CASE STUDY   LOW BATTERY

"Man down, CPR in progress." The feet hit the floor before the tones had finished. Down South Pearl to Main and up two blocks. Total response time was 4 minutes.

Looking ahead one could see that CPR was in progress. A middle-aged male was lying on the ground obviously unconscious. After apnea and pulselessness had been confirmed, the automated external defibrillator (AED) pads were applied and the "analyze" pressed.

The AED warning light came on reading "low battery." Miguel's heart sank. He was sure he had checked out the AED at the start of the tour of duty. Miguel quickly replaced the battery with a fresh spare found in the side pocket and proceeded with the defibrillation.

Taking a minute to look up, Miguel saw several family members looking down with a puzzled look on their faces. He proceeded with the shocks and CPR and loaded the patient for the trip to the hospital.

ADDITIONAL CASE STUDY

"Quick, roll him," cried out Daphne as the patient started to vomit. The firefighters grabbed the patient at the shoulders and hips and rolled him onto his side. Fortunately, the backboard straps and the head immobilization device kept the patient in neutral alignment.

Reaching for the portable suction, she pressed the on button only to hear a low moan as the battery quit. While the firefighters held the patient on his side, Daphne rummaged through the jump-kit and pulled out a turkey baster. "Better than nothing," she declared and went about clearing the airway.

STOP AND THINK

1. Should the low battery be reported? To whom?
2. Should it be reported on the PCR?
3. What information should be included in a report?
4. Is this information "discoverable" in a court of law?

ANSWERS TO STOP AND THINK

1. Any mechanical failures that impact patient care should be reported to an officer or manager. In some cases, a mechanical failure must be reported to the state health department or the federal Food and Drug Administration.

2. Most EMS agencies restrict reporting of equipment/mechanical failure to special reports only. The patient care report should only reflect patient care information.

3. The PCR contains pertinent information on the patient. The special incident report contains information on the failure of any device.

4. With cause, the court can obtain, via a subpoena, any reports. In some states, reports of quality-improvement(QI) committees are not discoverable under normal conditions.

CASE STUDY   CRIME SCENE

"Unit 15, man shot, police on scene, proceed to the corner of Moyers and Onondaga and stand by." Proceeding with no lights or siren to the staging area, Mark, the EMT, is approached by Officer Stevens, who advises him that the scene is safe and he may proceed in to care for the patient.

Mark introduces himself to the patient, Marvin, who is lying on the couch, and starts to treat him. Rolling Marvin over, Mark uncovers a bag of what appears to be marijuana. Officer Stevens, who is standing nearby, reaches over and picks up the bag.

After the call is over and the patient has been properly turned over to the emergency department, Officer Stevens calls and asks Mark to report to the police substation to make a statement.

ADDITIONAL CASE STUDY

"Stinking drunk," Matt muttered under his breath. "What? Do you think he's drunk?" asked the police officer. Even as the answer came from his mouth, Matt wished he had kept his mouth shut. Did he breach his duty to maintain patient confidentiality, or had he simply been acting as a good citizen? Regardless of the correct answer, Matt wished he had not said anything to the officer. Now, he would have to complete a special report and explain himself to his supervisor.

STOP AND THINK

1. Is a statement required?
2. Does this incident need to be reported to Mark's supervisor?
3. Does Mark's agency need additional paperwork?

ANSWERS TO STOP AND THINK

1. Legally, the EMT may be required by law to make a statement called a *deposition.* Ethically, the EMT may be compelled to make a statement to law enforcement in the role as a citizen.

2. Most EMS agencies require that an EMT report, usually in writing, any unusual contact with another emergency service. In this case, serious issues of privacy and patient confidentiality have been raised.

3. In this case, the EMT should report that drugs were found on-scene and that the police confiscated those drugs. The EMT should also consider notifying his or her immediate superior whenever police request a statement.

CASE STUDY   MULTICAR PILE-UP

On a foggy Tuesday morning, the police report that twenty-seven cars and two trucks are involved in a chain-reaction motor vehicle collision.

The 9-1-1 communications center dispatches ten ambulances from three townships to respond to the incident. Upon arrival, about 30 minutes later, most of the patients have either been transported or are being staged in a field hospital.

The EMTs are directed to report to the field hospital to take vital signs and perform reassessments.

ADDITIONAL CASE STUDY

The word *triage* rang through Tu's head as he was given his assignment. When the incident commander was done with the briefing, Tu was handed a fistful of triage tags and directed to stand by the gate awaiting the first victims. Almost immediately, firefighters started to drag victims of the plant fire to the triage post and deposit them at Tu's feet.

STOP AND THINK

1. Is a PCR needed for each patient?
2. What minimum information would be required?
3. Does this information become part of the patient record?

ANSWERS TO STOP AND THINK

1. A PCR for each patient in a multiple-casualty incident would be impractical. Instead, a triage tag would be used for each patient.

2. A triage tag typically contains demographic information, a minimal injury, and vital signs. See figure 21–14 for an example.

3. Once the patient has arrived at the hospital, the triage tag is usually included in the patient's medical record like the PCR.

CASE STUDY   PATIENT REFUSAL

"Ambulance one-five, rescue ten, and engine fifty-one, respond to the front of Albertson's for a man down, possible diabetic reaction. Time out is 15:33."

Arriving on-scene, EMT Shelley sees several people huddled around a twentyish-looking male. He is drinking orange juice from a carton.

As Shelley approaches, he says, "Oh no, I'm not going to no hospital. I'm fine. My sugar is giving me a little trouble that's all."

ADDITIONAL CASE STUDY

A disheveled man was speaking to the beat cop when the ambulance pulled up. Disembarking from the ambulance, the EMT, Joe, could her the patient say to the officer, in a slurred voice, "I don't want to go to no hospital."

As the EMT approached, the man turned on his heels as if to leave, and said, "I don't want your help," and fell down. Rushing to his side Joe was immediately aware of the stench of stale beer and body odor. Despite his urge to retreat, he knelt down and held manual stabilization of the patient's head.

Blood was gushing out of the new cut on the side of his head when he was overheard to say again, " I don't want to go to no hospital."

STOP AND THINK

1. How is a patient's refusal documented?
2. What critical elements must be contained in the medical warning?
3. Should anybody be notified before this patient is allowed to sign himself off?

ANSWERS TO STOP AND THINK

1. Some EMS agencies document the patient's refusal on the PCR. Others have an additional form that leads the EMT through the entire process.

2. Every documentation of refusal must show that the patient was capable of refusing, that is, that the patient was of the age of majority and was capable of understanding the consequences of refusal.

3. Some patients, with a minor complaint, will refuse medical attention (RMA). Other more seriously injured patients will refuse medical care or transportation, even against medical advice (AMA). Some EMS systems require that a supervisor witness an RMA. In the case of an AMA, the EMT should consider contacting medical control for advice and further instruction.

FURTHER STUDY

Anderson, C. (1999). Patient care documentation. *Emergency Medical Services, 28*(3) , 59–61.

Burstein, J. L., Hollander, J. E., Delagi, R., Gold, M., Henry, M. C., & Alicandro, J. M. (1998). Refusal of out-of-hospital medical care: Effect of medical-control physician assertiveness on transport rate. *Academic Emergency Medicine, 5*(1), 4–8.

Joyce, S. M., Dutkowski, K. L., & Hynes, T. (1997). Efficacy of an EMS quality improvement program in improving documentation and performance. *Prehospital Emergency Care, 1*(3), 140–144.

Krafsur, J.& Nagorka, F. (2000) . Prehospital rounds: Documentation in a two-tiered system. *Emergency Medical Services, 29*(3), 106–8.

Ornato, J. P., Doctor, M. L., Harbour, L. F.,Peberdy, M. A., Overton, J., Racht, E. M., Zauhar, W. G., Smith, A. P., & Ryan, K. A. (1998). Synchronization of timepieces to the atomic clock in an urban emergency medical services system. *Annals of Emergency Medicine, 31*(4), 483–487.

Weaver, J., Brinsfield, K. H., & Dalphond, D. (2000). Prehospital refusal-of-transport policies: Adequate legal protection? *Prehosptial Emergency Care, 4*(1), 53–56.

ANSWERS TO TEST YOUR KNOWLEDGE

1. The patient care report (PCR) is used to convey historical information about a patient to other health care providers. The PCR is also used to support and defend an EMT's actions in a court of law should an allegation be made.

2. Every PCR should minimally contain the patient's demographic information, the patient's chief complaint, the patient's history of present illness, and the patient's pertinent past medical history. Furthermore, every PCR should document the EMT's physical examination, including vital signs, as well as treatments provided to the patient.

3. The PCR is a part of the emergency department's record within the patient's medical record.

4. Four purposes of the PCR include medico-legal documentation, quality improvement, research, and EMS system administration.

5. A minimum data set contains the smallest amount of information that is still acceptable for a complete PCR. For example, one system may set, as a standard, that the patient's full name and address plus age or date of birth is the minimally accepted data set for demographic information.

6. SOAP means Subjective, Objective, Assessment, and Plan.

7. CHEATED means Chief complaint, History of present illness, Examination, Assessment of the problem, Treatments initiated for the problem, Evaluation of those treatments, and the patient's final Disposition or discharge.

8. The PCR is a medical document that is read by other health care providers. Nonstandard abbreviations may lead to confusion or even errors in patient care predicated on the PCR's information.

9. All PCRs should be legibly written with black ink on an accepted standard PCR form. Errors should

be crossed out once and never covered. Only standard abbreviations should be used during documentation, and the EMT should always date and time the PCR, at time of documentation.

10. When an error is made on a PCR, the EMT should cross the error out once and then initial and note the time next to the error.

11. Additional entries are permitted on the PCR provided that the entry is dated, timed, and initialed by the writer.

12. Any time an unusual incident occurs, the EMT should consider writing a special incident report. The special incident report serves to explain the EMT's observation of the event at the time that it occurred.

13. The use of PCR during a mass casualty incident would be time-consuming and impractical. In those instances an abbreviated report, called a *triage tag*, is used.

14. Minimally, the refusal of medical assistance (RMA) documentation should state, convincingly, that the patient was capable of refusing care, that is, of age and mental capacity, as well as capable of understanding the results of refusal.

15. The best witnesses to any refusal of medical assistance are uninvolved or disinterested parties who are without financial or other interest. The witness should be capable of testifying to the mental state of the patient at the time of refusal as well as to his or her willingness (lack of coercion) to sign the refusal documentation.

CHAPTER 22

Pharmacology for the Street

OBJECTIVES

Upon completion of this chapter, the reader should be able to:

1. Discuss the importance of basic pharmacology to the EMT.
2. Explain the difference between the generic name and the trade name of medications.
3. Define the terms *indication* and *contraindication*.
4. List the different forms that medications may come in.
5. List at least three routes of drug administration used by the EMT.
6. Review the "Five Rights" verified prior to drug administration.
7. Discuss the importance of reassessment after drug administration.
8. Explain how drug administration is documented.
9. Explain the importance of the role of medical control in the administration of medication by the EMT.
10. Describe the indications, contraindications, actions, side effects, dose, and route of the following medications: activated charcoal, oral glucose, oxygen, prescribed inhaler, nitroglycerin, epinephrine.
11. Discuss the difference between an EMT's administering a drug and an EMT's assisting a patient to take a previously prescribed medication.

GLOSSARY

action   The effect of a medication on the person who takes it.

activated charcoal   A suspension of charcoal in a liquid that has the ability to bind most ingested toxins and prevent their absorption.

angina   Pain or discomfort that is a result of insufficient oxygenated blood flow to the heart muscle.

bronchodilator   A medication that specifically opens up narrowed airways.

dose   The amount of a substance; usually refers to the amount of a medication given.

epinephrine   A medication that dilates the airways and constricts the blood vessels.

expiration date   The last day that a medication is guaranteed by the manufacturer to be safe and effective as expected.

generic name   The initial name given to a drug that is shorter than the actual chemical name and is listed in the *U.S. Pharmacopoeia*.

glucose   A substance used by the body for fuel.

hypoglycemia   A condition of low blood glucose levels.

intramuscular Administration of medication into the muscular layer under the subcutaneous layer of soft tissue.

intravenous Administration of medication into the veins.

metered dose inhaler A handheld device that carries a form of medication that may be aerosolized upon discharge of the inhaler device.

nebulizer A device that creates a fine mist of a liquid medication so that it can be inhaled.

nitroglycerin A medication that dilates, or opens, blood vessels.

oral Administration of medication into the mouth.

oxygen A colorless gas that the body needs in adequate amounts to function normally.

pharmacology The study of medications and their interactions.

side effect An effect of a medication that was not intended.

subcutaneous The space just under the skin that is made up of fat and tiny blood vessels.

sublingual Referring to under the tongue.

suspension A powder suspended in a liquid so that it may be more easily ingested.

topical On the surface; administration of medication by placing it on the surface of the skin so that it can be absorbed slowly.

trade name The brand name given to a medication by the manufacturer.

PREPARATORY:

Materials: None.

Personnel: Primary Instructor-Advanced-level provider who ha administered medications. Assistant Instructor: The instructor-to-student ratio should be 1:6 for psychomotor skill practice. Individuals used as assistant instructors should be knowledgeable in general pharmacology.

Recommended Minimum Time to Complete: 1 hour

STUDENT OUTLINE

I. Overview
- A. Terminology
  - 1. Drug Name
    - a) Generic
    - b) Trade
  - 2. Indication
  - 3. Contraindication
  - 4. Actions
  - 5. Side Effects
- B. Prescribing Information
- C. Forms of Medications
  - 1. Compressed Powders/Tablets
  - 2. Liquids
  - 3. Gels
  - 4. Suspensions
  - 5. Powder for inhalation
  - 6. Gases
  - 7. Aerosols
- D. Routes of Administration
  - 1. Inhaled
  - 2. Sublinqual
  - 3. Injection
    - a) Subcutaneous
    - b) Intramuscular
    - c) Intravenous
  - 4. Oral
  - 5. Topical
- E. Medication Administration Procedure
  - 1. Patient Assessment
  - 2. The "Rights" of Drug Administration
    - a) Right Patient
    - b) Right Medication
    - c) Right Route
    - d) Right Dose
    - e) Right Date
  - 3. Reassessment
  - 4. Documentation
- F. Medical Control
  - 1. Off-Line
    - a) Standing Order Protocols
  - 2. On-Line
- G. Specific Drugs Administered by the EMT
  - 1. Med Notes: Oxygen
    - a) Administration Procedure
  - 2. Med Notes: Glucose
    - a) Administration Procedure
  - 3. Activated Charcoal
    - a) Administration Procedure
- H. Specific Assisted Medications
  - 1. Definitions
    - a) Prescribed Inhalers
      - i) Bronchodilator Inhalers
      - ii) Administration Procedure
        - (a) Med Notes: Prescribed Inhalers
    - b) Nitroglycerin
      - i) Administration Procedure
        - (a) Med Notes: Nitroglycerin
    - c) Epinephrine
      - i) Administration Procedure
        - (a) Med Notes: Epinephrine

II. Conclusion

LECTURE OUTLINE

I. Overview
    A. Pharmacology—defined
    B. Terminology
        1. Key Terms Only
        2. Drug Name
            a) Thousands of Drugs
                (1) Use a Handbook/
                      Guidebook
            b) Generic
                (1) Government Name
                    (a) *U.S. Pharmacopoeia*
                        (USP)
            c) Trade
                (1) Company Name
                    (a) Advertising
        3. Indication
            a) Why something is given
        4. Contraindication
            a) Why something should not be
               given
        5. Actions
            a) Primary or Intended Effect of
               Medicine
        6. Side Effects
            a) Secondary or Unintended
               Effects of Medicine
    C. Prescribing Information
        1. Physician's Order
            a) Name
            b) Dose
            c) Frequency
            d) Number of Tablets to Be Dis-
               pensed
            e) As written
                (1) Generic
    D. Forms of Medications
        1. Compressed Powders/Tablets
            a) Easier to Swallow or Dissolve
        2. Liquids
            b) Injection
                (1) Intramuscular
                (2) Subcutaneous
        3. Gels
            a) Melt with Warmth
        4. Suspensions
            a) Solid Held in Liquid
        5. Powder for Inhalation
            a) Finely Pulverized for Absorp-
               tion

        6. Gases
            a) Inhalation
         7. Aerosols
            a) Liquid for Inhalation
    E. Routes of Administration
        1. Inhaled
            a) Via the Lung
        2. Sublingual
            a) Buccal Pocket
        3. Injection
            a) Subcutaneous
                (1) Under the Skin
                    (a) Capillary Beds
            b) Intramuscular
                (1) Within the Muscle
                    (a) Near Venous
                        Blood Flow
            c) Intravenous
                (1) Directly into Blood-
                    stream
                    (a) Rapid to Target
                        Organ
        4. Oral
            a) Directly Absorbed by
               Stomach
        5. Topical
            a) Slow Absorption Through the
              Skin
    F. Medication Administration Procedure
        1. Patient Assessment
            a) Complete SAMPLE
                (1) Allergies Important
        2. The "Rights" of Drug
          Administration
                (1) Prevent Procedural
                    Errors
            a) Right Patient
                (1) Prescribed
            b) Right Medication
                (1) Proper Drug
            c) Right Route
                (1) Correct Method of
                    Administration
            d) Right Dose
                (1) Correct Amount of
                    Drug
            e) Right Date
                (1) Not Expired
        3. Reassessment

a) Effects/Impact of Medication
4. Documentation
   a) All of the above
G. Medical Control
   a) Medication Administration
      Controlled by Physician
   1. Off-Line
      (1) Orders in Anticipation
         of Patient Problem
      a) Standing Order Protocols
         (1) No Direct Needed
            (a) Criteria
   2. On-Line
      a) Direct Order to Admininster
H. Specific Drugs Administered by the EMT
   1. Med Notes: Oxygen
      (1) Colorless
      (2) Life-giving
      a) Administration Procedure
         (1) Ventilation
            (a) Bag-valve
               mask(BVM)
         (2) Respiration
            (a) Nonrebreather
               Mask (NRB)
   2. Med Notes: Glucose
      (1) Life-giving
         (a) carbohydrate
      a) Administration Procedure
         (1) Orally
         (2) Caution
            (a) Airway
   3. Med Notes: Activated Charcoal
      (1) Poisoning
      a) Adminsistration Procedure
         (1) Orally
         (2) Caution
            (a) Airway
I. Specific Assisted Medications
   1. Definitions
      a) Assist versus Administer
         (1) Locally defined

b) Prescribed Inhalers
   (a) Preexisting Condi-
      tion/Disease
      (i) Asthma
      (ii) Emphysema
      (iii) Bronchitis
   (1) Bronchodilator Inhalers
      (a) Mist Medications
      (b) Administration
         Procedure
         (i) Inhalation
         (ii) Aerosol
            Chambers
   (2) Med Notes: Prescribed
      Inhalers
      (a) Two puffs a
         minute apart
   (3) Nitroglycerin
      (a) Coronary Artery
         Dilator
      (b) Venous Dilator
         (i) Hypotension
            (1) Gloves
   (4) Administration Proce-
      dure
      (a) Med Notes: Nitro-
         glycerin
         (i) One
            Puff/Tablet
            Sublingual
c) Epinephrine
   (a) Venous Constric-
      tor
      (i) Anaphylaxis
   (1) Administration Proce-
      dure
      (a) Med Notes: Epi-
         nephrine

II. Conclusion
   A. Lifesaving
   B. Responsibility

TEACHING STRATEGIES

1. Obtain a placebo bronchodilator inhaler and a practice epinephrine auto-injector (both available from the drug companies), as well as a breath spray. Using these simulated medications, have the students take a SAMPLE history from a mock patient, then administer the appropriate medication. The student should be able to discuss the indications, contraindications, dosages, and side effects of each medication.

FURTHER STUDY

Gonsoulin, S., & Raynovich W. (2000). *Prehospital Drug Therapy*. Philadelphia: Mosby.

CASE STUDY   FIREFIGHTER DOWN

Bill, a firefighter in his forties, is dragged out of the fire by two firefighters. They drop him on the front lawn. One firefighter, pulling his face mask up, yells, "Medic." Turning about-face, the two firefighters walk back into the smoke and disappear from sight.

Greg, the first EMT on-scene, helps half-carry, half-drag Bill to the backstep of the pumper. Bill is coughing vigorously and spitting out soot-laden sputum. Apparently, his face mask had blown off his face when the fire flashed over his head and knocked him backward.

Bill yells out, "Somebody got a cigarette?" while Greg starts his assessment.

ADDITIONAL CASE STUDY

"I" "Can't" "Breathe," sputtered Ray in monosyllabic answers. The patient was a sixty-five-year-old male with a forty-five-year history of smoking two packs of cigarettes a day. He was diagnosed with emphysema ten years ago and just last year he was placed on home therapy oxygen. Today he called EMS because his breathing was worse than normal.

STOP AND THINK

1. What are some indications for oxygen administration?
2. What is the dose of oxygen that would be appropriate for this patient?
3. Are there any contraindications to oxygen administration?

ANSWERS TO STOP AND THINK

1. Any patient with altered mental status, shortness of breath, or signs of hypoperfusion should be administered oxygen. Other specific indications include possible carbon monoxide poisoning.

2. Smoke can hid the odorless, colorless gas carbon monoxide. Every patient exposed to potentially toxic fumes or smoke should receive high-flow oxygen via nonrebreather mask.

3. There are no contraindications for oxygen in the field provided there is an indication.

CASE STUDY   DIABETIC EMERGENCY

The call came out over the air: "Man acting strangely, meet the security officer, Golden Oaks Tower Building break room. Police also en route." Sean looked at his watch; it was 10 o'clock. He gave a knowing glance to his partner, Nick. Both EMTs had been to the Tower Building before for the patient "acting strangely."

It was old Tom, the housekeeper. Tom was a "bad diabetic" who never seemed to keep his sugar under control. They guessed that Tom hadn't eaten breakfast again and his blood sugar was dropping like a stone. When Tom hit a low, he would start to act strangely, and sometimes he would even get violent. The key to Tom's care was to get there quickly and treat him before he passed out.

Once Tom passed out, the paramedics would have to start an IV and Tom's veins were terrible. Several times Tom had to be rushed to the hospital with lights and sirens while the medic made repeated attempts at starting an IV. This could all be avoided if Sean and Nick could get to Tom while he was still awake.

STOP AND THINK

1. What are indications for administration of oral glucose?
2. What are contraindications to administration of oral glucose?
3. Why does the patient with low blood glucose act confused?

ANSWERS TO STOP AND THINK

1. Oral glucose is indicated when a known diabetic, who is conscious, is suspected of being hypo-glycemic.

2. Oral glucose should not be administered if the patient is not awake and capable of controlling her or his own airway.

3. The patient with low blood sugar is confused because the brain needs glucose, almost as much oxy-gen, to operate.

CASE STUDY   POSSIBLE POISONING

Putting the phone down, Alisha went to see what her three-year-old daughter, Desiree, was doing. Look-ing in the bedroom, then in the family room, she couldn't find the child. Calling out "Desiree" she heard a faint call from the bathroom: "Mommy." Rushing into the bathroom, Alisha found Desiree sitting on the floor, with pill bottles strewn around her and a handful of pills.

Quickly Alisha knocked the pills from the little girl's hand and swept out her mouth with her fingers. Pill fragments fell to the floor. Scooping the child up in her arms, the young mother ran to the kitchen and called Poison Control. While speaking to Poison Control, Alisha pulled the poison kit from the kitchen cabinet. Poison Control proceeded to ask Alisha a series of questions.

STOP AND THINK

1. What are indications for activated charcoal administration?
2. What are contraindications to giving any medication by mouth?
3. Are there any issues surrounding the administration of an activated charcoal suspension?

ANSWERS TO STOP AND THINK

1. There are many indications for use of activated charcoal. In every case, the EMT must follow the instructions from the manufacturer, Poison Control, or medical control.

2. Activated charcoal should not be administered if the patient is not awake and capable of controlling her or his airway for at least the next 20 minutes.

3. Aspirated activated charcoal can lead to a serious respiratory illness—hence the contraindication for an unconscious patient. Activated charcoal suspension is a slurry that when spilled can stain.

CASE STUDY ASTHMA ATTACK

"Squad 23 out, Pinebush School." EMT-Firefighters Seigel and Sorenson step off the pumper and pro-ceed to the school nurse's office. After being ushered into the room, the firefighters note a teen-aged girl with apparent shortness of breath. The nurse explains that the girl's wheezing started right after gym class. The nurse had called the girl's mother, but the girl was getting progressively worse, even after one treat-ment with her prescribed inhaler. So the nurse decided to call EMS.

STOP AND THINK

1. What are indications to assist a patient to use his or her own prescribed inhaler?
2. What are contraindications to prescribed inhaler use?

ANSWERS TO STOP AND THINK

1. A prescribed inhaler should be used whenever the patient feels the need and/or its use is clinically indicated.

2. An inhaler should not be used if the patient has a decreased level of consciousness, and cannot cooperate with care, or if the patient requires ventilatory assistance.

CASE STUDY   REPEAT ATTACK

Mr. Moon, an older man living alone in a studio apartment in the upper westside, calls EMS when he starts to feel a bout of chest pain coming on. He relates to the two EMTs, Matt and Forrest, that he recently had a heart attack and that he is currently experiencing feelings in his chest just like that, only worse. He has been prescribed nitroglycerin but is not sure if he should use it. When Matt asks where the medicine is, Mr. Moon points to the cabinet over the kitchen sink.

Matt, opening the cabinet, finds a little brown bottle with the label marked "Nitroglycerin" but no prescription. He carries the bottle over to Mr. Moon, and asks if this is his medicine. "Yes, that's my medicine," Mr. Moon can be heard to say through the oxygen mask.

STOP AND THINK

1. What are the indications for using nitroglycerin?
2. What are the contraindications?
3. What are some of the more common side effects of this medication?

ANSWERS TO STOP AND THINK

1. An EMT can assist a patient with nitroglycerin any time the patient has potentially cardiac-related chest pain.

2. Nitroglycerin is not indicated if the patient is hypotensive or has already taken the maximum dosage of drug.

3. Nitroglycerin is a potent vasodilator. Nitroglycerin can lead to profound hypotension. The patient should always be seated whenever nitroglycerin is administered and the EMT should always wear gloves to avoid accidental contact with the nitroglycerin.

CASE STUDY   BEE STING

Eric dutifully climbs up the ladder and starts to clean out the leaves in the rain gutter, thinking to himself what a pain this chore is when suddenly a swarm of bees rises. Scrambling down the ladder, Eric runs away from the bees.

Too late, Eric is stung by one of the bees on the back of the neck. Recalling his nearly fatal reaction the last time he was stung, he yells for his wife Bette to call 9-1-1. "Tell them to hurry, I've been stung by a bee!" Bette grabs the portable phone, dials 9-1-1, and starts talking to the communicator, while looking through the medicine cabinet. She remembers that Eric's doctor had prescribed an Epi-pen™ just in case an emergency like this arose.

Finding the Epi-pen™ in the back of the cabinet, she grabs it and starts to run outside. The rescue squad crew is already with Eric, loosening his shirt and listening to his lungs. His chest is bright red with a rash, and his speech sounds like he's drunk, it's so thick. Bette thrusts the Epi-pen™ into an EMTs hands and says, "Use this!"

STOP AND THINK

1. What are the indications for epinephrine injection?
2. Are there any contraindications?
3. What are some special concerns the EMT should have about handling needles after injections?

ANSWERS TO STOP AND THINK

1. Epinephrine is indicated whenever a patient has a known allergy and is experiencing an anaphylactic reaction.

2. There are no contraindications to epinephrine administration if the patient is experiencing an anaphylactic reaction.

3. While most auto-injectors automatically cover the needle after the injection, the EMT should handle the spent auto-injector as if it were a sharp needle. This includes use of a sharps container.

ANSWERS TO TEST YOUR KNOWLEDGE

1. Before EMTs can assist a patient with a medication, they must have a basic understanding of how certain drugs work, how they are administered, and what the precautions are.

2. The generic name is the shortened chemical name that is listed in the *U.S. Pharmacopoeia.* The trade name is the name that the drug is marketed under to the public.

3. An indication is a reason to give a drug. A contraindication is a reason why a drug should not be given.

4. There are many forms that a medication can come in. Some of the more common forms include tablet, gel, spray, inhaled liquid, and gas.

5. Three common routes of drug administration that an EMT can assist a patient with are inhaler, sublingual, and injection.

6. Before any medication is administered, the EMT should confirm that it is the right patient (the one named on the prescription), the right medication (for the condition at that time), the right dosage (appropriate), right route (will it be effective given this way?), and right date (is the drug fresh?).

7. A reassessment of the patient after a drug has been administered is important to verify that the drug had its intended action and that the patient did not have an unintended (untoward) reaction.

8. Documentation of medication administration should include a complete SAMPLE history, the five rights of administration, and a reassessment of the patient afterwards.

9. The following are the Med notes for the listed drugs:

Med Notes: Oxygen
Generic Name: Oxygen
Trade Name: Oxygen
Indications: Many. Any respiratory or cardiac complaint, stroke or seizure, altered mental status, abdominal pain, bleeding, or any evidence of shock.
Contraindications: No contraindications in the prehospital setting.
Dose: 1–6 lpm by nasal cannula, 10–15 lpm by nonrebreather mask
Route: Inhaled via nasal cannula or nonrebreather face mask

Med Notes: Glucose
Generic Name: Oral glucose
Trade Name: Insta-glucose, and others
Indications: Suspected low blood glucose

Contraindications: Patients who cannot control their own airway and swallow their own secretions should NOT be given oral medications.
Dose: One tube, or container
Route: Orally only

Med Notes: Activated Charcoal
Generic Name: Activated charcoal
Trade Name: Acti-dose, Super-char, and more
Indications: Recent ingestion of susceptible poison.
Contraindications: Patients who cannot control their own airway and swallow their own secretions should NOT be given oral medications.
Dose: 1 gram/kg (50–100 gm for typical adult)
Route: Orally

Med Notes: Prescribed Inhalers
Generic Name: Albuterol
Trade Name: Ventolin, Proventil
Indications: Signs and symptoms of respiratory distress in a patient who has a physician-prescribed hand-held inhaler.
Contraindications: The nonalert patient cannot cooperate with administration of an inhaler.
Dose: Two puffs given one minute apart.
Route: By inhalation

Med Notes: Nitroglycerin
Generic Name: Nitroglycerin
Trade Name: Nitrostat
Indications: Cardiac-related chest pain or angina
Contraindications: Hypotension, infants and children, patient has already taken maximum dosage prior to EMS arrival.
Dose: 0.4 mg tablet or metered dose spray
Route: Sublingual

Med Notes: Epinephrine
Generic Name: Epinephrine
Trade Name: Epi-Pen
Indications: Life-threatening allergic reaction
Contraindications: None in the presence of an indication
Dose: 0.5 milligrams
Route: Intramuscular

10. When an EMT assists a patient with his medications, he is ensuring the patient properly administers a drug to himself that has been prescribed for him. When an EMT administers a medication, he is giving the patient a medication that the patient has not previously been prescribed by a physician.

Skill 22–1 Use of Metered Dose Inhaler

Student Name: _____   Date: _____

Purpose: To administer a dose of prescribed bronchodilator medication to the patient.

Standard Precautions: Icon—Gloves—Goggles—Mask

Equipment needed:
Prescribed Metered Dose Inhaler
Oxygen

Procedural Steps:

Step 1. Assure scene safety and apply appropriate personal protective equipment prior to assessing the patient.

YES: _____   RE-TEACH: _____   RETURN: _____   INSTRUCTOR INITIALS _____

Step 2. Assess patient and apply oxygen as appropriate.

YES: _____   RE-TEACH: _____   RETURN: _____   INSTRUCTOR INITIALS _____

Step 3. Confirm "rights."

YES: _____   RE-TEACH: _____   RETURN: _____   INSTRUCTOR INITIALS _____

Step 4. Shake inhaler.

YES: _____   RE-TEACH: _____   RETURN: _____   INSTRUCTOR INITIALS _____

Step 5. Remove mouthpiece cover.

YES: _____   RE-TEACH: _____   RETURN: _____   INSTRUCTOR INITIALS _____

Step 6. Ask patient to exhale, then inhale slowly and deeply. Remove oxygen mask.

YES: _____   RE-TEACH: _____   RETURN: _____   INSTRUCTOR INITIALS _____

Step 7. Place inhaler to patient's mouth and at onset of inhalation, depress canister to release one puff of aerosolized medication.

YES: _____   RE-TEACH: _____   RETURN: _____   INSTRUCTOR INITIALS _____

Step 8. Remove inhaler from patient's mouth. Reapply oxygen and instruct the patient to continue the inhalation and hold his or her breath for several seconds.

YES: _____   RE-TEACH: _____   RETURN: _____   INSTRUCTOR INITIALS _____

Step 9. Wait one minute, then repeat procedure.

YES: _____   RE-TEACH: _____   RETURN: _____   INSTRUCTOR INITIALS _____

Step 10. Reevaluate patient.

YES: _____   RE-TEACH: _____   RETURN: _____   INSTRUCTOR INITIALS _____

Skill 22–2 Epinephrine Auto-Injector Administration

Student Name: _____   Date: _____

Purpose: To assist the patient with administration of epinephrine by auto-injector in a case of anaphylaxis.

Standard Precautions:
Icon — Handwashing—Gloves

Equipment needed:
Oxygen
Airway and Ventilation Equipment (standing by)
Prescribed Epinephrine Auto-Injector

Procedural Steps:

Step 1. Assure scene safety and apply appropriate personal protective equipment prior to assessing patient.
YES: _____   RE-TEACH: _____   RETURN: _____   INSTRUCTOR INITIALS _____

Step 2. Assess patient and apply oxygen as appropriate.
YES: _____   RE-TEACH: _____   RETURN: _____   INSTRUCTOR INITIALS _____

Step 3. Determine need for epinephrine and confirm presence of auto-injector.
YES: _____   RE-TEACH: _____   RETURN: _____   INSTRUCTOR INITIALS _____

Step 4. Bare patient's lateral thigh.
YES: _____   RE-TEACH: _____   RETURN: _____   INSTRUCTOR INITIALS _____

Step 5. Follow instructions on auto-injector to remove safety mechanism.
YES: _____   RE-TEACH: _____   RETURN: _____   INSTRUCTOR INITIALS _____

Step 6. Press auto-injector firmly against the patient's lateral thigh, midway between knee and hip, and allow 10 seconds for medication administration.
YES: _____   RE-TEACH: _____   RETURN: _____   INSTRUCTOR INITIALS _____

Step 7. Remove the injector and properly dispose of it.
YES: _____   RE-TEACH: _____   RETURN: _____   INSTRUCTOR INITIALS _____

Step 8. Initiate transport if not already done and reassess patient.
YES: _____   RE-TEACH: _____   RETURN: _____   INSTRUCTOR INITIALS _____

CHAPTER 23

Shortness of Breath

OBJECTIVES

Upon completion of this chapter, the reader should be able to:

1. List the structures and functions of the respiratory system.
2. State the signs and symptoms of a patient with difficulty breathing.
3. Describe the emergency medical care of the patient with difficulty breathing.
4. Recognize the need for medical direction to assist in the emergency medical care of the patient with difficulty breathing.
5. Recognize the patient in need of airway management and ventilatory assistance.
6. List the signs of adequate air exchange.
7. Identify when administration of a prescribed inhaler is indicated.
8. Identify the key elements in management of patients with epiglottitis, croup, asthma, COPD, and CHF.

GLOSSARY

alveolar-capillary gas exchange   The movement of gases between alveoli and adjacent capillaries.

asthma   A disease characterized by a hyperreactive airways; also known as reactive airway disease.

bronchospasm   Constriction of the lower airways in the lungs.

cellular respiration   The process that allows the exchange of gases in the periphery.

chronic obstructive pulmonary disease (COPD)   A group of diseases characterized by chronic airway obstruction and bronchospasm.

congestive heart failure (CHF)   A condition in which there is a backup of pressure from the left ventricle, allowing fluid to leak out of the pulmonary capillaries into the alveoli.

crackles   A popping sound heard in the lungs that is created as tiny air spaces that are stuck together by abnormal fluid accumulation pop open.

croup   A swelling and inflammation of the larynx, trachea, and, to some extent, the bronchi, usually caused by a viral infection.

diffusion   The movement of oxygen and carbon dioxide across a membrane from an area of higher concentration to an area of lower concentration.

epiglottitis   A swollen, inflamed epiglottis, usually caused by a bacterial infection.

hypoxic drive   The stimulus to breathe becomes low oxygen levels instead of the usual stimulus, high carbon dioxide levels.

pulmonary embolus   A blockage in the pulmonary arterial circulation resulting in an area of lung that does not allow alveolar capillary gas exchange.

rhonchi A coarse sound that is heard over the lungs when mucus or other foreign material accumulates in the larger airways.

PREPARATORY

Materials: Utilize various audiovisual materials relating to respiratory emergencies. The continuous design and development of new audiovisual materials relating to EMS requires careful review to determine which best meet the needs of the program. Materials should be edited to assure meeting the objectives of the curriculum.

EMS Equipment: Handheld inhaler suitable for training purposes and various spacer devices.

Personnel: Primary Instructor: One advanced-level provider or EMT-Basic instructor who is knowledgeable in respiratory diseases and handheld inhalers. Assistant Instructor: The instructor-to-student ratio should be 1:6 for psychomotor skill practice. Individuals used as assistant instructors should be knowledgeable in respiratory emergencies.

Recommended Minimum Time to Complete: 2.5 hours

I. Overview
II. Anatomy Review
    A. Upper Airway
    B. Respiratory Tree
    C. Musculature
        1. Diaphragm
        2. Chest Wall Muscles
III. Physiology Review
    A. Respiratory Drive
    B. Ventilation
        1. Inhalation
        2. Exhalation
    C. Respiration
        1. Pulmonary Respiration
        2. Cellular Respiration
IV. Normal Breathing
    A. Patient Appearance
    B. Lung Sounds
    C. Rates and Patterns
    D. Vital Signs
    E. Color
V. Respiratory Distress
    A. Signs and Symptoms
    B. Assessment
        1. Initial Assessment
        2. Focused History and Physical
           Examination
           a) Responsive Patient
               (1) History
               (2) Focused Physical Exam
               (3) Vital Signs
           b) Unresponsive Patient
               (1) Rapid Physical
                    Examination
               (2) Vital Signs
    C. History from Others
    D. Transport
        1. Destination Decisions
        2. Advanced Life Support
        3. Ongoing Assessment
VI. Causes of Shortness of Breath
    A. Airway

        1. Foreign Body Obstruction
        2. Epiglottitis
            a) Signs and Symptoms
            b) Management
        3. Croup
            a) Signs and Symptoms
            b) Management
    B. Breathing
        1. Bronchospasm
            a) Asthma
                (1) Signs and Symptoms
               (2) Management
            b) Chronic Obstructive Pul-
               monary Disease
               (1) Acute Exacerbation of
                    COPD
               (2) Signs and Symptoms
                  (a) Hypoxic Drive
                  (b) Management
        2. Respiratory Infection
            a) Signs and Symptoms
            b) Management
        3. Chronic Lung Diseases
    C. Circulation
        1. Pulmonary Embolus
            a) Signs and Symptoms
            b) Management
        2. Pulmonary Edema
            a) Signs and Symptoms
            b) Management
        3. Shock
VII. General Management of a Respiratory
    Emergency
    A. Oxygen
        1. Spontaneously Breathing Patient
        2. Assisting Ventilations
        3. Intubation
    B. Positioning
    C. Prescribed Medications
        1. Bronchodilator Inhalers
    D. Reassessment
VIII. Conclusion

LECTURE OUTLINE

I. Overview
    A. Vital System for Survival
II. Anatomy Review
    A. Upper Airway
        1. Conduit for Air Passage
    B. Respiratory Tree
        1. Gaseous Exchange
    C. Musculature
        1. Diaphragm
            a) Nervous Control
        2. Chest Wall Muscles
            a) Accessory Muscles of
               Breathing
III. Physiology Review
    A. Respiratory Drive
        1. Carbon Dioxide Primary Drive
    B. Ventilation
        1. Inhalation
            a) Negative Inspiratory Pressure
        2. Exhalation
            a) Passive Exchange
    C. Respiration
        1. Pulmonary Respiration
            a) Exchange of Gases at Alveoli
        2. Cellular Respiration
            a) Exchange of Gases at Cellular
               Level
IV. Normal Breathing
        1. Minimal Effort
    A. Patient Appearance
        1. Normal
            a) Appears Relaxed
        1. Distress
            a) Effort
    B. Lung Sounds
        1. Normal
            a) Clear
        2. Abnormal
            a) Wheezes
               (1) Narrowed Airways
            b) Crackles
               (1) Fluid in Airways
            c) Coarse, Gurgly Sound
               (1) Rhonchi
                  (a) Mucus/
                     Pneumonia
    C. Rates and Patterns
    D. Vital Signs

    E. Color
        1. Poorly Oyxgenated
            a) Cyanosis
V. Respiratory Distress
    A. Signs and Symptoms
        1. Increased Respiratory Rate
        2. Cyanosis
        3. Accessory Muscle Use
    B. Assessment
        1. Initial Assessment
        2. Focused History and Physical
           Examination
            a) Responsive Patient
               (1) History
                  (a) SAMPLE
                  (b) OPQRST
               (2) Focused Physical Exam
                  (a) JVD
                  (b) Dependent Periph-
                     eral Edema
                     (i) Ankles
               (3) Vital Signs
                  (a) Pulse Oximetry
            b) Unresponsive Patient
               (1) Rapid Physical
                  Examination
                  (a) Vital Clues
                     (i) Hives/
                       Uticaria
               (2) Vital Signs
    C. History from Others
    D. Transport
        1. Destination Decisions
            a) Closest Facility
        2. Advanced Life Support
            a) Lifesaving Treatments
        3. Ongoing Assessment
VI. Causes of Shortness of Breath
    A. Airway
        1. Foreign Body Obstruction
            a) Café Coronary
        2. Epiglottitis
               (1) Infectious Process
            a) Signs and Symptoms
               (1) Stridor
               (2) Drooling Saliva
            b) Management
               (1) No Probing Airway

(2) Calm Child
(3) 100% O$_2$
    (a) Blow-by
(4) Rapid Transport
3. Croup
    a) Signs and Symptoms
       (1) Barking, Seal-like Cough
    b) Management
       (1) Similar to Epiglottitis
B. Breathing
  1. Bronchospasm
    a) Asthma
       (a) Hyperreactive Airway
       (b) Stimulant
          (i) Smoke
          (ii) Pollen
          (iii) Cold Air
          (iv) Exercise
       (1) Signs and Symptoms
          (a) Diffuse Wheezes
          (b) Silence
             (i) Ominous Pre-arrest Finding
       (2) Management
          (a) Inhaled Bronchodilator
          (b) 100% Oxygen
    b) Chronic Obstructive Pulmonary Disease
       (a) Primarily Emphysema
       (b) Chronic Bronchitis
       (1) Acute Exacerbation of COPD
          (i) Increased Mucous Plugs
          (ii) Flu-like Symptoms
       (a) Signs and Symptoms
          (i) Quiet Lungs
             (1) Destroyed Lung Tissue
       (b) Hypoxic Drive
          (i) Secondary "Survival" Drive

(c) Management
       (ii) Oxygen Deprivation
          (1) Oxygen Administration
  2. Respiratory Infection
    a) Signs and Symptoms
    b) Management
  3. Chronic Lung Diseases
C. Circulation
  1. Pulmonary Embolus
       (1) Blockage of Pulmonary Circulation
       (2) At-Risk Populations
    a) Signs and Symptoms
       (1) Severe Hypoxia
    b) Management
       (1) High-Flow Oxygen
  2. Pulmonary Edema
    a) Heart Failure
       (1) Backwards Failure
    b) Signs and Symptoms
       (1) Fluid in Lungs
          (a) Crackles
    c) Management
       (1) High-Flow Oxygen
  3. Shock
    a) Respiratory Failure
VII. General Management of a Respiratory Emergency
  A. Oxygen
    1. Spontaneously Breathing Patient
    2. Assisting Ventilations
      a) Severe Hypoxia
    3. Intubation
      b) Airway Control
         (1) Unconscious
  B. Positioning
    1. High-Fowlers Position
  C. Prescribed Medications
    2. Bronchodilator Inhalers
  D. Reassessment
VIII. Conclusion

TEACHING STRATEGIES

1. Invite a patient with asthma, a patient with chronic obstructive pulmonary disease, and a patient with heart failure to class. First, have the patients describe their experiences with EMS and the issues/problems that they may have encountered. Then have the students break into groups to obtain a medical history and perform a physical on the patients.

2. Obtain a breath sounds audiotape. First play the tape and identify the following breath sounds: stridor, wheezing, crackles, and rhonchi. Then play the tape in an asynchronous order and ask the students to identify the sounds heard.

3. Ask a respiratory therapist from the local hospital to speak on the leading respiratory diseases seen in the community, emphasizing asthma, emphysema, and pulmonary edema.

FURTHER STUDY

Scott, A. S., & Fong, E. (1998). *Body structures and functions* (9th ed.). Albany, NY: Delmar-Thompson Learning.

CASE STUDY   BREATHING DIFFICULTY

EMTs Bell and McCall arrive on-scene to find an approximately seventy-year-old thin male sitting hunched over at a small table. His eyes are half open. A half empty cup of coffee, an ashtray overflowing with cigarette butts, a half dozen prescription medicine bottles, and two inhalers are on the table.

"Good afternoon, Mr. Coyne. How can we help you today?" asks Bell. Mr. Coyne strains to say the words, "Trouble . . . Breathing." Looking more closely, the EMTs note that Mr. Coyne's lips are bluish.

ADDITIONAL CASE STUDY

Mrs. White greeted the EMTs at the open door. "Hello, gentleman, please come in. My daughter has cystic fibrosis and is having trouble breathing." The EMTs were ushered into a small bedroom where a little girl was sitting bolt upright in bed and obviously struggling to breath. She was grossly cyanotic. As the EMTs entered the room, they noticed a humidifier, an electric suction machine, and a large number of inhalers on a bedside table. As they proceeded to the bedside, the little girl's eyes rolled back into her head and she went unconscious.

STOP AND THINK

1. What signs of respiratory distress are present?
2. What environmental clues may suggest respiratory disease?
3. What assessment findings would the EMTs likely discover?
4. What are the treatment priorities?

ANSWERS TO STOP AND THINK

1. The physical signs of respiratory distress include the cyanosis and the monosyllabic answers.

2. The environmental clues include the prescription bottles, including the inhalers, as well as the ashtray overflowing with cigarette butts.

3. The EMTs can expect to find a patient who is using his accessory muscles to breath, who has quiet lungs, and who has trouble taking a deep breath.

4. Oxygen therapy is immediately indicated for this patient. The EMTs should support the patient in the position of comfort and transport immediately. Use of the metered dose inhalers may be indicated.

CASE STUDY   CHOKING

The public safety officer was using the security camera and panning the lunch room for activity when he noticed a crowd of people around someone on the floor. The person on the floor appeared to be unresponsive to the people shaking her. While keeping the camera trained on the crowd he called 9-1-1 for an "unknown, woman down." Shortly afterward, a call came into the security office. "Listen, we need an ambulance. Some woman passed out. She appeared to be choking, then passed out." The security officer responded, "Sir, an officer has been dispatched and should be there any minute now and I have called for an ambulance."

ADDITIONAL CASE STUDY

"My baby is having trouble breathing!" the woman at the door told the EMTs. The child, a two-year-old by appearance, was seated on the toilet seat in a mist-filled bathroom coughing loudly. The EMT immediately recognized the sound of the child's cough from his own youth. His mother used to take him into the bathroom and turn on the hot water in the shower until the room was filled with steam.

After introducing himself to the patient, the EMT turned to the mother and asked her how long had he been like this.

STOP AND THINK

1. On the basis of the limited information provided, is this patient a high- or low-priority patient?
2. What is the first priority in this patient's assessment?
3. What techniques could be used to manage this situation?

ANSWERS TO STOP AND THINK

1. The fact that the patient is unconscious and unresponsive makes her a high-priority patient.
2. Assuming that there was no trauma, the first priority for this patient would be to control the airway.
3. The case suggests that the patient has experienced a foreign body airway obstruction (FBAO). The EMT should proceed with standard basic life support airway maneuvers until the airway clears.

CASE STUDY   SHORTNESS OF BREATH

Practice was going as usual until one of the swimmers appeared to be having some trouble with her strokes. The coach advised her to rest for a minute. She stopped her practice, went to take her medicine, and then resumed swimming. Shortly after resuming swimming, she started to experience even greater difficulty breathing and she had to be helped out of the pool. Her coach immediately sent two swimmers to the coach's office to get more help and to call 9-1-1.

After what seemed hours, but was actually only a few minutes, EMS arrived. The coach gave the EMT a quick description of what had happened and then left to call the swimmer's parents.

ADDITIONAL CASE STUDY

"Peanuts," thought Kyle as soon as the brownie hit his lips. Kyle had a severe allergy to peanuts and even the smell of peanuts would send him into a fit of wheezing. Motioning to the school aide, he got up and ran out the door to the school nurse's office. The school nurse had specific instructions for Kyle's care. If he was wheezing she was to give him his inhaler, call 9-1-1, and then call his mother. In the event Kyle got worse before the ambulance arrived, she was to use the epinephrine auto-injector.

STOP AND THINK

1. What are the patient care priorities?
2. On the basis of this limited information, what is the likely cause of her shortness of breath?
3. How should an EMT proceed with treatment?

ANSWERS TO STOP AND THINK

1. The patient should be immediately assisted to a position of comfort and then administered high-flow oxygen via a non-rebreather mask (NRB).
2. Exercise and an unnamed medication would make the EMT suspect that the patient is an asthmatic.
3. Assuming that the initial patient care treatments are in place, the EMT should consider assisting the patient with her metered dose inhaler.

CASE STUDY   HEART PROBLEMS

The family had just finished the holiday ham dinner and were sitting down to watch the football game on television. Grandma was busy washing the dishes in the kitchen when she suddenly became short of breath. Sitting down at the kitchen table to rest, she called out to Junior. Junior had seen Grandma like this before and immediately dialed the fire station.

"Grandma's having troubling breathing again. You'd better get up here. She's got heart problems you know," Junior reported to the emergency hotline operator. "End of Canyon Road, second farm house on the right past the bridge, we'll turn the porch light on for you."

ADDITIONAL CASE

The patient had been loaded into the back of the ambulance and was being transported to the hospital. A paramedic intercept had been called for and the ambulance was expected to meet them about 4 miles ahead. The patient was complaining of severe chest pain, like an elephant sitting on his chest, and had not gotten relief from his nitroglycerin. Now his blood pressure was too low to give more nitroglycerin.

Suddenly the patient's respiratory rate started to pick up and he became more ashen. A quick listen to his lungs confirmed the EMT's fear: crackles. The patient was starting to go into heart failure. The EMT picked up the microphone and advised the paramedic that the patient had developed pulmonary edema.

STOP AND THINK

1. What are the priorities in this patient's assessment?
2. What physical findings might be expected?
3. What are the treatment priorities?
4. What differs between the treatment of this patient and the treatment of an asthmatic patient?

ANSWERS TO STOP AND THINK

1. The patient's apparent respiratory distress mandates that the EMT immediately administer high-flow oxygen via nonrebreather mask (NRB).
2. With the history of heart problems it can be anticipated that the patient is experiencing heart failure again and will have evidence of pulmonary edema, specifically crackles in the lungs.
3. After getting the patient to a position of comfort and administering high-flow oxygen, the EMT should prepare to transport the patient rapidly. It may be appropriate to ask the patient if she is experiencing any chest pain, then assist her with her nitroglycerin.
4. The treatment of an asthmatic patient and a heart failure patient is very similar. First, assist the patient to a position of comfort. Second, administer high-flow oxygen while performing an initial assessment. Third, consider assisting the patient with medications as appropriate. Last, initiate immediate transport while calling for an ALS intercept.

ANSWERS TO TEST YOUR KNOWLEDGE

1. Starting at the mouth, the first portion of the airway is the pharynx. The pharynx leads to the trachea, which is protected by the epiglottis, and then into the bronchus. The airway below the larynx, or voicebox, is called the lower airway and is essentially sterile and farther than the reach of an EMT's suction. The lower airway subdivides, first into the two bronchi, repeatedly until it reaches the alveolar level. In the alveoli the process of gas exchange, called *respiration,* occurs and the blood picks up oxygen.

2. The symptoms of difficulty breathing range from a declaration, "I can't breathe," to monosyllabic answers like "Yes" or "O.K." to silence, indicating complete airway obstruction. The signs of respiratory failure include a diminished level of consciousness, nasal flaring, open-mouth breathing, cyanosis around the lips and the conjunctiva, neck-strap muscle use, rapid breathing, abdominal muscle use, and low pulse oximetry readings.

3. The patient with difficulty breathing needs immediate attention to ventilation and oxygenation. Immediate emergency medical care should focus on lifesaving procedures such as ventilation and oxygenation, in that order. Then the EMT should consider assisting the patient with medications as appropriate. Last, the EMT should initiate immediate transport while calling for an ALS intercept.

4. Many respiratory aliments are chronic diseases with acute flare-ups or exacerbations. The EMT is part of the therapeutic team during the acute phase, but long-term survival depends on continual medical surveillance. From the standing orders in the EMT's protocols to on-line supervision, the patient's care must remain under the control of a physician to be effective in the long term.

5. Ventilatory support should begin as soon as the patient shows signs of respiratory failure. The EMT should not wait for the patient to become apneic before assisting the patient's breathing. A decreased level of consciousness, slowing breathing in the face of cyanosis, or cyanosis in the presence of high-flow oxygen administration should alert the EMT to the need for assisted ventilation and possible intubation.

6. The patient with adequate air exchange will be awake and alert, breathing through the nose effortlessly, without any adventitious breath sounds. Oxygen saturation should be above 95% and the patient should be able to speak in full sentences.

7. The EMT should assist the patient with a prescribed inhaler whenever the patient exhibits symptoms for which the inhaler was prescribed. For example, if the patient is an asthmatic and an inhaler has been prescribed, then whenever the patient wheezes the EMT should consider the use of the inhaler.

8. The key elements of managing any respiratory disease are essentially the same. First, assist the patient to a position of comfort. Second, administer high-flow oxygen while performing an initial assessment. Third, consider assisting the patient with medications as appropriate. Last, initiate immediate transport while calling for an ALS intercept. In the case of the epiglottis/croup, the EMT should not probe the pharynx.

CHAPTER 24

Chest Pain

OBJECTIVES

Upon completion of this chapter, the reader should be able to:

1. Describe the importance of early cardiac care.
2. List the risk factors of heart disease.
3. Describe the circulatory system in terms of systemic and pulmonary circuits.
4. Describe the disease process that causes coronary artery disease.
5. List the signs and symptoms of cardiac-related disorders.
6. List important historical questions to ask the patient with chest pain.
7. Describe the focused physical examination of the patient with chest pain.
8. List the appropriate prehospital treatments for chest pain.
9. List the indications, contraindications, side effects, and precautions that are taken when administering nitroglycerin.
10. Describe the transportation considerations for a patient with chest pain.

GLOSSARY

acute myocardial infarction (AMI)   The death of heart muscle due to an inadequate supply of oxygen-rich blood (hypoperfusion).

angina   The pain produced by injured or dying heart muscle.

atherosclerosis   The process of fatty build-up on the walls of blood vessels.

bradycardia   A decreased heart rate below 50 beats per minute.

coronary arteries   The two arteries that supply blood to the heart muscle.

diaphoretic   Excessive perspiration due to stress or pain.

hypertension   An abnormally high blood pressure.

myocardium   The heart muscle.

pulmonary edema   Swelling of the pulmonary blood vessels.

sudden cardiac death (SCD)   The death of a patient early in the course of a heart attack, usually due to an arrhythmia.

tachycardia   Increased heart rate above 100 beats per minute.

PREPARATORY

Materials: EMS Equipment: CPR mannequins, artificial ventilation mannequins, automated external defibrillator, NTG training bottle, defibrillation mannequin.

Personnel: Primary Instructor: One advanced-level provider with knowledge and experience in out-of-hospital cardiac resuscitation. Assistant Instructor: The instructor-to-student ratio should be 1:6 for psychomotor skill practice. Individuals used as assistant instructors should be knowledgeable in cardiac emergencies.

Recommended Minimum Time to Complete: 7 hours

STUDENT OUTLINE

I. Overview

II. Anatomy and Physiology Review
- A. The Left Heart
- B. The Right Heart
- C. Coronary Circulation

III. Coronary Artery Disease
- A. Pathophysiology
- B. Risk Factors
- C. Signs and Symptoms
- D. Noncardiac Chest Pain
- E. Assessment
  - a) Initial Assessment
    - (1) Unresponsive Cardiac Patient
    - (2) Responsive Cardiac Patient
  - b) Focused History
    - (1) Onset
    - (2) Provocation
    - (3) Quality
    - (4) Radiation
    - (5) Severity
    - (6) Time of Onset
  - c) Focused Physical Examination
  - d) Baseline Vital Signs
- F. Management
  - a) Nitroglycerin
- G. Transport
  - a) Aeromedical Transportation
  - b) ALS Intercept
- H. Ongoing Assessment
  - a) Thrombolytics
  - b) Interventional Cardiology

IV. Conclusion

LECTURE OUTLINE

I. Overview
- A. Cardiovascular Disease
  - 1. Leading Cause of Mortality
- B. Risk Factors
  - 1. Controllable
  - 2. Uncontrollable
- C. Presenting Symptoms
  - 1. Chest Pain
    - a) Leading EMS Call

II. Anatomy and Physiology Review
- A. Heart
  - 1. Pair of Pumps in Parallel
- B. The Left Heart
  - 1. Systemic Circuit
    - a) Efficiency
      - (1) Blood Pressure
        - (a) Systolic
        - (b) Diastolic
- C. The Right Heart
  - 1. Pulmonary Circuit
    - a) Low Pressure
- D. Coronary Circulation
  - 1. Supplies Heart Muscle

III. Coronary Artery Disease
- A. Pathophysiology
  - 1. Atherosclerosis
    - a) Plaques (Atheromas)
- B. Risk Factors
  - 1. Nonmodifiable
    - a) Sex
    - b) Family History
    - c) Diabetes
  - 2. Modifiable
    - a) Diet
    - b) Weight
    - c) Exercise
- C. Signs and Symptoms
  - 1. Signs
    - a) Tachycardia
    - b) Bradycardia
  - 2. Symptoms
    - a) Chest Pain
      - (1) Radiation
        - (a) Jaw
        - (b) Left Shoulder
    - b) Nausea
    - c) Atypical Presentations
      - (1) Shortness of Breath
      - (2) Unexplained Syncopy
- D. Noncardiac Chest Pain
  - 1. Muscular
  - 2. Skeletal
  - 3. Gastrointestinal
- E. Assessment
  - 1. Initial Assessment
    - a) Unresponsive Cardiac Patient
      - (1) CPR
      - (2) Defibrillation
    - b) Responsive Cardiac Patient
      - (1) Focused History
        - (a) Onset
        - (b) Provocation
          - (i) Activity at Time
        - (c) Quality
        - (d) Radiation
        - (e) Severity
          - (i) Scale of 0–10
        - (f) Time of Onset
          - (i) Denial
  - 2. Focused Physical Examination
    - a) Sluggish Pupillary Reaction
    - b) Jugular Venous Distention
    - c) Pulmonary Edema
      - (1) Crackles
      - (2) Wheezes
  - 3. Baseline Vital Signs
- F. Management
  - 1. Position of Comfort
  - 2. Oxygen Therapy
    - a) High-Flow Oxygen via Non-rebreather Mask (NRB)
  - 3. Nitroglycerin
    - a) Caution—Hypotension
- G. Transport
  - 1. Carried
  - 2. Position of Comfort
  - 3. Ground
    - a) No Lights or Siren
  - 4. Aeromedical Transportation
    - a) Remote Locales to Cardiac Centers
  - 5. ALS Intercept
    - a) Advanced Cardiac Life Support
- H. Ongoing Assessment
  - 1. Thrombolytics
    - a) Time is Muscle
  - 2. Interventional Cardiology
    - a) Designated Heart Centers

IV. Conclusion
- A. Omnipresent Threat
  - 1. Sudden Cardiac Death
  - 2. EMS = Improved Survival

TEACHING STRATEGIES

1. Using an unlabeled map of the cardiovascular system, have the students label and trace the path of blood through the circulatory system.

2. Have a patient-model mimic a heart attack. Ask the students to obtain a complete history, using SAMPLE as OPQRST, as well as perform a complete physical examination; including an initial assessment then a detailed physical examination.

FURTHER STUDY

Criss, E. (1997). An unrecognized epidemic: Women and heart disease. *Journal of Emergency Medical Services,* *22*(5), 58–63.

Dernocoeur, K. (1997) A page from history: Prehospital use of aspirin. *Journal of Emergency Medical Services,* *22*(9), 42–48.

Henry, M., & Stapleton, E. (1998). A voyage to chest pain. *Journal of Emergency Medical Services, 23*(5), 74–79.

Wilcox, D. (1997). *Angina: Improving the outcome. RN, 60*(7), 34–40.

CASE STUDY   HEART ATTACK

Sandy kneels in front of Mr. Williams and asks, "What's bothering you today, sir?" "It's my wife," Mr. Williams replies. "She got all nerved up and started saying that this could be a heart attack. Look, I'm not having a heart attack. It's just a little indigestion. It'll go away after a while."

While Mr. Williams is talking, Sandy is doing a quick assessment. Mr. Williams is in his forties and is overweight. He appears anxious, and is covered in sweat. "Can you tell me the kinds of symptoms you are experiencing?" Sandy asks. Mr. Williams relates that he has had indigestion for the past 12 hours. He took some antacids, Pepto-Bismol™, he thinks, but it didn't get better. When he started to get a little lightheaded and could feel his pulse race, his wife, Dianne, called 9-1-1.

Just as he says, "Look I really don't need any help . . ." Mr. Williams passes out.

ADDITIONAL CASE STUDY

Mr. Williams was sitting in the front seat of the car. His wife had pulled into the ambulance station after he complained that he was going to pass out. He had a heart attack just last year and had nearly died. Frightened, Mrs. Williams honked the horn repeatedly until someone came out.

"What's wrong, ma'am?" asked Del. "It's my husband. I think he's having a heart attack." Del leapt into action. He immediately called out to the crew to the pull the ambulance out and then bring the jump-kit over. "Mr. Williams, what kind of discomfort are you having?" asked Del. Mr. Williams clutched his fist to his chest and said, "It feels like an elephant is sitting on my chest." Just then Mr. Williams passed out.

STOP AND THINK

1. What immediate actions should the EMT take in this case?
2. What risk factors does Mr. Williams have that might lead the EMT to think he is a candidate for heart disease?
3. What symptoms does Mr. Williams have that would lead the EMT to suspect a heart attack?
4. What treatments would be in order for Mr. Williams?

ANSWERS TO STOP AND THINK

1. The EMT needs to immediately determine if the patient is unconscious, apneic, and pulseless. If so, the EMT needs to start CPR until a defibrillator is available. If the patient is unconscious but still alive, the EMT needs to control the airway and administer oxygen. It may be appropriate to place the patient on the AED; that action is dependent on local protocols.

2. First, being a male puts Mr. Williams at increased risk of heart disease. He is also obese, making him a candidate for heart disease.

3. Mr. Williams' indigestion would make the EMT suspicious that he may be having a cardiac event. The fact that antacids are not relieving his indigestion also suggests a cardiac event.

4. Assuming that the patient is not in cardiac arrest, Mr. Williams should immediately be placed in a position of comfort and administered oxygen. If Mr. Williams has a prescription for nitroglycerin, the EMT may want to consider assisting the patient with self-administration.

ANSWERS TO TEST YOUR KNOWLEDGE

1. Early cardiac care can reduce or eliminate the potential for sudden cardiac death secondary to ventricular fibrillation. Furthermore, early cardiac care, including rapid transportation to definitive care, permits the patient access to new medical treatments that can prevent further damage and even reverse the myocardial infarction.

2. Risk factors for heart disease can be divided into two categories: modifiable and nonmodifiable. The modifiable risk factors include diet, weight, and exercise. The nonmodifiable risk factors include sex, familial history, and diabetes.

3. Starting at the left ventricle, blood is ejected out of the heart and into the aorta. From the aorta the blood travels through the systemic circuit, through the various organs of the body, returning to the central circulation, from the capillary beds, via the venous circulation, to the great vein, the vena cava. From the vena cava the blood is returned to the right side of the heart to be pumped through the pulmonary circuit and back to the left side of the heart.

4. Typically, the patient having a heart attack will experience substernal chest pain, often associated with radiation into the jaw and/or left shoulder. Patients with shortness of breath, unexplained syncopy, and inexplicable fatigue should also be suspected of having a heart attack. Signs of a heart attack include pallor, diaphoresis, tachycardia, irregular pulse, tachypnea, and hypertension.

5. The patient possibly experiencing a cardiac event should be placed in a position of comfort and given oxygen. If the patient has a prescription for nitroglycerin, the EMT should consider assisting the patient with self-administration.

6. Nitroglycerin is a potent vasodilator that can lead to profound hypotension and syncopy. In every case where the EMT is administering nitroglycerin, the patient should be either seated or lying down.

7. The patient experiencing a possible cardiac event should be transported immediately, without lights or use of the siren, to the emergency department, preferably a cardiac center.

8. Most coronary occlusions, leading to myocardial infarction, are secondary to a blood clot (thrombus). Thrombolytics are drugs that dissolve these clots. If a patient can be transported rapidly to an emergency department, thrombolytics can be administered and damage to the heart prevented.

CHAPTER 25

Cardiac Arrest

OBJECTIVES

Upon completion of this chapter, the reader should be able to:

1. Describe the assessment of the patient in cardiac arrest.
2. Describe the importance of early defibrillation.
3. Describe the importance of CPR to cardiac arrest survival.
4. List the indications for AED.
5. List the contraindications for AED.
6. Differentiate between a semiautomated and a fully automated defibrillator.
7. Describe the fundamentals of AED operation.
8. Describe the safety considerations for AED use.
9. Describe the importance of advanced life support to patient survival.
10. Discuss postresuscitative care of the arrested patient.
11. Discuss the function of the physician and AED use.
12. Discuss the importance of quality improvement for AED programs.

GLOSSARY

all clear   An order that means that nothing, not even the bag-valve mask, should touch the patient.

artificial pacemaker   A man-made electronic device that creates the electrical impulse signaling the heart to beat.

asystole   The flatline ECG of the heart in cardiac standstill.

automated external defibrillator (AED)   A defibrillator that can "read" the ECG, using a logic algorithm stored in a microprocessor, advise the EMT to "shock," or defibrillate, then deliver that shock to the patient.

automatic implantable cardioverter/defibrillator (AICD)   An AED that can be placed within the body.

automaticity   The ability of the myocardium to self-pace.

cardiac standstill   A condition in which the heart lies flaccid and unable to respond to any stimulus.

chain of survival   The important steps that must be taken to improve cardiac arrest survival.

defibrillation   The application of an electrical shock to the heart in ventricular fibrillation.

defibrillator   A device that can deliver an electric shock to the heart through the use of cables and electrodes.

dysrhythmia   Any disruption of the normal sinus rhythm.

electrocardiogram (ECG) The recording of the electrical activity of the heart graphically displayed on an oscilloscope or printed on paper; also abbreviated EKG.

escape rhythm The special ability of the myocardium to function independently when the electrical system fails.

hypothermia A condition in which the body temperature drops below 95°F.

motion artifact A false ECG reading created by vibration.

normal sinus rhythm (NSR) The predominant natural pacemaker of the heart.

premature ventricular complex (PVC) A small group of irritated cells in the ventricles that fire earlier than expected.

public access defibrillation (PAD) Public training in the use of an AED.

pulseless electrical activity (PEA) A situation in which pulse is not created but the ECG will show a rhythm.

rhythm A regularly repeating ECG complex.

semi-automatic defibrillator (SAD) An AED that requires the EMT/operator to determine pulselessness as well as to manually trigger the shock.

ventricular fibrillation The uncoordinated and spontaneous contraction of individual heart muscle fibers.

ventricular tachycardia A cardiac event in which a small group of irritated cells in the ventricles start to fire automatically at rates of 100 bpm to 250 bpm.

PREPARATORY

Materials: EMS Equipment: CPR manikins, artificial ventilation mannequins, automated external defibrillator, NTG training bottle, defibrillation mannequin.

Personnel: Primary Instructor: One advanced-level provider with knowledge and experience in out-of-hospital cardiac resuscitation. Assistant Instructor: The instructor-to-student ratio should be 1:6 for psychomotor skill practice. Individuals used as assistant instructors should be knowledgeable in cardiac emergencies.

Recommended Minimum Time to Complete: 7 hours

STUDENT OUTLINE

I. Chapter Overview
II. The History of Defibrillation
    A. Chain of Survival
        1. Early Access
        2. Early CPR
        3. Early Defibrillation
        4. Early Advanced Cardiac Life Support
        5. Survival from Cardiac Arrest
III. The Automated External Defibrillator
    A. The Use of the AED
        1. Batteries
        2. Supplies
IV. Cardiac Arrest
    A. Signs and Symptoms
        1. Normal Sinus Rhythm
        2. Escape Pacemakers
        3. Dysrhythmia
        4. Pulseless Electrical Activity
    B. Assessment
        1. Scene Size-Up
            a) General Impression
        2. Initial Assessment
    C. Management
    D. Special Situations
        1. Artificial Pacemakers
        2. Automatic Implantable Cardioverter/Defibrillator (AICD)
        3. Medication Patches
            a) Hypothermia
    E. Transport
        1. Postarrest Care
        2. Ongoing Assessment
    F. Field Termination
V. Postcall
    A. Competency Assurance
    B. Critical Incident Stress Debriefing
VI. Conclusion

I. Chapter Overview
  A. Past—CPR only
  B. Advent of Defibrillation
    1. Improved Survival
II. The History of Defibrillation
    1. Cause of Sudden Cardiac Death
      a) Ventricular Fibrillation
    2. Treatment—Defibrillation
      a) Invention of Portable
        Defibrillators
      b) Utilization of Automated
        External Defibrillators (AEDs)
  A. Chain of Survival
    1. Time to Defibrillation Critical
    2. Early Access
      a) Universal Number (9-1-1)
    3. Early CPR
      a) Citizen CPR
    4. Early Defibrillation
      a) Public Access Defibrillation
    5. Early Advanced Cardiac Life Support
      a) Stabilization of Patient
    6. Survival from Cardiac Arrest
      a) Defibrillation less than 8
        minutes
        (1) 43 percent survival
III. The Automated External Defibrillator
    1. The Heart of the AED
      a) Computer
        (1) Rhythm Analysis
          (a) Advisory to Shock
  A. The Use of the AED
    1. Batteries
      a) Types
        (1) Rechargeable Battery
        (2) NiCad Battery
    2. Supplies
      a) Back-up Battery
      b) Electrodes
      c) Scissors or Safety Razor
      d) Towel/Gauze
IV. Cardiac Arrest
    1. Sudden Cardiac Death
      a) Within 2 hours of symptoms
      b) 50 percent out-of-hospital
  A. Signs and Symptoms
    1. Substernal Chest Pain
    2. Cardiac Conduction System
      a) SA Node

      b) AV Node
      c) Bundle Branches
      d) Purkinje Fibers
    3. ECG
      a) Normal Sinus Rhythm
        i) Primary Pacemaker
      a) Escape Pacemakers
        (1) Failure of Primary Pace-
          maker
      a) Dysrhythmia
        (1) Irregularity in Conduc-
          tion
          (a) Indicates Ventricu-
            lar Irritability
        (2) Ventricular Tachycardia
        (3) Cardiac Standstill
          (a) ECG Shows Asystole
      b) Pulseless Electrical Activity
        (1) Positive ECG Without
          Pulse
          (a) CPR Needed
  B. Assessment
    1. Scene Size-Up
      a) Danger
        (1) Fluids on Scene
        (2) Metal Surfaces
      b) General Impression
        (1) Sudden Collapse
          (a) Risk of Spinal
            Trauma
        (2) Grossly Cyanotic
        (3) Position
          (a) Movement to Facili-
            tate CPR
    2. Initial Assessment
      a) Standard CPR "ABC Check"
        (1) Call for Defibrillator
  C. Management
    1. Start CPR
    2. Defibrillation as Soon as Possible
      a) Place Electrodes
      b) Follow Procedure
      c) Shock as Advised
  D. Special Situations
    1. Artificial Pacemakers
      a) Move AED Electrodes to Left
    2. Automatic Implantable
      Cardioverter/Defibrillator (AICD)
      a) Automatically Defibrillates

                b) Patient Unconscious
                    (1) Use AED
        3. Medication Patches
            a) Remove Patches
                (1) Medication Medium/Aluminum Backing Reactive
        4. Hypothermia
            a) One Set of Shoc, Then Transport
    E. Transport
            a) Closest Hospital
            b) ALS Intercept
        1. Postarrest Care
            a) Pulsed—Nonbreathing
                (1) Assist Ventilations
                b) Breathing
                    (1) Recovery Position
        2. Ongoing Assessment
            a) Recurrence of Ventricular Fibrillation
    F. Field Termination
        1. Fruitless Effort
        2. Medical Control Decision
V. Postcall
    A. Competency Assurance
        1. Physican Oversight
            a) AED Read-out
    B. Critical Incident Stress Debriefing
VI. Conclusion
    A. AED Permits Definitive Care in the Field

TEACHING STRATEGIES

1. Using an ACLS-type mannequin, have the students practice in teams the following scenarios: CPR first, then AED arrives; AED arrives with team; team using AED and ALS arrives; and team uses AED but no shock advised.

2. Discuss the typical outcome of an out-of-hospital cardiac arrest. Ask students to define criteria for termination of resuscitation, then review local or state protocols regarding termination in the field.

FURTHER STUDY

Newman, M. (1998). The chain of survival revisited. *Journal of Emergency Medical Services, 23*(5), 46–52. The critical moment. (1997). *Journal of Emergency Medical Services, 22*(1), Supplement.

CASE STUDY   CPR IN PROGRESS

"Unit 24, man down, CPR in progress, Eagle Hills Office, Tower Lobby, time out 16:45." As he put the ambulance in gear and turned on the lights and siren, Tony thought, "The timing couldn't be worse. Five o'clock traffic is a mess and we are at least 15 minutes from the scene." As Tony passed by stopped cars on the road, he thought of the minutes that were flying by for the patient.

As he pulled up to the curb in front of the Tower Building, Tony looked in the window. Clearly CPR was in progress. One security officer was using a pocket mask to ventilate while another was doing compressions. Then he saw it: an AED was attached to the patient. "Maybe the patient has a chance after all," he thought. Tony quickly grabbed the response kit and ran in the front door.

ADDITIONAL CASE STUDY

"Stand clear," cried the woman. Looking across the airport terminal, Nanci could see a flight attendant kneeling next to a man. The man had apparently collapsed. On the wall next to the man was a blinking blue light and below it a recess where a public access defibrillation (PAD) unit was once stored. That PAD was now on the ground next to the patient, electrodes attached to his chest.

Running toward the scene, Nanci quickly reviewed what she had learned in CPR class. Kneeling next to the flight attendant, Nanci said, "Hi, I'm Nanci. I know CPR. Can I help?" The flight attendant passed her hand over the body once more and called clear. "In just a minute," said the flight attendant, "I think I'll need help with CPR. Do you know how to do compressions?"

STOP AND THINK

1. What factors are working against this man's survival?
2. What factors are working for this man's survival?
3. Why is time important to this patient's survival?
4. What can an EMT do to reverse the cardiac arrest?

ANSWERS TO STOP AND THINK

1. Prolonged downtimes are the single greatest factor to poor outcomes with defibrillation.

2. Rapid response by responders and CPR help to improve the chances of survival. In this scenario it is possible that bystanders may have used the public access defibrillator.

3. Each minute the heart goes without circulation, it becomes more resistant to defibrillation and a return to normal sinus rhythm.

4. An EMT can reverse a cardiac arrest, and restore normal circulation, using an AED.

ANSWERS TO TEST YOUR KNOWLEDGE

1. Initially, as the EMT establishes that the scene is safe, he or she should consider whether the patient may have experienced a trauma. If no evidence of trauma is present, the EMT should proceed with a quick check of the ABCs. If the patient is unresponsive, apneic, and pulseless, the EMT should start CPR until an AED is ready. Once the AED has arrived, the electrodes should be placed on the patient's chest and the AED turned on. Following the AED operating instructions, the EMT should ensure that everyone is safe (clear) and defibrillate as advised.

2. Early defibrillation is critical to patient survival. Every minute of delay makes the heart more resistant to defibrillation.

3. The AED should be attached to any patient in cardiac arrest.

4. The only shockable rhythms are ventricular fibrillation and pulseless ventricular tachycardia. All other rhythms, including asystole, are nonshockable rhythms.

5. A semi-automatic defibrillator requires the operator to confirm pulselessness before administering the defibrillation. The automatic defibrillator functions entirely independently once attached to the patient.

6. The AED should not be used when the patient is either lying on a metal surface or in a pool of liquid.

7. An AED is not useful if a pediatric patient is in cardiac arrest or the patient has a do not resuscitate order.

8. The postarrest patient is prone to recurrence of ventricular fibrillation. ALS providers can provide medications and treatments that can stabilize the patient's condition and prevent such a recurrence.

9. The physician, as medical control, oversees the operation of the AED and ensures that the team uses the AED according to protocols as well as national standards.

10. Whenever a resuscitative effort is unsuccessful, members of the team may feel responsible for the outcome. A critical incident stress debriefing provides team members an opportunity to discuss the arrest management and how it impacted them psychologically.

Skill 25-1 Operation of an Automated External Defibrillator

Student Name _____ Date_____

Purpose: To perform an external defibrillation, when indicated, on a patient in cardiac arrest.

Standard Precautions: Icon—Handwashing—Gloves

Equipment:

Automated External Defibrillator

Procedural Steps:

Step 1. The EMT confirms the patient is in cardiac arrest.

YES: _____   RE-TEACH: _____   RETURN: _____   INSTRUCTOR INITIALS _____

Step 2. The EMT applies the electrode pads to the anterior chest wall, one to the apex of the heart and the other to the left sternal border below the clavicle.

YES: _____   RE-TEACH: _____   RETURN: _____   INSTRUCTOR INITIALS _____

Step 3. The EMT turns on the power to the AED while calling for "all clear." The EMT must ensure that no one is touching the patient.

YES: _____   RE-TEACH: _____   RETURN: _____   INSTRUCTOR INITIALS _____

Step 4. The EMT presses the analyze button and the "shock" button, as advised. Again, the EMT must ensure that no one is touching the patient.

YES: _____   RE-TEACH: _____   RETURN: _____   INSTRUCTOR INITIALS _____

Step 5. After the series of shocks have been performed, the EMT checks for the presence or absence of a pulse. If the pulse is absent, CPR must be continued for another minute.

YES: _____   RE-TEACH: _____   RETURN: _____   INSTRUCTOR INITIALS _____

Step 6. If the patient's pulse returns, the EMT should check for breathing. If the patient's pulse does not return, another round of shocks may be indicated.

YES: _____   RE-TEACH: _____   RETURN: _____   INSTRUCTOR INITIALS _____

CHAPTER 26

Altered Mental States

OBJECTIVES

Upon completion of this chapter, the reader should be able to:

1. Define the terms *awake* and *oriented*.
2. Define the term *altered mental state*.
3. List several causes of an altered mental state.
4. Describe the general underlying conditions that create altered mental status.
5. Describe how insulin works.
6. Describe the treatment of diabetes.
7. Describe the signs and symptoms of hypoglycemia.
8. Define the term *seizure*.
9. Differentiate between a generalized and a partial seizure.
10. Describe the care of the seizing patient.
11. Describe the care of the postictal patient.
12. Describe the most common causes of seizures.

GLOSSARY

AEIOU TIPS   A mnemonic used to remember the causes of altered mental states: **A**lcohol, **E**pilepsy, **I**nsulin, **O**xygen/overdose, **U**remia, **T**rauma, **I**nfection, **P**sychiatric, and **S**troke.

altered mental state   A change in behavior due to illness or disease.

Alzheimer's disease   A progressive, irreversible deterioration of intellectual function.

anticonvulsant drug   Any drug intended to control or prevent seizures.

aura   The sensation or awareness that a seizure is about to begin.

clonic phase   The stage in a seizure in which the body paroxysmally stiffens and relaxes.

diabetes mellitus   A disease in which the pancreas fails to produce insulin.

diabetic coma   The condition of an unconscious, hyperglycemic diabetic patient.

diabetic ketoacidosis (DKA)   The result of excessive fat metabolism seen in diabetic patients.

diet-controlled diabetes   The condition of a person whose blood sugar is controlled by modification of diet.

epilepsy   A disease characterized by recurrent seizures of a similar nature.

generalized seizure   A seizure that involves the entire brain and results in loss of consciousness; also known as grand mal.

gestational diabetes   A form of diabetes that occurs only in pregnant women and usually only for the duration of the pregnancy.

grand mal seizure   The old term for a generalized seizure.

hyperglycemia   A high amount of sugar in the blood.

insulin-dependent diabetes A condition for which the diabetic patient must inject insulin into her or his body to survive.

insulin shock A condition resulting from low blood sugar because of either too much insulin or too little sugar.

keto-acid An organic acid that is the by-product of ineffective metabolism; also called a ketone.

Kussmaul's respiration Deep, almost sighing, respiration.

non-insulin-dependent diabetes A condition of a diabetic patient whose blood sugar is controlled by diet or drugs and not by insulin injections.

partial seizure A malfunction in the brain isolated to a small portion of the brain; also known as a petit mal.

petit mal seizure The old term for a partial seizure.

postictal phase The recovery period immediately after a seizure.

seizure An event that begins within the brain and results in involuntary movements and sometimes loss of consciousness.

seizure paroxysms Involuntary muscle contractions.

status epilepticus One continuous seizure or one or more seizures without an intervening period of consciousness.

tonic The stage in a seizure in which the entire body stiffens.

PREPARATION

Materials: EMS Equipment: Exam gloves, stethoscope (6:1), blood pressure cuff (6:1), penlight, tube of glucose, suitable glucose substitute.

Personnel: Primary Instructor: One EMT-Basic instructor knowledgeable in treatment of diabetic emergencies. Assistant Instructor: The instructor-to-student ratio should be 1:6 for psychomotor skill practice. Individuals used as assistant instructors should be knowledgeable in diabetic emergencies.

Recommended Minimum Time to Complete: 2 hours

STUDENT OUTLINE

I. Overview
II. Mental States
    A. Altered Mental Status
III. Causes of Altered Mental States
    A. Specific Causes of Altered Mental States
IV. Diabetes Mellitus
    A. Insulin-Dependent Diabetes
        1. Supplemental Insulin
    B. Non-Insulin-Dependent Diabetes
    C. Other Forms of Diabetes
    D. Signs and Symptoms
    E. Acute Diabetic Problems
        1. Hyperglycemia
            a) Signs and Symptoms of Diabetic Ketoacidosis
            b) Management of DKA
        2. Hypoglycemia
            a) Signs and Symptoms of Hypoglycemia
            b) Management of Hypoglycemia—Unconscious Patient
        3. Treatment of Hypoglycemia—Conscious Patient
            a) Glucose Administration
V. Seizure Disorders
    A. Causes of Seizures
    B. Types of Seizures
    C. Phases of a Generalized Seizure
        1. Tonic-Clonic Phase
        2. Postictal Phase
    D. Management of the Patient with a Seizure
        1. The Actively Seizing Patient
            a) Status Epilepticus
        2. The Postictal Patient
        3. Anticonvulsant Medications
    E. Refusal of Care
VI. Conclusion

LECTURE OUTLINE

I. Overview
  A. Concerned Citizens/Family Members
  B. Altered Mental Status Defined
    1. Abnormal Change in Behavior
II. Mental States
  A. Normal
    1. Awake and Alert
      a) Aware of Person, Place, and Time
      b) A on AVPU Scale
  B. Altered Mental Status
    1. Confusion—Disorientation
      a) Amnesia
III. Causes of Altered Mental States
    1. Medical Conditions
      a) Chronic
        (1) Alzheimer's Disease
      b) Acute
        (1) Causes of Hypoxia
        (2) Hypoglycemia
        (3) Hypoperfusion
  A. Specific Causes of Altered Mental States
    1. Alcoholism
    2. Epilepsy
    3. Insulin
    4. Overdose/Oxygen
    5. Uremia
    6. Trauma—Occult
    7. Infection
    8. Psychosis
    9. Stroke
IV. Diabetes Mellitus
  A. Insulin as Carrier
  B. Insulin Insufficiency
  C. Insulin-Dependent Diabetes
    1. Supplemental Insulin
      a) Peak of Effect
        (1) Long-Acting
        (2) Short-Acting
  D. Non-Insulin-Dependent Diabetes
    1. Oral Hypoglycemic Agents
  E. Other Forms of Diabetes
    1. Diet-Controlled Diabetes
    2. Gestational Diabetes
  F. Signs and Symptoms
    1. Hyperglycemia
      a) Polyuria
        (1) Spilling Sugar
      b) Polydipsia
      c) Polyphagia
        (1) Unexplained Weight Loss
  G. Acute Diabetic Problems
    1. Hyperglycemia
      a) Signs and Symptoms of Diabetic Ketoacidosis
        (1) Gradual Onset
        (2) Kussmaul Respiration
          (a) Deep, Rapid, Sighing Respiration
        (3) Altered Mental Status
          (a) Diabetic Coma
      b) Management of DKA
        (1) High-Flow Oxygen
        (2) High Priority
    2. Hypoglycemia
      a) Insulin Overdose
        (1) Missed Meal
        (2) Overexercise
      b) Signs and Symptoms of Hypoglycemia
        (1) Insulin Shock
          (a) Rapid Onset
          (b) Signs of Hypoperfusion
            (i) Effects of Epinephrine
          (c) Combativeness
          (d) Seizures
      c) Management of Hypoglycemia—Unconscious Patient
        (1) Conscious versus Unconscious
          (a) Unconscious
            (i) Medical Emergency
              (1) Closest ALS
                (a) IV Glucose
    3. Treatment of Hypoglycemia—Conscious Patient
      a) Patent Airway
        (1) Glucose Administration
V. Seizure Disorders
  A. Causes of Seizures
    1. Acute

a) Hypoxia
b) Hypoglycemia
c) Fever
d) Poison
e) Toxemia of Pregnancy
f) Alcohol Withdrawal
   (1) Delirum Tremens
2. Chronic
  a) Epilepsy
B. Types of Seizures
  1. Partial Seizures (Petit Mal)
  2. Generalized Seizures (Grand Mal)
C. Phases of a Generalized Seizure
  1. Aura
   a) Awareness
    (1) Visual/Olfactory Clue
  2. Tonic-Clonic Phase
   a) Loss of Consciousness
   b) Loss of Motor Function
  3. Postictal Phase

a) Recovery
D. Management of the Patient with a Seizure
  1. The Actively Seizing Patient
   a) Protect the Patient
   b) Status Epilepticus
    (1) One Prolonged Seizure
    (2) Repeated Seizure without intervening period of lucidity
  2. The Postictal Patient
   a) Airway Patency
   b) Assessment—Detailed Physical Exam
  3. Anticonvulsant Medications
   c) Compliance
E. Refusal of Care
  1. Capacity
VI. Conclusion
  A. Manage ABCs
  B. Effective Treatment Key to Survival

TEACHING STRATEGIES

1. Consider asking a speaker from the American Epilepsy Society or local foundation to relate the experiences of patients who have experienced epilepsy. These organizations have prepared educational materials, for example, "Seizures . . . a medical emergency," that can be distributed to students.

2. Consider having the students assess and treat a model/victim for hypoglycemia, using cake frosting as an oral glucose substitute.

3. Consider asking a patient with epilepsy to speak to the class about his or her experiences with EMS.

FURTHER STUDY

Cobaugh, D. (1999). *Inhalant abuse. Journal of Emergency Medical Services, 24*(10), 66–69.

Goss, J. (1999). Clinical clues to illicit drug use. *Journal of Emergency Medical Services, 24*(3), 110–118.

LeDuc, T. (1997). Alcoholism: America's pervasive disease. *Journal of Emergency Medical Services, 22*(5), 76–79.

Meade, D., & Fending, D. (1996). PCP. *Emergency Medical Services, 25*(6), 29–34.

Murphy, P., & Alfaro, S. (1999). Meningitis. *Journal of Emergency Medical Services, 24*(5), 74–79.

Murphy, P. (1995). Brain storm. *Journal of Emergency Medical Services, 20*(11), 58–60.

Nicholl, J. (1999). Prehospital management of the seizure Patient. *Emergency Medical Services, 28*(5), 71–79.

CASE STUDY   STRANGE BEHAVIOR

"Officer, I was stopped and I thought he started up, so I started up, then he suddenly stopped again and I slammed into him," Darryl related as he shifted through the glove compartment looking for the car's registration. "I immediately got out of my car and asked him if he was all right and he mumbled something crazy."

"Sir, I'm not a police officer and I don't need to see your registration. I'm an EMT with the quick response team," Andy replied.

"Whatever man, I'm telling you he's not right," Darryl countered. "He's acting weird, man."

"We'll check him out, sir. Please remain seated in your car until we can get back to you," Andy instructed.

As Andy approached the car, he started to survey the vehicle for damage. Clearly it was a minor fender-bender with minimal rear-end damage. "Sir, are you alright?" Andy called out. The driver, an elderly male, looked up at him and said, "What happened? How come the fire department's here?"

Andy couldn't help but notice the smell of cigarettes and stale urine. On the floorboard of the car were several empty beer cans. As Andy continued to survey the scene, he listened to the driver. His speech was slurred, as though he was drunk, and he repeated his questions over and over.

STOP AND THINK

1. What are the probable causes of this patient's altered mental state?
2. What important medical history should an EMT obtain in this case?
3. What are the immediate treatment priorities?

ANSWERS TO STOP AND THINK

1. The EMT should immediately suspect a possible head injury in light of the mechanism of injury (a motor vehicle collision).

2. The case provides insufficient data to make a determination. The EMT should focus on obtaining a medical history using the AEIOU-TIPS mnemonic.

3. The EMT should immediately take cervical spine immobilization in this case and then proceed with a complete initial assessment.

CASE STUDY   SUGAR SICKNESS

"Police unit twelve and ambulance three. Meet the party, Yellowstone rest area, Interstate 85. Possible EMS."

As Claire slowly pulled the ambulance into the rest area, she noticed a new-model car with the passenger side door wide open and a woman attending to a man sitting in the front seat.

Turning off her emergency lights to prevent drawing undue attention to the situation, Claire listened to Charlie, the highway patrolman, who was first on-scene.

"Claire, the woman says that it's her husband. Something about his sugar sickness acting up again," Charlie started to say when suddenly the woman cried out, "Can someone help him before he passes out!" The woman appeared to be struggling with her husband.

STOP AND THINK

1. What is the nature of this emergency?
2. What actions should the EMT take immediately?
3. Would the actions be different if the patient were unconscious?

ANSWERS TO STOP AND THINK

1. The case presentation would indicate that this is a diabetic emergency.

2. After making a determination of a diabetic emergency, the EMT should consider administering oral glucose.

3. If the patient lapses into unconsciousness, the EMT should package the patient and rapidly transport him to ALS.

CASE STUDY   SEIZURE

"9-1-1, what is your emergency?" Darlene, an emergency communications specialist, asked the caller as she noted that the caller was using one of the new cell-phones that gave her his exact location by coordinates. "We are in the park, near the swings. This girl, she fell down."

"Is she conscious?" asked Darlene in a calm voice.

"She's shaking and jerking and stuff," replied the caller.

"Please stay on the phone, it's a free call. I am dispatching the park police to your location now."

STOP AND THINK

1. What is the likely nature of this emergency?
2. What are the assessment priorities for this patient?
3. What are the treatment priorities for this patient?
4. What special concerns should the EMT have for this patient?

ANSWERS TO STOP AND THINK

1. The case presentation would suggest that this is a seizure disorder.

2. Provided that the patient is still seizing, the EMT should protect the patient from striking objects. If possible, the patient should be turned to the recovery position.

3. As soon as the seizure is done, the EMT should clear the airway and then begin an assessment of the patient.

4. The EMT should be alert to the possibility that the patient will seize again. Another seizure, without an intervening period of lucidity, would demonstrate that the patient is status epilepticus, a medical emergency.

ANSWERS TO TEST YOUR KNOWLEDGE

1. A patient who is awake and alert is conscious and aware of himself, his surroundings, and the time.

2. A patient who is not awake and alert has an altered state of mind.

3. The general causes of an acute altered mental status include hypoxia, hypoglycemia, and hypoperfusion.

4. The common conditions for an altered mental state can be remembered by the acronym AEIOU-TIPS: alcohol, epilepsy, insulin, overdose/oxygen, uremia, trauma/occult, infection, psychosis, and stroke.

5. Insulin is the carrier for glucose from the blood, across the cell membrane, and into the cell for metabolism into energy.

6. Diabetes is a lack of insulin in the body. The treatment for diabetes is to inject insulin into the body.

7. Untreated diabetes leads to a gradual build-up of glucose in the bloodstream. Hyperglycemia can lead to diabetic coma.

8. A generalized seizure occurs when the entire brain fires chaotically, leading to overall body convulsions.

9. A generalized seizure involves the entire brain whereas a partial seizure, or petit mal, only affects a portion of the brain and thus only a portion of the body.

10. An EMT must protect the actively seizing patient. While seizing the patient may inadvertently strike surrounding objects, inflicting bodily injury.

11. The airway of a postictal patient is the first and immediate concern of the EMT. Thereafter, the EMT should proceed with the rest of the initial assessment and then a detailed physical examination.

12. While traumatic head injury and fever are common cause of seizures, the most common causes of seizures is noncompliance with anticonvulsant medication for a previously diagnosed epileptic condition.

CHAPTER 27

Abnormal Behavior

OBJECTIVES

Upon completion of this chapter, the reader should be able to:

1. Define what constitutes a behavioral emergency.
2. Describe several functional reasons for a behavioral emergency.
3. Describe several mental illnesses that could result in a behavioral emergency.
4. List several signs and symptoms of severe or clinical depression.
5. List several symptoms, or features, of psychotic behavior.
6. Describe how substance abuse withdrawal can lead to a behavioral emergency.
7. List signs and symptoms of a behavioral emergency.
8. Describe several concerns an EMT should have about safety on the scene of a behavioral emergency.
9. Describe the general approach to a call involving a behavioral emergency.
10. Describe how a person might be verbally persuaded to accept medical care.
11. Describe how a person would be safely restrained.
12. Discuss the medical-legal issues surrounding restraint by EMTs.
13. Describe the dangers, for the patient as well as the crew, during a patient restraint.
14. List unacceptable restraint devices and techniques for patient restraint.
15. Describe the important elements in an ongoing assessment of the medically restrained patient.

GLOSSARY

addiction   The physical need the body has for a drug

anxiety disorder   An inappropriate or exaggerated response that is abnormal in relation to the situation; formerly called neurosis.

auditory hallucination   A false perception of the sensation of the ears.

behavioral emergency   Any situation in which a patient exhibits a behavior that is unacceptable or intolerable to one's self, the family, or the community.

bipolar disorder   A psychiatric disorder characterized by cyclic mood changes ranging from extreme elation to severe depression; same as manic-depressive disorder.

command hallucinations   Auditory hallucinations coming from a false or imaginary figure or persona that tell a person what to do.

delirium   A sudden, erratic change in behavior.

delirium tremens (DTs)   The symptoms associated with the sudden withdrawal of alcohol from an alcohol-dependent person.

dementia   The gradual loss of cognitive function (thinking).

dependency   The psychological need a person has for a drug.

depression   A psychiatric condition characterized by sad mood and lack of interest in usual life pleasures.

excited delirium   A state of hyperactive, irrational behavior.

hallucination   A sensation or perception that has no basis in reality.

hobble restraint   The tying of wrists to ankles behind the patient.

medically necessary restraint   Used when a patient must be confined in order to prevent him from harming himself or others.

mental illness   Any disorder that impairs the brain's function that is without a firm physical (organic) cause.

organic disorder   Any disease or condition that causes the brain to malfunction.

positional asphyxia   Suffocation that results from the patient's inability to take a deep breath.

psychiatry   The medical study of mental illness.

show of force   A demonstration of determination.

substance abuse   The misuse of a drug in order to alter the perception or mood of the person.

suicide   The voluntary taking of one's own life.

tactile hallucination   A false perception of a sensation of the skin; a false feeling.

takedown   A planned, orderly restraint of a patient for a medical purpose.

visual hallucination   A false perception of the sensation of the eyes; a false visualization.

withdrawal symptoms   The unpleasant physical and/or psychological effects experienced by an addicted patient when a drug is kept from her or him.

PREPARATORY

Materials: EMS Equipment: Stretcher, restraints.

Personnel: Primary Instructor: One EMT-Basic instructor knowledgeable in behavioral emergencies. Assistant Instructor: none required.

Recommended Minimum Time to Complete: 1.5 hours

I. Overview
II. Behavioral Emergency
    A. Organic Disorders
        1. Dangerous Assumptions
    B. Mental Disorders
    C. Signs and Symptoms
    D. Scene Size-Up
        1. Scene Safety
    E. Assessment
        1. Focused History and Physical Examination
    F. Management
        1. Verbal Persuasion
        2. Physical Restraint
            a) Medical Necessity
            b) Restraint Procedure
            c) Total Body Restraint
            d) Extremity Restraint
            e) Restraint Devices
            f) Safety
    G. Transport
        1. Ongoing Assessment
        2. Documentation
III. Psychiatric Disorders
    A. Depression
        1. Signs and Symptoms
        2. Assessment
        3. Management
    B. Suicide
        1. Signs and Symptoms
        2. Management
    C. Manic-Depressive Disorder
        1. Signs and Symptoms
        2. Management
    D. Schizophrenia
        1. Signs and Symptoms
        2. Management
    E. Anxiety Disorder
        1. Signs and Symptoms
    F. Substance Abuse
        1. Overdose
        2. Drug Withdrawal
            a) Alcohol Withdrawal
                (1) Signs and Symptoms
                (2) Management
IV. Conclusion

LECTURE OUTLINE

I. Overview
   A. Mental Illness Defined
      1. Disorder exhibited in behavior
      2. Patient is danger to self or others
      3. Socially unacceptable
II. Behavioral Emergency
      1. Intolerable Behaviors
   A. Organic Disorders
      1. Malfunction of the Brain
         a) Primary Cellular Disease
      2. Dangerous Assumptions
         a) Cause is medical until proven
            otherwise
   B. Mental Disorders
      1. Disordered thinking without organic
      cause
   C. Signs and Symptoms
      1. Inappropriate Anger/Violence
      2. Inappropriate Weeping/Crying
   D. Scene Size-Up
         a) Heads Up from Dispatch Infor-
            mation
      1. Scene Safety
         a) Never Enter Alone
         b) Sling Bags over Shoulders
         c) Think Escape
            (1) Clear Path
            (2) Cover
            (3) Concealment
         d) Radio Contact
   E. Assessment
         a) Approach
            (1) Stop, Look, and Listen
               (a) Angry Stances
               (b) Eye Contact
      1. Focused History and Physical Exami-
      nation
         a) Speech
            (1) Pressured
            (2) Angry Words
   F. Management
         a) One Contact—One Focus
      1. Verbal Persuasion
         a) Calm and Professional
         b) Personal Contact—First Name
         c) Repeative Persistence
         d) Hallucinations
            (1) Patient Protection

         e) Good Listener
      2. Physical Restraint
         a) When All Else Fails
            (1) Excited Delirium
               (a) Drug-Induced
                   Frenzy
               (b) Mental Illness
         b) Medical Necessity
            (1) Protection of Patient and
               Others
         c) Restraint Procedure
            (1) Talk-Down Then Take-
               Down
            (2) Show of Force
               (a) Signals
            (3) Extremity Control
         d) Total Body Restraint
            (1) Older/Weak
               (a) Papoose
            (2) Flexible Stretcher
         e) Extremity Restraint
            (1) Counterforces
         f) Restraint Devices
            (1) Cravats
            (2) Leather Restraints
            (3) Kling® or Kerlix®
            (4) Chest Harness
         g) Safety
            (1) Police Escort
   G. Transport
      1. Ongoing Assessment
         a) Distal Pulses Every 10 Minutes
      2. Documentation
         a) Order
            (1) Medical
            (2) Police
III. Psychiatric Disorders
      1. Loss of Touch with Reality
      2. Inappropriate Interactions with Envi-
      ronment
      3. Inabilty to Complete Activities of
      Daily Living (ADLs)
   A. Depression
         a) Overwhelming Melancholy
            (1) Situational
               (a) Self-Resolving
            (2) Mental Illness
               (b) Unpredictable

1. Signs and Symptoms
    a) Despondent
    b) Failure of ADLs
    c) Weight Loss
2. Assessment
    a) Description of Surroundings
3. Management
    a) Supportive
    b) Decision-Making
B. Suicide
    a) Voluntary Taking of One's Life
1. Signs and Symptoms
    a) Self-Inflicted Injury
    b) Mechanism of Injury Does Not
       Match Pattern of Injury
    c) Verbal Threats
2. Management
    a) Direct Questioning
    b) Refusal
        i) Firm Denial
C. Manic-Depressive Disorder
    a) Bipolar
1. Signs and Symptoms
    a) Violent Mood Swings
2. Management
    a) Protection
    b) Transportation
D. Schizophrenia
    a) Fantasic Thought
1. Signs and Symptoms
    a) Hallucinations
        i) Tactile
        ii) Visual
        iii) Auditory
            (a) Command

2. Dangerous
3. Management
    a) Protection
E. Anxiety Disorder
    a) Abnormal Response to Stressors
1. Signs and Symptoms
    a) Overreaction
F. Substance Abuse
    a) Dependency
        (1) Psychological
    b) Addiction
        (1) Physical
1. Overdose
    a) Poisoning
        (1) Life-Threatening
2. Drug Withdrawal
        (1) Marked Bodily Reactions
    a) Alcohol Withdrawal
        (a) Delirium Tremens
           (Rum Fits)
            (i) Seizure Activity
    (1) Signs and Symptoms
        (a) Tremors (Shaking)
        (b) Mental Confusion
        (c) Visual Hallucinations
        (d) Life-Threatening
           Seizures
    (2) Management
        (a) ABCs
        (b) Transportation
IV. Conclusion
    A. Unique Challenge
        1. Affronts to Personal Dignity
        2. Medical Urgency

TEACHING STRATEGIES

1. Consider inviting a defensive tactics Instructor from the local police or correctional academy to teach the students how to protect themselves and how to restrain a patient safely.

2. Consider inviting the local psychiatric crisis team to discuss suicide, mental illness, and other behavioral emergencies. Ask the crisis workers to discuss their techniques for dealing with a behavioral emergency.

FURTHER STUDY

Abdon-Beckman, D. (1997). An awkward position: Restraints and sudden death. *Journal of Emergency Medical Services, 22*(3), 88.

Ball, R. (1998). Waiting to exhale—Treatment of hyperventilation. *Journal of Emergency Medical Services, 23*(1), 62–69.

Doyle, T., & Vissers, R. (1999). An EMS approach to psychiatric emergencies. *Emergency Medical Services,* *28*(6), 87–88.

Goss, J. (1997). Somatoform disorders. *Journal of Emergency Medical Services, 22*(12), 58–64.

LeDuc, T. (1997). Depression. *Journal of Emergency Medical Services, 22*(11), 84–88.

CASE STUDY AGGRESSIVE BEHAVIOR

Tom regularly checked on his father every other day just to make sure that he was alright and that he had everything he needed. Smitty was a widower, and since his wife had died five years ago he was prone to "hitting the bottle."

Today Tom just had a feeling something wasn't right. The front door was open and the window was broken. Approaching carefully, he could see the old man sitting in his overstuffed chair. He had a crazy look in his eyes.

Calling out to Smitty, Tom asked, "Hey, are you alright?" That's when the old man got out of his chair and charged at Tom. Tom, being younger and quicker, easily ducked the old man's fist and headed straight to his truck. Calling 9-1-1, he told them "Smitty's out of his head. Better send the Sheriff up here."

ADDITIONAL CASE STUDY

The stench from the house could be smelled from the road. The call was for a woman who had fallen and needed help. The neighbors met EMS at the end of the driveway. "Watch her, she's crazy," they advised. They called her the cat lady. Once inside the house, it was apparent why they did.

There were literally dozens of cats all around. The floor was littered with old urine-soaked newspapers and bowls of rotting cat food. The old woman cried out weakly, "In here, I'm in here."

Finding the woman on the floor, her leg grossly distorted under her, all she could talk about was her cats. "Don't let them out, they are my precious."

STOP AND THINK

1. What signs and symptoms of a potential behavioral emergency are present in this case?
2. What are some of the potential causes of this abnormal behavior?
3. What are the EMT's first priorities?

ANSWERS TO STOP AND THINK

1. The signs and symptoms of a potential behavioral emergency include a history of alcohol abuse, death of a loved one, changes in behavior patterns, and outward aggression.

2. Utilizing the acronym AEIOU-TIPS, a number of potential causes must be investigated. The EMT should initially attribute the abnormal behavior to medical causes before assuming that it is psychotic in origin.

3. Initially, the EMT should be concerned with hypoxia, hypoglycemia, and hypoperfusion.

CASE STUDY   ATTEMPTED SUICIDE

The woman caller on the phone was frantic. "Please hurry, I think my son may be trying to kill himself." "Ma'am, were is your son now? Does he have any weapons?" asked the communications specialist.

As emergency units were being dispatched, the caller gave the whole story. Her son had recently completed his junior year of high school and didn't do as well as he had hoped. In fact, he would probably have to repeat the year. Coping with the fact that his father had recently died, her son had become increasingly more withdrawn and solitary.

Today, however, he seemed up-beat for at change and went up to his room to listen to his music. That was at two o'clock. At five o'clock she called up to him to come down for dinner. When she got no answer, she went and knocked on his door. When he failed to answer her calls, she tried the door only to find that it was locked from the inside. Frightened, she called the emergency number for help.

ADDITIONAL CASE STUDY

The upstairs neighbor called the building's super because of the stench of car exhaust had permeated his apartment from the first-floor garages.

Going into the garage the super, George, saw a car running with the door down and a figure slumped over the steering wheel. He called 9-1-1 immediately and then proceeded to evacuate the building.

By the time EMS had arrived, a first-due engine was on-scene and the patient had been dragged out of the car. They were preparing to ventilate the building.

STOP AND THINK

1. What are the clinical signs and symptoms evident in this case?
2. What would be the EMT's priorities on this scene?
3. How should an EMT respond to a despondent patient?

ANSWERS TO STOP AND THINK

1. The clinical signs in this case include the recent death of the father, a poor year in school, and a change in behavior (withdrawn and solitary).

2. The EMT's first priority is personal safety. Males often use violent means, including handguns, in their suicide attempts. The EMT would next concern himself with securing the scene and preventing the patient from harming himself.

3. The EMT should respond to the despondent patient in a caring manner, being direct in his questions.

CASE STUDY MENTALLY ILL

"Meet the officer, front of the coffee shop, Madison at Lark," was all the information that Maggie was given. She knew the spot. Just down the road from the psychiatric center and across from the park, it was a favorite gathering place.

Maggie pulled up next to the curb and got out. She immediately recognized Bret, the beat cop, and Mr. Gibbons, who liked to be called "Michael the archangel."

Today, it seems that Michael had tangled with a customer from the doughnut shop. The customer, frightened, had insisted that the cashier call the police for that "strange man out there." Although Michael was indeed loud, cursing and shaking his fist skyward, he was not acting any differently than normal. That was until Bret had asked him to quiet down and move along.

When Michael refused, stating he had his orders from God, Bret called for EMS. "Maggie, take him back in, and get him tuned up again," Bret ordered.

ADDITIONAL CASE STUDY

"Ma'am, all your credit cards are max'ed out. You have no more credit," explained the sales clerk. "No credit, no credit!" yelled Mrs. Snyder. With those words, she began to pound on the countertop. Frightened, the sales clerk called for security and then retreated.

When the first security officer arrived, he found Mrs. Snyder, a handsomely dressed woman, sitting on the floor in the middle of the aisle crying like a baby. "Better call EMS," the officer whispered over the radio. Mrs. Synder's purse had spilled all over the floor and as the officer helped her pick up her belongings, he found an empty prescription bottle labeled Lithium.

STOP AND THINK

1. What signs and symptoms of a psychiatric disorder are evident?
2. What past medical history might be important?
3. What would be the EMT's treatment priorities in this case?

ANSWERS TO STOP AND THINK

    1. Acts like cursing and shaking a fist skyward and making statements like a person has orders from God are all psychotic features.

    2. The patient's previous psychiatric admissions are germane to the current situation.

    3. The first priority of every EMT is to assess the patient for possible medical causes of abnormal behavior.

CASE STUDY   WITHDRAWAL

    The war monument was a favorite hangout for the local street alcoholics and a frequent place for EMS calls. Tonight was no different. Joel was usually unkempt but he normally was not disagreeable. Joel was what people call a "nice drunk."

    Today, he was arguing with everybody and telling them all, "I can kick it. I don't need no help from nobody." But he confided in a friend that he did need some help, and that's how EMS appeared at the old war monument.

    Approaching the scene, careful not to step on the wine bottles strewn about the ground, EMTs Campion and Hilts knelt down and asked Joel what was wrong. Joel reluctantly spoke up and said, " I've got the shakes, man, can you help me out?"

ADDITIONAL CASE STUDY

"Over here, he's over here," a voice called out from the dark. Slumped in the corner was the figure of a man. As Charlie, an EMT, approached the patient, he could see that he was shaking violently. He smelled of vomit and one look at his arms told the tale. Angry red track marks, some scarred over, ran up his arms.

"Just one fix, to get me over and I swear I'll go to detox," the voice sputtered. Taking a quick pulse, after donning his gloves, Charlie felt a rate almost too fast to count.

STOP AND THINK

1. What signs and symptoms of substance abuse are evident?
2. What past medical history might be important?
3. What would be the EMT's treatment priorities in this case?

ANSWERS TO STOP AND THINK

1. The patient readily admits to efforts to try to stop abusing a substance.

2. A past history of detoxification, and especially delirium tremens, would be helpful.

3. The EMT must assess the patient and transport the patient to a drug rehabilitation center for detoxification.

ANSWERS TO TEST YOUR KNOWLEDGE

1. A behavioral emergency is whenever a patient is a danger to self or others or exhibits socially unacceptable behavior.

2. A patient can have a behavioral emergency due to some organic cause, for example, Alzheimer's disease.

3. Depression, schizophrenia, anxiety attacks, or any mental disorder that causes the person to lose contact with reality.

4. Typical signs and symptoms of depression include melancholy, mood swings, unexplained weight loss, and a failure to complete activities of daily living.

5. A psychotic feature is a behavior that is specific mental illness, for example, feelings of grandeur or invincibility.

6. The most common drug of abuse is alcohol. Cocaine, heroin, and designer drugs like ecstasy are other drugs of abuse.

7. The EMT should always ensure that there is a clear exit path. The EMT should never enter a scene alone. When approaching a scene, the EMT should observe for cover and/or concealment in case of attack. Finally, the EMT should maintain radio contact with an outside person.

8. A person is restrained out of medical necessity whenever the patient is a danger to self or others and a physician orders the patient restrained and transported for medical and psychiatric evaluation.

9. When an EMT is unsuccessful in convincing a patient to cooperate without a show of force, a group of individuals prepared to restrain the patient is brought in and one last appeal is made to the patient before force is used.

10. When a patient is restrained on a stretcher, he should be face-up, one hand secured to a rail at his side and the opposing hand secured to a rail over his head. Straps should then be placed across the chest, pelvis, and just above the knees. Ankle restraints should be applied only as needed.

11. Whenever an EMT restrains a patient, he or she should check the patient's distal pulses, movement, and sensation every 10 minutes.

CHAPTER 28

Environmental Emergencies

OBJECTIVES

Upon completion of this chapter, the reader should be able to:

1. Describe the various mechanisms by which the body loses heat.
2. Describe the various mechanisms by which the body generates heat.
3. Identify local cold injuries and describe the proper treatment for these conditions.
4. List signs and symptoms of generalized hypothermia.
5. Describe the emergency medical care of the patient with generalized hypothermia.
6. List signs and symptoms of heat exhaustion and heat stroke and differentiate between the two.
7. Describe the emergency medical care of the patient with heat exhaustion and heat stroke.
8. Identify the complications of near-drowning.
9. Describe the emergency medical care of the near-drowning victim.
10. Identify signs and symptoms of diving-related emergencies.
11. Describe the emergency medical care of diving-related emergencies.
12. Identify signs and symptoms of altitude emergencies.
13. Describe the emergency medical care of altitude emergencies.
14. Identify the priorities in caring for the victim of a lightning strike.
15. Describe the emergency medical care of a victim of a bite or a sting.

GLOSSARY

active rewarming Actions taken to actively try and increase body temperature.

acute mountain sickness An illness that is seen at altitude in unacclimated individuals.

afterdrop A drop in core body temperature as a result of peripheral vasodilation and shunting of cool blood to the body center during active rewarming of the severely hypothermic patient.

air embolism Air that has gotten into a blood vessel, resulting in a blockage of blood flow.

black widow spider A poisonous spider that is black and has a red hourglass mark on the abdomen.

Boyle's law The law stating that volume of a gas varies indirectly with the surrounding pressure.

brown recluse spider A poisonous spider that is brown and has a classic violin-shaped mark on its back.

chilblains Painful, inflamed skin lesions resulting from chronic exposure of skin to cool, windy, damp weather.

conduction Transfer of heat from a warm object to a cool object by direct contact.

convection Heat loss to air currents passing by a warm surface.

coral snake   A venomous snake identified by its red and yellow bands directly opposed.

decompression sickness   A diving injury that occurs during a rapid ascent, resulting in expansion of gases that become trapped in tissues; also known as the bends.

evaporation   Transfer of heat into body fluids, such as sweat, for dissipation into the environment.

frostbite   Tissue damage resulting from exposure to freezing and subfreezing temperatures.

frostnip   A mild local skin injury resulting from exposure to freezing temperatures.

heat cramps   Painful, involuntary muscle spasms caused by exposure to heat and dehydration.

heat exhaustion   The mildest form of generalized heat-related illness, characterized by multiple symptoms and often by dehydration.

heat stroke   A life-threatening form of heat illness that involves a rise in body temperature and altered mental status.

high altitude cerebral edema (HACE)   Swelling of the brain as a result of hypoxia at high altitudes; characterized by altered mental status, difficulty walking and decreased level of consciousness.

high altitude pulmonary edema (HAPE)   Pulmonary edema as a result of hypoxia at high altitudes; characterized by a dry cough and dyspnea on exertion.

hyperbaric chamber   A device that creates a simulated dive to allow for recompression of air in a diver suffering from decompression sickness or other diving-related illnesses.

hyperthermia   Overall heat gain greater than heat loss, resulting in a rise in body temperature.

near-drowning   Water submersion that does not result in death within a 24-hour period.

nitrogen narcosis   A reversible condition caused by the anesthetic effect of nitrogen at high partial pressures seen in divers at depth.

passive rewarming   Treatment that is geared toward preventing any further body heat loss.

pit viper   A venomous snake that can be recognized by the pits that are seen in front of each eye.

pulmonary overpressurization syndrome (POPS)   Expanding air within the lungs as pressure decreases and the volume of air proportionally increases, resulting in rupture of alveoli.

radiation   The transfer of heat from the warm body into the cooler environment just by the fact that a temperature gradient exists.

thermoregulation   An attempt to balance the amount of heat lost and heat gained in order to maintain a constant body temperature.

trenchfoot   An injury to tissue resulting from prolonged exposure of the skin to cool, wet conditions.

PREPARATORY

Materials: EMS Equipment: Exam gloves, stethoscopes, blood pressure cuffs, penlight

Personnel: Primary Instructor: One EMT-Basic instructor knowledgeable in heat, cold, and aquatic emergencies. Assistant Instructor: None required.

Recommended Minimum Time to Complete: 2 hours

STUDENT OUTLINE

I. Overview
II. Temperature Regulation
   A. Heat Loss
      1. Radiation
      2. Convection
      3. Conduction
      4. Evaporation
      5. Maximizing Heat Loss
   B. Heat Gain
      1. Internal
         a) Routine Cellular Metabolism
         b) Muscle Contraction
      2. External Sources
   C. Preservation of Body Heat
   D. Individual Factors
      1. Extremes of Age
   E. Pediatric Considerations
      1. Other Medical Conditions
      2. Drugs
III. Cold Exposure
   A. Local Cold Injuries
      1. Chilblain
      2. Trenchfoot
      3. Frostnip
      4. Frostbite
      5. Management of Local Cold Injuries
   B. General Hypothermia
      1. Spectrum of Illness
      2. Management
   C. Prevention Among Health Care Workers
IV. Heat Exposure
   A. Heat Cramps
      1. Management
   B. Heat Exhaustion
      1. Management
   C. Heat Stroke
      1. Management
   D. Prevention among Health Care Workers
V. Water-Related Emergencies
   A. Near-Drowning
      1. Series of Events

      2. Cold Water
      3. Management
   B. Diving Emergencies
      1. Boyle's Law
      2. Descent
         a) Squeeze
         b) Management
      3. Ascent
         a) Decompression Sickness
         b) Pulmonary Overpressurization
            Syndrome (POPS)
         c) Air Embolism
         d) Management
      4. Nitrogen Narcosis
         a) Management
VI. Altitude Emergencies
   A. Acute Mountain Sickness (AMS)
   B. High Altitude Cerebral Edema (HACE)
   C. High Altitude Pulmonary Edema (HAPE)
   D. Management
VII. Lightning Strikes
   A. Minor Injuries
   B. Severe Injuries
   C. Management
VIII. Bites and Stings
   A. Snakes
      1. Pit Viper
      2. Coral Snakes
      3. Management
   B. Spiders
      1. Brown Recluse
      2. Black Widow
      3. Management
   C. Scorpions
      1. Management
   D. Marine Animals
      1. Management
IX. Conclusion

LECTURE OUTLINE

I. Overview
- A. Increasing frequency with increasing out-of-door activities

II. Temperature Regulation
- 1. Hypothalmus
- A. Heat Loss
    - 1. Radiation
        - a) Accounts for 60 percent of heat loss
        - b) Cooler environment
    - 2. Convection
        - a) Air Currents
    - 3. Conduction
        - a) Direct Contact
    - 4. Evaporation
        - a) Sweat heat
            - (1) 30 percent loss
    - 5. Maximizing Heat Loss
        - a) Vasodilation
            - (1) Flushing of Skin
        - b) Sweat
- B. Heat Gain
    - 1. Internal
        - a) Routine Cellular Metabolism
            - (1) Exercise increases heat
        - b) Muscle Contraction
            - (1) Shivering
    - 2. External Sources
        - a) Environmental
- C. Preservation of Body Heat
    - 1. Shivering
    - 2. Shunting
    - 3. Piloerection
- D. Individual Factors
    - 1. Extremes of Age
        - a) Elderly
            - (1) Less Lean Muscle Mass for Shivering
        - b) Pediatric
            - (1) Immature Hypothalamus
        - c) Other Medical Conditions
            - (1) Systemic Infection
            - (2) Burns
            - (3) Injuries to Spinal Cord
        - d) Drugs
            - (1) Antihypertensive
                - (a) Blunts Reflexive Tachycardia

III. Cold Exposure
- A. Local Cold Injuries
    - a) Skin and Musculoskeletal
    - 1. Chilblain
    - 2. Trenchfoot
        - a) Prolonged Cold, Wet Feet
    - 3. Frostnip
        - a) Mild Form of Frostbite
            - (1) Comparable to Partial Thickness Burn
    - 4. Frostbite
        - a) Tissue Damage
            - (1) Comparable to Full Thickness Burn
    - 5. Management of Local Cold Injuries
        - a) Warm Water Immersion
- B. General Hypothermia
    - a) Heat Loss Greater Than Heat Gain
    - 1. Spectrum of Illness
        - a) Mild
            - (1) Shivering
            - (2) Impaired Judgment
                - (a) Paradoxical Undressing
        - b) Severe Hypothermia
            - (1) Muscle-Joint Stiffness
            - (2) Shivering Stops
            - (3) Decreasing Level of Consciousness
            - (4) Pupils Sluggish
    - 2. Management
        - a) Remove Patient from Environment
        - b) Mild Hypothermia
            - (1) Passive External Rewarming
                - (a) Remove Wet Clothing
                - (b) Dry Blankets
            - (2) Active External Rewarming
                - (a) Hot Packs at Pulse Points
                - (b) Hot Caloric Beverage
        - c) Severe Hypothermia
            - (1) Passive External Rewarming
            - (2) Transport for Active Internal Rewarming

C. Prevention Among Health Care Workers
IV. Heat Exposure
  A. Heat Cramps
      a) Loss of Fluids and Salts
      b) Involuntary, Painful Spasms
    1. Management
      a) Oral Rehydration
  B. Heat Exhaustion
    1. Mild Heat Illness
      a) Dizziness/Lightheadedness
      b) Headache
      c) Nausea and Vomiting
      d) Fatigue
    2. Management
      a) Remove from Heat
        (1) Remove Clothing Layers
      b) Rehydration
        (1) Intravenous Fluids
      c) External Cooling
        (1) Mist Tents
        (2) Cold Packs at Pulse
          Points
          (a) Avoid Shivering
  C. Heat Stroke
    1. Life-threatening Medical Emergency
      a) Loss of Thermoregulatory Center of Hypothalamus
        (1) High Body Temperature (>105°F)
        (2) Decreased/Loss of Consciousness
        (3) Loss of Sweat (50%)
        (4) Seizures
    2. Management
      a) Remove from Heat
        (1) Strip Clothing
      b) Active Cooling
        (1) Mist Cooling
        (2) Ice Packs at Pulse Points
      c) High-Flow Oxygen
  D. Prevention Among Health Care Workers
    1. Rehabilitation Stations
V. Water-Related Emergencies
  A. Near-Drowning
      a) Immersion in Water with Death within 24 hours
    1. Series of Events
      a) Breath-holding Stage
      b) Larnygospasm
      c) Bronchospasm
        (1) Dry Drownings (25%)
          (a) Asphyxiation

      d) Bronchorelaxation
        (1) Swallowing Water
          (a) Suffocation
    2. Cold Water
      a) Hypothermia
    3. Management
      a) Reach
      b) Throw
      c) Row
      d) Go
        (1) Last Resort—When Trained
  B. Diving Emergencies
    1. Boyle's Law
      a) Law of Gases
        (1) Volume of Gas Varies Inversely with the Surrounding Pressure
    2. Descent
      a) Squeeze
        (1) Sinus and Ears
      b) Management
        (1) No Dive Order Until Medically Cleared
    3. Ascent
        (1) Rapid Expansion of Lung Volume
      a) Decompression Sickness
        (1) Also Called the Bends
      b) Pulmonary Overpressurization Syndrome (POPS)
        (1) Rupture of Alveoli
      c) Air Embolism
        (1) Bubbles in Blood
          (a) Pulmonary Embolism
          (b) Stroke
      d) Management
        (1) 100% Oxygen
        (2) Reverse Trendelenburg
        (3) Hyperbaric Chamber
    4. Nitrogen Narcosis
      a) Rapture of the Deep
        (1) Anesthetic Effect
      b) Management
        (1) Transport and Medical Evaluation
VI. Altitude Emergencies
    1. Low Partial Oxygen Pressure
      a) Hypoxia
  A. Acute Mountain Sickness (AMS)
    1. Lightheadedness

2. Headaches
B. High Altitude Cerebral Edema (HACE)
    1. Brain Swelling
        a) Headache
        b) Trouble Walking
        c) Coma
C. High Altitude Pulmonary Edema (HAPE)
        a) Rales
        b) Hypoxia
D. Management
    1. Oxygen Therapy
    2. Transportation to Lower Elevation
VI. Lightning Strikes
    1. Survival Possible
A. Minor Injuries
    1. Ruptured Eardrums
B. Severe Injuries
    1. Cardiac Arrest
C. Management
    1. Reverse Triage
        a) Stunned Myocardium
            (1) CPR
            (2) Defibrillation
        b) Phrenic Nerve Paralyzed
            (1) Ventilatory Assistance
VII. Bites and Stings
    1. Envenomations
        a) 25 percent Dry Bites

A. Snakes
    1. Pit Viper
        a) Retractable Fangs
    2. Coral Snakes
        a) Red on Yellow, Kill a Fellow
    3. Management
        a) Limb below Heart
        b) Transportation
B. Spiders
        a) Rarely Fatal
        b) Symptomatic Relief of
           Discomfort
    1. Brown Recluse
    2. Black Widow
    3. Management
        a) Supportive Care
        b) Transportation
C. Scorpions
    1. Management
        a) Pain Control
D. Marine Animals
    1. Management
IX. Conclusion
    A. Further Training for Specific Local Hazards

TEACHING STRATEGIES

1. National and state hiking organizations and college outdoor clubs often have speakers willing to discuss environmental emergencies.

2. Consider having a Wilderness EMT (WEMT) speak to the students regarding environmental emergencies.

3. Consider using educational programming from groups like PBS and TLC. These groups periodically run special educational presentations such as lightning strikes and snake bites and have tapes available.

FURTHER STUDY

Gurr, D., & Brown, T. (1998). Zapped. *Journal of Emergency Medical Services, 23*(12), 66–69.
Margolis, G. (1998). Immersion hypothermia. *Journal of Emergency Medical Services, 23*(9), 66–70.
Schulmerich, S. (1999). When nature turns up the heat. *RN, 62*(8), 35–39.
Stewart, C. (2000). When lightning strikes. *Emergency Medical Services, 29*(3), 57–59.

CASE STUDY   COLD EMERGENCY

On a cold December morning around Christmas, EMS is called to meet the local forest ranger. Ranger Pete reports that he is caring for a hunter who was brought out of the woods by his friends because "he was acting drunk." The hunting buddies swear that they hadn't been drinking, so Pete, sensing something might be amiss, called EMS to check the hunter out.

The patient's buddies report that he had been with them all morning standing on watch waiting for deer. Then he suddenly got up, slowly walked a few feet from his stand, and sat down in the middle of a snowbank. He then started taking off his winter coat. When he answered their questions about what he was doing, they noticed he had notably slurred speech. His only complaint was pain in his feet and tingling in his hands.

Using a C-B radio, they had contacted Ranger Pete and told him that they would meet him at the end of the old logging road just north of the river fork. They complained that they had had a difficult time getting their buddy out of the woods because he was becoming increasingly uncooperative.

ADDITIONAL CASE STUDY

"Ma'am, are you all right?" asked Marilyn. Marilyn was an EMT with the commercial ambulance service. She and her partner had been asked to meet the police officer at the corner of Parkwood Street and Washington Avenue. The officer had investigated a welfare complaint and discovered an elderly woman, covered in urine, lying on the kitchen floor. Apparently, she had broken her hip sometime the day before and was unable to get up. A neighbor, noticing that the window blinds were still closed, called 9-1-1.

The elderly woman was shivering uncontrollably and could only utter the word, "Cold." Pale and frail, she didn't seem to notice that her leg was twisted under her at a grotesque angle.

STOP AND THINK

1. What could be wrong with this hunter?
2. What are the priorities in management of this condition?
3. What signs and symptoms should the EMT attempt to elicit?
4. What are the short- and long-term consequences of this condition?

ANSWERS TO STOP AND THINK

1. The presentation is consistent with hypothermia.

2. The first priority of care in this patient is to get him out of the cold.

3. Because the patient is still conscious, the next question would be is the patient shivering. The EMTs should also obtain a full set of vital signs, remembering to take a full minute to count the pulse.

4. Active rewarming of this patient may create afterdrop, which could, in turn, result in ventricular fibrillation. However, the more likely scenario is that this patient has concurrent cold injury, either frostnip or frostbite. Cold injuries can take months to resolve even with good medical care.

CASE STUDY   HEAT EMERGENCY

The local Miracle Marathon draws hundreds of runners from all over the region. Some runners train for months in preparation for this race; others are pure amateurs.

Today, race day, is an oppressively hot summer day with temperatures running in the 90s and the humidity almost as high.

Race officials have provided aid stations at one-mile intervals along the route as well as a small field hospital at the finish line in anticipation of the large number of athletes who might become ill or injured.

EMTs Hsiung and Weatherby volunteered for duty and have been assigned to the treatment sector of the field hospital. As soon as they arrive patients start to be brought in.

"This runner went down at the halfway point," yells the race volunteer over the din inside the tent, "and we brought her here in the back of a pickup."
The patient is disoriented, thrashing about and grossly diaphoretic. Her pulse seems to be racing as well. The physician in charge orders the EMTs to assess the patient and start basic life support treatment, then report their findings.

ADDITIONAL CASE STUDY

"Almost finished," Bryan thought to himself as he stood up on top of the roof. Although it was over 100 degrees in the shade, Bryan had promised his dad that he would get the roof done before he went away to college. As soon as he stood up, he felt lightheaded and faint. Trying to sit down quickly, he lost his footing and rolled down the roof. Landing on the overhang, he lay there feeling too weak to get up.

His mother Marion, hearing the clatter, ran outside to see what was the matter. "Bryan," she called out. "Bryan!" she shrieked when she saw his prostate figure on the overhang. "Stay put," she yelled out and ran inside the house to call the fire department.

STOP AND THINK

1. What could be wrong with this runner?
2. What are the priorities in management of this patient?
3. What signs and symptoms should the EMT look for to determine whether the patient is suffering from heat exhaustion or heat stroke?
4. What will be the short- and long-term consequences of this patient's condition?

ANSWERS TO STOP AND THINK

1. This runner could be suffering from either heat exhaustion, or, likely, heat stroke.

2. The first priority is to get the runner out of the heat and to remove sweat-soaked clothing.

3. The EMT should assess first, for level of consciousness. If the patient is disoriented and hot to the touch, the EMT should immediately proceed with cooling measures.

4. If the patient is experiencing heat stroke, the immediate complications include cardiac arrest. Long term, the patient may suffer injury to her brain and kidneys.

CASE STUDY   POSSIBLE DROWNING

The first police unit arrived at the private residence of Ms. Roberta Freeman within minutes. She had called 9-1-1 and reported that her two-year-old had wandered away. She was frantic at the door, screaming over and over, "My baby, my baby, where's my baby!"

Officer Lee calmly asked the mother to look upstairs in the house and under the beds and he would start to look outside. As Ms. Freeman stepped inside the doorway, Officer Lee made his way around to the backyard.

He immediately noticed an in-ground pool and remembered that small children are often attracted to pools. As soon as he entered the backyard, his worst fear was confirmed. Lying face down in the shallow end of the pool was Justin.

He quickly entered the pool and carried Justin to the deck, then using his radio, he called in "Infant submerged, unknown downtime."

ADDITIONAL CASE STUDY

The addition was almost finished and just in time. The baby was growing fast and the new parents needed a spare bedroom quickly. The construction equipment was scattered around the room. Sheet rock, studs, and paint cans indicated a work in progress.

Jenann had gone to answer the telephone, leaving two-year-old Bryan to play in the living room. When she returned, Bryan was nowhere to be found. Searching from room to room, she entered the new room last.

There he was, head first in a plastic bucket. Pulling his lifeless body from the bucket, she ran into the kitchen to call 9-1-1.

STOP AND THINK

1. What is the definition of near-drowning?
2. What are the priorities in management of this child?
3. Does the temperature of the water make a difference in long-term outcome?
4. What are the short- and long-term consequences of this condition?

ANSWERS TO STOP AND THINK

1. Near-drowning occurs when a patient has survived a submersion incident for 24 hours.
2. The first priority of management of a near-drowning patient is to remove the patient from the water.
3. Submersion in cold water has a neuroprotective effect, improving the patient's long-term prognosis.
4. Provided that the patient is not in cardiac arrest, the long-term consequences of near-drowning can include severe neurological injury. The usual short-term consequences include aspiration and hypothermia.

CASE STUDY   DIVING ACCIDENT

EMTs Lorento and Alfonso were enjoying their first day on beach patrol. Both EMTs had requested a transfer from South-Central to Beach Patrol for a change of pace and a little relaxation.

Their first call of the day was at a local beach resort where scuba diving lessons are offered to tourists. The dive-master had called EMS for a woman who claimed she was unable to walk after surfacing from a dive.

As Lorento starts his initial assessment of the patient, Alfonso questions the dive-master about the events preceding the call. They discover that the patient is a novice diver who had dived to a moderate depth. Immediately upon surfacing from her dive, she was unable to support herself or control her legs.

ADDITIONAL CASE STUDY

"EMS meet security, exit 2C, ramp 81, sick passenger, flight 691," squawked the portable radio. The flight was coming in from the Florida Keys. Sometimes these calls are pregnancy-related and sometimes a passenger is having a heart attack.

The EMTs were ushered into the first-class section of the plane by the airline attendants. Seated in row two was a young woman who appeared cyanotic around the lips. An oxygen mask was dangling in front of her face as she said, "I can't breathe." Her boyfriend quickly explained that they had been on vacation in the Keys and had decided to go diving that morning before coming home. He remembered the dive-master telling them not to fly for 24 hours, but he didn't think he was serious.

STOP AND THINK

1. What might be the cause of the patient's symptoms?
2. How should the EMTs treat her?
3. What considerations in transport are relevant to this condition?

ANSWERS TO STOP AND THINK

1. The patient may be suffering from an ascent-related problem called *decompression sickness*.

2. The EMT should support the patient's airway, breathing, and circulation as needed. This includes high-flow oxygen.

3. The patient should be transported to a hyperbaric chamber as soon as possible.

CASE STUDY   ALTITUDE EMERGENCY

The alert tones went out. "Southern Tier Blue Team, assemble at Black Mountain trailhead. All team members prepare for a possible backcountry rescue."

EMTs Yates and Butts had just completed their wilderness EMT course and were prepared for this first mission. The patient was a young woman who was visiting the high country for the first time. She was complaining of a headache, a nonproductive cough, and severe shortness of breath. Her shortness of breath had started right after she had arrived from Miami and had become progressively worse. Initially, the trouble breathing occurred only when she exerted herself, but now it had become so severe that she could not tolerate lying flat.

ADDITIONAL CASE STUDY

How ironic. Jon had finally gotten to the top of the Grand Teton and couldn't enjoy the view because of a splitting headache. He recognized the symptoms and told his buddy, "We had better get down today, I'm not getting any better." With those words the two picked up their packs and made their way down the mountain toward the glen.

At first Jon thought he was just tired from the walk up the mountain then he realized something was terribly wrong. He couldn't walk right. His legs felt like they were going to buckle under him any minute. Stopping at the glen to rest, he said, "Look, Bill, I can't go any farther. Please go get help from the Park Service."

STOP AND THINK

1. What could be wrong with this young woman?
2. What are the priorities in emergency medical care of this condition?
3. What are the potential consequences of not treating this type of illness?

ANSWERS TO STOP AND THINK

1. The patient is likely suffering from acute mountain sickness. The associated symptom, shortness of breath, suggests she may have high-altitude pulmonary edema. Her headache may be due to hypoxia or due to high-altitude cerebral edema.

2. High-flow oxygen should be immediately administered to the patient while she is transported to a lower elevation.

3. Cardiac arrest from hypoxia is the worse-case scenario from acute mountain sickness. Pulmonary edema and cerebral edema with coma are two other serious conditions.

CASE STUDY LIGHTNING STRIKE

"Rescue nine, ambulance nine-five-two, and engine twenty-one respond to the municipal golf course, at the thirteenth hole, for a possible lightning strike."

Emergency crews arrive at the thirteenth hole to find a man in cardiac arrest with CPR being performed by a caddie. Three other patients are lying around the hole. They have various complaints, but all appear to be minor.

"At first we just tingled, then all of a sudden, swish, boom, and crash," remarks one golfer, "and I looked over and poor Harry was down and the caddie was doing CPR. I used my cell phone to call the EMS."

The thunderstorm continues as the captain calls for backup to assist in caring for the multiple victims.

ADDITIONAL CASE STUDY

"Attention," yelled the scoutmaster as the bugler stopped to play reveille. "Better make this quick or we are going to get wet," thought the scoutmaster as he saw the dark clouds overhead. Finally, the flag was down and the scoutmaster yelled, "Dismissed."

Suddenly, the air crackled and the scoutmaster's skin felt like there was a thousand ants all over him. Then came the boom. Stunned by the sudden silence, he got up and put his hands to his ears and felt blood trickling. Looking around he could see five, maybe six, bodies lying on the ground, very still.

STOP AND THINK

1. What are the priorities in management of these patients?
2. How is the triage concept different in lightning strikes than any other situation?
3. What are some of the consequences of a lightning strike?

ANSWERS TO STOP AND THINK

1. After assuring that the scene is safe from downed limbs and the like, the EMT should immediately triage the patients into high- and low-priority categories.

2. Because of the nature of a lightning strike, EMTs usually perform reverse triage, managing the cardiac-arrested patients first.

3. Long-term consequences of a lightning strike can include permanent neurological damage.

CASE STUDY   ANIMAL BITE

Camping in the High Country of the Sierras had always been a dream of Matt's, and when he had an opportunity to take a group of scouts into the wildlands, he jumped on it.

The first day was grueling and Matt slept like a log that night. The next morning Matt rolled out of bed, slipped his feet into his boots, thinking he was ready for the trail ahead, and suddenly felt a sharp pain on the bottom of his left foot.

He violently threw the boot off his foot and yelled out, "Ouch! Something just bit me!" Examining his foot, Matt noted that it had started to swell and he was wondering how he was going to hike the 20 miles back out if he needed to.

ADDITIONAL CASE STUDY

Looking around Paul thought to himself, "What a beautiful New Mexico sunset." Then he knelt down and picked up the bag of trash. Almost immediately, a sharp pain shot up his arm and he dropped the bag. Looking down, he saw a black spider crawl under another bag. "Shoot, I think I've been bitten," Paul thought as he opened the kitchen door and picked up the phone to call emergency services.

STOP AND THINK

1. What is the likely source of the pain and swelling?
2. What would be the immediate treatment?
3. Are all bites treated the same?

ANSWERS TO STOP AND THINK

1. Any number of creatures could have crawled into the boot during the night. Likely candidates include snakes, spiders, and scorpions.

2. The immediate treatment would be to examine and then dress the wound. The wound should be kept below the level of the heart and the patient transported to the hospital for further evaluation.

3. Essentially, all animal/insect bites are treated the same; supportive care and transportation to a medical facility for further evaluation.

ANSWERS TO TEST YOUR KNOWLEDGE

1. The body loses heat from radiation, convection, conduction, and evaporation.

2. The body generates heat by shunting, shivering, and cellular metabolism as well as conduction from the environment.

3. Frostbite and frostnip, as well as trenchfoot, are all forms of local cold injury. Generally, these distal cold injuries are warmed in lukewarm water until thawed, then dressed. Rewarming is not performed if there is a chance of refreezing.

4. Hypothermia starts with slowing of coordination and profound shivering and proceeds to slowing of the all bodily functions and a decreasing level of consciousness.

5. If the patient is mildly hypothermic, passive external rewarming is appropriate. However, if the patient has a decreased level of consciousness, or is unconscious, the EMT should avoid efforts at rewarming and transport the patient to the nearest appropriate medical facility.

6. Heat exhaustion lies on one end of the continuum of heat illness and heat stroke lies on the other end. Symptoms start with nausea, fatigue, lightheadedness, and syncopy. Symptoms continue and the patient becomes hypertensive, tachycardiac, and eventually loses consciousness. Ultimately, heat illness can result in seizures, coma, and death.

7. All patients with suspected heat illness must be removed from the source and unnecessary clothing removed. If the patient is conscious, the EMT can assist the patient with cool liquids. Active cooling, using mist fans, should begin. If the patient is not conscious or is deteriorating, the EMT should consider ALS, initiate active cooling measures, and consider immediate transportation.

8. Complications of near-drowning include hypoxia-induced cerebral injury, aspiration, and hypothermia.

9. The near-drowning victim should be aggressively treated with high-flow oxygen and ventilation, as needed, and then transported to an emergency facility.

10. The entire spectrum of diving-related emergencies revolve around the compression and expansion of gases in the lungs. Signs and symptoms of diving-related emergencies include hypoxia (from POPS), embolisms resulting in stroke, or pulmonary embolism (from the bends).

11. Medical care of diving-related emergencies is high-flow oxygen and transportation to a hyperbaric chamber.

12. The signs and symptoms of high-altitude illness (acute mountain sickness) revolve around hypoxia and include headache, cerebral edema (HACE), and pulmonary edema (HAPE).

13. The emergency medical care of acute mountain sickness includes high-flow oxygen and transportation to lower altitudes.

14. Care of multiple injured patients at a lightning strike involve a concept called *reverse triage*. The patients in cardiac arrest, usually P-O, are resuscitated with CPR and ventilatory support while others await treatment.

15. The medical care of the insect or snake bite revolves around resting the patient, giving symptomatic relief when possible, and transporting to an emergency department.

CHAPTER 29

Poisoning and Allergic Reactions

OBJECTIVES

Upon completion of this chapter, the reader should be able to:

1. List various ways that poisons can enter the body.
2. Describe signs and symptoms associated with different types of poisoning.
3. Discuss the emergency medical care of the patient who has been poisoned.
4. Discuss the special considerations required in the emergency medical care of the intentional overdose patient.
5. Identify the potential airway issues in the poisoned patient.
6. Discuss the indications and contraindications for activated charcoal in the poisoned patient.

7. Recognize the need for medical control and advanced life support in the poisoned patient.
8. Recognize the patient experiencing an allergic reaction.
9. Describe the emergency medical care of the patient with an allergic reaction.
10. Differentiate between a simple allergic reaction and anaphylaxis.
11. Describe the implications of anaphylaxis in regard to airway management.
12. State the indications and contraindications for the epinephrine auto-injector.
13. Identify the importance of medical control and advanced life support in the care of the patient with anaphylaxis.

GLOSSARY

allergen A substance that causes an exaggerated response of the immune system (allergic reaction).

allergic reaction An exaggerated response of the immune system upon exposure to a particular substance.

overdose Intentional exposure to, usually ingestion, of a potentially harmful substance.

Poison Control Center A regional center that serves as a resource for laypersons and health care providers regarding poisons and the management of the poisoned person.

poisoning Exposure to a substance that results in illness.

PREPARATORY

Materials: EMS Equipment: Activated charcoal, suction equipment.

Personnel: Primary Instructor: One EMT-Basic instructor knowledgeable in this area. Assistant Instructor: None required.

Recommended Minimum Time to Complete: 2 hours

STUDENT OUTLINE

I. Overview
II. Poisoning
    A. General Assessment
        1. Specific History
    B. General Management
        1. Scene Safety
        2. Life-Threatening Problems
        3. Medical Direction
C, Transport
        1. Ongoing Assessment
    D. ALS Intercept
III. Ingested Poisons
    A. Intentional Ingestions
    B. Signs and Symptoms
    C. Specific Management
        1. Charcoal
IV. Inhaled Poisons
    A. Signs and Symptoms
    B. Specific Management
V. Injected Poisons
    A. Signs and Symptoms
    B. Specific Management
VI. Absorbed Poisons
    A. Signs and Symptoms
    B. Exposure
    C. Specific Management
VII. Allergic Reactions
    A. Anaphylaxis
        1. Pathophysiology
            a) Skin
            b) Respiratory
            c) Cardiovascular
    B. Signs and Symptoms
    C. Assessment
        1. Initial Assessment
        2. Focused History and Physical Examination
    D. Management
        1. Epinephrine
    E. Transport
VII. Conclusion

LECTURE OUTLINE

I. Overview
   A. Poison Defined
      1. A substance with deadly ingredients
   B. Allergic Reaction
      1. Unexpected activation of the immune system
II. Poisoning
   A. General Assessment
         a) Scene Safety
      1. Specific History
         a) Poison and Container
         b) Time of Exposure
         c) Treatments Prior to Arrival
   B. General Management
      1. Scene Safety First
      2. Life-Threatening Problems
      3. Medical Direction
   C. Transport
      1. Ongoing Assessment
   D. ALS Intercept
III. Ingested Poisons
      1. Common Route of Poisoning
   A. Intentional Ingestions
      1. Referred to as an Overdose
      2. Medical Problem Compounded with Psychiatric Disorder
   B. Signs and Symptoms
      1. Constitutional Symptoms
      2. Specific Signs
         a) Peri-oral Burns
         b) Chemical Odors
   C. Specific Management
      1. Charcoal
         a) Absorbs Poison
IV. Inhaled Poisons
   A. Signs and Symptoms
      1. Respiratory Complaints
   B. Specific Management

V. Injected Poisons
   A. Signs and Symptoms
      1. Insect Bites
         a) Scorpions
         b) Spiders
      2. Snakes
   B. Specific Management
VI. Absorbed Poisons
   A. Signs and Symptoms
      1. Exposure
   B. Specific Management
      1. Flushing
VII. Allergic Reactions
   A. Anaphylaxis
         a) Allergic Reaction
      1. Pathophysiology
         a) Skin
            (1) Hives (Uticaria)
         b) Respiratory
            (1) Wheezes
         c) Cardiovascular
            (1) Hypotension
   B. Signs and Symptoms
   C. Assessment
      1. Initial Assessment
      2. Life-Threatening Airway Constriction
      3. Hypotension
   D. Focused History and Physical Examination
      1. History
         a) Previous Exposure
         b) Previous Reaction
      2. Facial Swelling
      3. Hives
      4. Wheezes
   D. Management
      1. Epinephrine
   E. Transport
VIII. Conclusion

TEACHING STRATEGIES

1. Consider a call or visit to the local Poison Control Center. Encourage the students to enact a mock scenario and see how the personnel at Poison Control would react.

2. Consider having a physician, whose practice deals with allergies, discuss anaphylaxis with the students.

FURTHER STUDY

Fortenberry, J. E., Laine, J., & Shalit, M. (1995). Use of epinephrine for anaphylaxis by emergency medical technicians in a wilderness setting. *Annals of Emergency Medicine, 25*(6), 785–787.

Haynes, B. E., & Pritting, J. (1999). A rural emergency medical technician with selected advanced skills. *Prehospital Emergency Care, 3*(4), 343–346.

Hellman, M. (1996). Pediatric poisonings. *Emergency Medical Services, 25*(6), 21–29.

Hunt, D. (1997). Curse of the black scorpion. *Emergency Medical Services, 26*(10), 37–44.

Marciano, S. (1997). Mammalian animal bites. *Emergency Medical Services, 26*(10), 50–55.

Phillips, K. (1997). Nicotine poisoning. *Emergency Medical Services, 26*(9), 38–40.

Shepard, S. (1996). Plant exposures. *Emergency Medical Services, 25*(6), 39–40.

CASE STUDY   ACCIDENTAL POISONING

An elderly woman meets EMS at the door and ushers the two EMTs into her living room. She explains that she called the emergency number after she found her four-year-old grandson playing with her heart pills.

The grandmother explains, "But I only left him for a moment." While EMT Rodriguez attempts to calm the visibly distraught grandmother, EMT Ruoff notes that the child is happily playing on the floor and wonders just how much trouble those pills can cause.

ADDITIONAL CASE STUDY

"Mary, Mary, you'll be late to school," cried her mother up the stairs as she proceeded to Mary's room. Opening the door, she found Mary still in bed. "Wake up Mary, it's time for school," the mother said as she shook Mary's arm. Mary was cold and unresponsive. Looking over to the bedside stand, Mary's mother saw her pill bottle, empty on its side, and a pint of rum. Gasping, Mary's mother ran to the door and yelled, "George, call 9-1-1. Mary's taken some pills!"

STOP AND THINK

1. What signs and symptoms should the EMT look for in this child?
2. What are the management priorities in the patient after the suspected ingestion of a poison?

ANSWERS TO STOP AND THINK

1. The EMT should immediately focus attention on potentially life-threatening complications.

2. After completing the initial assessment and obtaining both a set of vital signs and a SAMPLE history, the EMT should contact either Poison Control or medical control, as local protocols dictate.

CASE STUDY   INHALATION POISONING

"I couldn't get the sink clean, so I mixed the green stuff with the bleach," explained the dishwasher. The initial call was for an odor or gas in a local restaurant.

When EMS arrived, people were streaming out of the building coughing and acting as if they were choking. Several more complained of trouble breathing.

While the paramedic was establishing EMS command and calling for more resources, EMT Butler proceeded to corral the patrons into one area so they could all be treated.

ADDITIONAL CASE STUDY

It smelled like rotten eggs. That was all the driver could tell the dispatcher over the radio, then grabbed his clipboard and climbed out of the cab and ran away from the ever-enlarging cloud of yellow gas. Looking back at the tanker truck, with its placards, he realized this might be a bigger problem than he had originally thought and wondered if he should call 9-1-1.

STOP AND THINK

1. What are the immediate priorities for responding emergency personnel?
2. What are the priorities in the emergency medical care of these patients?
3. What are signs and symptoms characteristic of inhaled poisons?

ANSWERS TO STOP AND THINK

1. Whenever emergency personnel respond to a report of odors or chemicals, they should suspect a hazardous materials incident and take appropriate precautions to safeguard themselves.

2. Assuming that care can be rendered safely, these patients should be given high-flow oxygen and evaluated further.

3. Inhaled poisons typically present as a respiratory ailment. Coughing, complaints of shortness of breath, and associated signs and symptoms should make the EMT suspect an inhaled poison.

CASE STUDY OVERDOSE

"I don't feel well," complained Mary, a pale thin young woman probably in her early twenties. She was found on the front stoop of a known crack house and police were standing by as the crew started their work.

"Mary, can you tell me what you were doing?" asks Lieutenant McGreevy.

"Doing, doing," Mary spits out. "I've been doing whatever I can score, that's what I've been doing."

The track marks on the inside of her forearms were prominent, with long, angry-looking streaks running up into her armpit.

"He told me," she continued, "that it was some fine Horse. But I think he lied to me."

ADDITIONAL CASE STUDY

"Pass the lighter," Anatov asked. Carefully, he put the flame under the spoon and watched his "stuff" melt. Taking the needle and syringe, he drew up about 1 cc. Using a leather belt as a tourniquet, he injected the first vein he could find.

Three hours later his "buds" decide they better move on before the police find them. Kicking him in the ribs, Georgi said, "Anatov, wake up, man. We got to go. Anatov?" But there was no movement. Just then a spotlight probed the room and everybody hurried ran for the door.

STOP AND THINK

1. What are the priorities in management of the patient with an injected poison?
2. What are some signs and symptoms commonly seen in patients who have been poisoned in this manner?

ANSWERS TO STOP AND THINK

1. After assuring that the scene is safe, the EMT's first priority is to assess and treat any life-threats during the initial assessment.

2. Many illicit drugs are respiratory depressants. Shallow breathing, cyanosis, and associated signs of hypoventilation are commonly seen with injected poisons.

CASE STUDY   ABSORBED POISONS

Jim was moving several barrels of cleaning chemicals from the warehouse to the storeroom, as he had been instructed to, when a couple of them tipped over, spilling their contents all over the floor.

Hoping to avoid embarrassment, Jim thought he could quickly mop up the chemicals with a couple of rags. So he set about to do just that, using his bare hands.

Shortly afterward, Jim's hands started to tingle and burn and turn bright red. Alarmed, Jim reported to the company's infirmary immediately. There he was cared for by an industrial nurse, Mary-Beth, who was assisted by EMT Baker.

Jim tried to explain what had happened and concludes his story with the statement, "I've burned my hands." Realizing the importance of his hands to a laborer like Jim, EMT Baker activated the company emergency battalion and requested the ambulance.

ADDITIONAL CASE STUDY

Reaching the top shelf in the shed, Chad attempted to pull down the bag of fertilizer for the lawn. Unfortunately, the entire shelf, bag and all, came crashing down on his head and he was covered in a layer of powder. Springing to his feet he immediately started to brush the powder off.

Leaning out the door, he yelled, "Chris, call the fire department. I've spilled this bag of fertilizer all over myself."

STOP AND THINK

1. What are the priorities in the management of the patient who has been exposed to a topical poison?
2. What signs and symptoms might be seen in such a situation?

ANSWERS TO STOP AND THINK

1. After assuring that the scene is safe, the EMT should proceed with determining what the material is and what decontamination procedures must be taken before caring for the patient.

2. The signs and symptoms of an absorbed poison depend on what that poison is. The EMT should turn to manufacturer's decontamination recommendations, as well as calling Poison Control.

CASE STUDY   ALLERGIC REACTION

"What luck!" thought seventeen-year old camp counselor-in-training Cathie. "First I pull latrine duty, then I get stung by a bee!"

Cathie proceeded directly to the camp office to report that she had been stung. By the time she got there, she was covered with raised red bumps and was itchy all over.

She was surprised when she heard her own voice, as she said, "I've been stung." Her speech was thick and her tongue felt swollen.

Realizing what might be happening, the camp director Mr. Otis immediately called the local emergency number and asked for EMS. Then he went outside to look for the camp's EMT.

ADDITIONAL CASE STUDY

His sore throat was killing him. The doctor had prescribed a generic penicillin for the infection. He hadn't had a sore throat like this since he was a kid. He rushed to the pharmacy and had his prescription filled. He then immediately took his first dose and made the decision to go home and go to bed.

Waking several hours later, he noted that his chest felt tight and he was wheezing audibly. Opening his shirt, he noted that his chest was covered by a red rash. He immediately recognized the rash as hives. Picking up the phone he dialed his doctor's office.

STOP AND THINK

1. What is an allergic reaction?
2. What differentiates an allergic reaction from life-threatening anaphylaxis?
3. What are the management priorities for a simple allergic reaction?

ANSWERS TO STOP AND THINK

1. An allergic reaction is the body's response to a foreign protein, called an antigen, in the body.

2. While allergic reactions are generally protective of the body, anaphylaxis is an extreme bodily reaction that can be life-threatening.

3. The first priority of an EMT assessing a patient with a possible allergic reaction is to assess the airway for patency. Then the EMT should listen to the lungs for wheezes and to obtain a set of vital signs to determine if the patient is hypotensive and tachycardiac. Any of the above signs may indicate an potentially life-threatening anaphylaxis.

ANSWERS TO TEST YOUR KNOWLEDGE

1. Poisons can be inhaled, ingested, absorbed, or injected into the body.

2. The signs and symptoms associated with different types of poisons is dependent on the poison.

3. The emergency medical care of a poisoned patient focuses on scene safety first, followed by an assessment for life-threats using the initial assessment.

4. The patient who has an intentional overdose is also a behavioral emergency.

5. Various poisons can threaten an airway by swelling surrounding tissues or causing the patient to lose nervous control of the airway.

6. Activated charcoal is indicated for specific susceptible poisons that have been recently ingested. Activated charcoal should not be given to a patient who cannot control his or her own airway.

7. Poisons have broad systemic effects. Therefore, complications can be anticipated. Medical control can alert the EMT to symptoms or signs to look for and respond to.

8. The patient with an allergic reaction may initially respond with respiratory symptoms, like a tightness in the chest or swelling in the airway, or cardiovascular symptoms, like a racing heart or lightheadedness.

9. The initial emergency care of an allergic reaction revolves around maintaining the airway, administering high-flow oxygen, and transporting the patient immediately. In some cases, the EMT may be expected to assist the patient with an epinephrine auto-injector.

10. A simple allergic reaction is usually self-limiting, meaning that it gets to a point and stops. Anaphylaxis is life-threatening, leading to hypotension, respiratory, and/or cardiac arrest, if left untreated.

11. Frequently, anaphylaxis involves a swelling of the airway to the point it is closed. High-flow oxygen and positive pressure ventilation can be helpful, but the patient needs epinephrine to reverse the effects of anaphylaxis.

12. The epinephrine auto-injector is indicated whenever the patient is experiencing an allergic reaction for which the epinephrine was prescribed. In light of those conditions, an epinephrine auto-injector is not contraindicated.

13. While epinephrine can reverse the effects of anaphylaxis, other medical issues remain that must be dealt with by either ALS personnel or the emergency department.

CHAPTER 30

Head Injuries

OBJECTIVES

Upon completion of this chapter, the reader should be able to:

1. Discuss the relevance of head injuries to trauma deaths.
2. Describe the anatomy of the scalp, skull, and brain.
3. Identify injuries that are commonly associated with head injuries.
4. Discuss the physical findings associated with a scalp injury, a skull injury, and a brain injury.
5. Describe the management priorities of the patient with a scalp injury, a skull injury, and a brain injury.
6. Describe the Glasgow Coma Scale.
7. Discuss the consequences of increased intracranial pressure.
8. Identify the physical findings associated with increased intracranial pressure.
9. Describe the appropriate treatment modalities used by the EMT that can help to decrease intracranial pressure.

GLOSSARY

basilar skull fracture A break at the base of the skull (the area behind the face).

CSF otorrhea A leaking of cerebrospinal fluid from the ear.

CSF rhinorrhea A leaking of cerebrospinal fluid from the nose.

Cushing's reflex Hypertension and bradycardia associated with serious head injury.

Cushing's triad Hypertension, bradycardia, and an altered respiratory pattern seen in serious head injuries.

epidural hematoma A collection of blood between the skull and the dura mater, often arterial in nature.

Glasgow Coma Scale (GCS) A scale that is used to quantify a patient's level of responsiveness.

hematoma A collection of blood.

intracranial pressure (ICP) The pressure within the skull.

mastoid process The bony prominence behind the ear.

post-traumatic seizure A seizure that occurs immediately after head trauma.

subdural hematoma A collection of blood between the surface of the brain and the dura mater, often venous in nature.

PREPARATORY

Materials: EMS Equipment: Long spine board, short spine immobilization device, cervical immobilization devices, helmet, head immobilization device, blanket roll, 2-inch tape.

Personnel: Primary Instructor: One EMT-Basic instructor knowledgeable in head and spinal injuries. Assistant Instructor: The instructor-to-student ratio should be 1:6 for psychomotor skill practice. Individuals used as assistant instructors should be knowledgeable in head and spinal emergencies and treatment.

Recommended Minimum Time to Complete: 4 hours (shared with spinal injury)

STUDENT OUTLINE

I. Overview
II. Anatomy Review
III. Types of Injuries
    A. Scalp
    B. Skull
        1. Basilar Skull Fracture
        2. Open Skull Fracture
            a) Penetrating Injury
    C. Brain
        1. Open
        2. Closed
            a) Subdural Hematoma
            b) Epidural Hematoma
        3. Intracranial Pressure
IV. Associated Injuries
    A. Neck
    B. Face
V. Patient Presentation
    A. Mechanism of Injury
    B. Signs and Symptoms
    C. History
        1. Loss of Consciousness
        2. Seizure
        3. Vomiting
    D. Assessment
        1. Initial Assessment
        2. Rapid Trauma Assessment
            a) Glasgow Coma Scale
            b) Vital Signs
    E. Management
        1. ABCs
        2. Spine Precautions
        3. Maintenance of Oxygenation
        4. Hyperventilation
        5. Controlling External Blood Loss
        6. Elevate Head of Bed
    F. Transport
        1. Ongoing Assessment
VI. Conclusion

LECTURE OUTLINE

I. Overview
  A. Half of Trauma Deaths Secondary Due to Head Injury
  B. Significant Morbidity
II. Anatomy Review
  A. Layers of the Meninges
III. Types of Injuries
  A. Scalp
    1. Tough Rug
    2. Scalp Wounds
  B. Skull
    1. Basilar Skull Fracture
      a) Threatens Brain
      b) Signs
        (1) Battle's Sign
        (2) Raccoon's Eyes (Bilateral Periorbital Ecchymosis)
        (3) CSF Leakage
          (a) Nose (Rhinorrhea)
          (b) Ears (Otorrhea)
    2. Open Skull Fracture
      (1) Gray Matter Exposed
      a) Penetrating Injury
      (2) Underlying Damage
  C. Brain
    1. Open
      a) Cover and Protect
    2. Closed
      a) Subdural Hematoma
        (1) Venous Bleed
          (a) Hours to Days
      b) Epidural Hematoma
        (1) Rapid Bleed
    3. Intracranial Pressure
      a) Decompensation
        (1) Surgical Decompression
IV. Associated Injuries
  A. Neck
    1. 5 percent of Head with Associated Neck
  B. Face
    1. Significant Bleeding
V. Patient Presentation
  A. Mechanism of Injury
    1. Motor Vehicle Collisions
      a) Starred or Spidered Windshield
    2. Sports
      a) Helmet Use
  B. Signs and Symptoms

    1. DCAP-BTLS
  C. History
    1. Loss of Consciousness
    2. Seizure
      a) 5 percent of Traumatic Head Injury
    3. Vomiting
      a) Projectile
  D. Assessment
    1. Initial Assessment
      a) Airway and Ventilation Critical
      b) Hypotension
        (1) Secondary Source
          (a) Identify and Control
    2. Rapid Trauma Assessment
      a) Glasgow Coma Scale
        (1) Baseline
      b) Vital Signs
        (1) Baseline
        (2) Cushing's Triad
          (a) Bradycardia
          (b) Altered Respiratory Pattern
          (c) Hypertension
  E. Management
    1. ABCs
    2. Spine Precautions
      a) Routine—Trauma above Clavicles
    3. Maintenance of Oxygenation
      a) Reduce Cerebral Hypoxia
    4. Hyperventilation
      a) Effect
        (1) Vasoconstriction
      b) Benefit
        (1) Reduces Bleeding
      c) Risk
        (1) Pancerebral Hypoxia
    5. Controlling External Blood Loss
    6. Elevate Head of Bed
      a) Facilitate Drainage
  F. Transport
      a) High Priority
      b) Trauma Center
    1. Ongoing Assessment
      a) Subtle Changes
VI. Conclusion
  A. Efficient Field Care Equals Improved Survival

TEACHING STRATEGIES

1. Take a clear gallon milk container and place rubber tubing inside. Then inflate a balloon inside the container. The container represents the rigid skull and the balloon the soft brain. Start to fill the container with red fluid, representing blood, until the balloon either ruptures or pushes the balloon through the opening. This process represents what occurs when bleeding happens inside the skull.

2. Consider inviting a trauma surgeon to class to discuss trauma and head injuries.

FURTHER STUDY

Armstrong, J. (1998). Bombs and other blasts. *RN, 61*(11), 26–35.

Jastemski, C. (1998). Trauma! Head injuries. *RN, 61*(12), 40–44.

Murphy, P., & Heightman, A. (1998). Head injuries. *Journal of Emergency Medical Services, 23*(4), 66–70.

Price. D., & Burns, B. (1999). Brain injuries. *Emergency Medical Services, 28*(6), 65–71.

Schultz, R. (1997). Eggs and brains. *Emergency Medical Services, 26*(4), 29–35.

CASE STUDY   BAR FIGHT

"The scene is safe," declared Sergeant McNally over the command frequency. "Have EMS enter. We have a man with a head injury." The call had originally been dispatched as a "fight in progress," and EMS had been ordered to stage around the block.

With all emergency lights shut down, the ambulance approached the scene. The EMTs saw the perpetrator sitting in the back seat of a police cruiser, and entered through the front door.

Immediately to the right of the door was a broken beer bottle and lots of blood, and immediately to the left stood the source of the blood, a twentyish male with a mean-looking cut over his left eye. His hair may have been blond before but it was red with blood now.

EMT Johnson immediately took spine stabilization, with gloves on, while EMT Murawski started his assessment. In the meantime, the patient began to complain loudly about the splitting headache he had and loudly declared, "I want something for my pain."

The patient was unsure if he had been knocked out, and he was also unsure whether the attacker had used any weapons, like a club or a bottle, or just his fists.

ADDITIONAL CASE STUDY

As Bonnie approached the motor vehicles involved in the collision, she was immediately impressed by the dome-shaped protrusion in the front windshield of the second car. "Must not have been wearing a seatbelt," she thought to herself. As she got closer to the car she noticed a lock of hair and a pair of glasses embedded in the windshield. Immediately behind the windshield was a man whose face was covered in blood. The patient appeared unconscious.

STOP AND THINK

1. What are the assessment priorities for this patient?
2. What is the significance of the patient's symptoms?
3. What are the treatment priorities for the patient?
4. What signs or symptoms will the patient display if he decompensates?

ANSWERS TO STOP AND THINK

1. In consideration of the mechanism of injury, the EMT should immediately take cervical spine stabilization and begin the initial assessment: airway, breathing, circulation.

2. The fact that the patient cannot remember being hit (amnesia) suggests that the patient may have sustained a head injury. Coupled with the fact that the patient has a headache and is somewhat uncooperative lends more support to the argument that the patient has sustained a head injury.

3. After immobilizing the cervical spine, the first treatment priority would be to administer high-flow oxygen to the patient.

4. Loss of consciousness, decreasing level of consciousness, projectile vomiting, or a generalized seizure are all indications that the patient is decompensating.

ANSWERS TO TEST YOUR KNOWLEDGE

1. Head injuries are the number one cause of trauma death in the United States. Secondarily, head-injured patients who survive initially must undergo years of expensive medical treatments and long-term care.

2. The scalp is a tough mat that overlies the skull. Immediately underneath the scalp is the skull, a porous bone made of two layers of bone and a gelatin-like substance in the middle. Below the skull are the three layers of the meninges that pad the brain from injury; pia mater, archnoid, and dura mater.

3. Common head injuries include the concussion (capillary bleeding), the epidural hematoma (arterial bleeding), and the subdural hematoma (venous bleeding).

4. The management of the three head injuries—scalp, skull, and brain—revolves around maintaining an airway, ensuring ventilation as well as oxygenation, and preventing hypoperfusion.

5. The first priority with assessing a scalp injury is to determine if there is an underlying open or closed skull injury. Then the bleeding from a scalp injury should be controlled. Skull injuries imply a significant force has been applied to the head. The EMT assessing a skull injury should suspect an underlying brain injury. A brain injury, whether a concussion, an epidural hematoma, or a subdural hematoma, is potentially serious and needs immediate medical attention. Signs of a brain injury include, headache, projectile vomiting, seizures, decreasing or loss of consciousness, and Cushing's triad.

6. The Glscow Coma Scale assesses the patient's neurological status by evaluating eye opening, speech, and movement. These complex activities involve different parts of the brain.

7. As the pressure within the skull rises (increasing intracranial pressure[ICP]), the brain is crushed against the walls of its rigid container, the skull. Eventually, the brain is crushed and the patient dies.

8. Classic findings of increased ICP include sluggish or nonreactive pupils (a blown pupil is a late finding), hypertension, bradycardia, and abnormal respiratory patterns. Other signs of increased ICP include decreased level or loss of consciousness, projectile vomiting, and seizures.

9. The most appropriate treatment for a patient with signs of increasing ICP is rapid transportation to a trauma center. En route, the EMT should focus on maintaining the airway, providing high-flow oxygen, assisting ventilations (per protocols), and treating/preventing hypoperfusion.

CHAPTER 31

Spine Injuries

OBJECTIVES

Upon completion of this chapter, the reader should be able to:

1. Describe the anatomy and physiology of the spinal column and spinal cord.
2. Describe different types of spine injuries.
3. Identify common injuries to the spine.
4. Identify the potential complications of spinal cord injuries.
5. Describe the patient presentation that would lead the EMT to suspect a spine injury.
6. Relate the mechanism of injury to potential injuries of the spine.
7. Describe the appropriate assessment techniques to use when the EMT suspects the patient has a spine injury.
8. Identify how airway management is different for patients with suspected spine injuries compared to other patients.

9. Identify the priorities in management of the spine-injured patient.
10. Identify when spinal immobilization is necessary.
11. Describe how to properly apply a cervical spine immobilization device.
12. Describe how to immobilize a patient using a short immobilization device.
13. Describe how to perform a rapid extrication from a vehicle.
14. Describe how to immobilize a patient to a long spine board from the standing and supine positions.
15. Identify the situations that would require helmet removal.
16. Describe different types of helmets and the preferred method for removing them.

GLOSSARY

cervical spine immobilization device A semirigid, collar-like device that is used to aid cervical spine immobilization.

neurogenic shock Hypoperfused state that can result from a serious spinal cord injury.

paralysis An inability to move.

paraplegia A condition characterized by paralysis involving the lower extremities.

paresthesia An inability to feel normal sensation.

priapism Painful penile erection that can be caused by an interruption in the nerves from the spinal cord.

quadriplegia A condition characterized by paralysis involving all four extremities.

standing takedown A technique of achieving spinal immobilization of the standing patient.

PREPARATORY

Materials: EMS Equipment: Long spine board, short spine immobilization device, cervical immobilization devices, helmet, head immobilization device, blanket roll, 2-inch tape.

Personnel: Primary Instructor: One EMT-Basic instructor knowledgeable in head and spinal injuries. Assistant Instructor: The instructor-to-student ratio should be 1:6 for psychomotor skill practice. Individuals used as assistant instructors should be knowledgeable in head and spinal emergencies and treatment.

Recommended Minimum Time to Complete: 4 hours

I. Overview

II. Anatomy Review

III. Types of Spine Injuries
- a) Without Neurologic Injury
- b) With Neurologic Injury
- c) Region of Spine
  - (1) Cervical
  - (2) Thoracic
  - (3) Lumbar
  - (4) Sacrococcygeal

IV. Patient Presentation
- a) Mechanism of Injury
  - (1) Motor Vehicle Crash
    - 1) Flexion/Extension/Rotation
  - (2) Falls
    - 1) Compression
  - (3) Firearms
  - (4) Recreation
  - (5) Associated Injuries
    - (a) Head
    - (b) Face
    - (c) Chest
    - (d) Abdomen
- b) Signs and Symptoms
  - (1) Limitations
    - (a) Intoxication
    - (b) Distracting Injury
    - (c) Altered Mental Status
  - (2) Neck or Back Pain
  - (3) Neurologic Abnormality
    - (a) Respiratory Failure
    - (b) Neurogenic Shock
    - (c) Paralysis
    - (d) Paresthesias
- c) Assessment
  - (1) Initial Assessment
  - (2) Focused History and Physical Examination
  - (3) Vital Signs
  - (4) History
- d) Management
  - (1) Save the Patient
  - (2) Protect the Cord
    - (a) Cervical Spine Immobilization Device
    - (b) Short Immobilization Device
    - (c) Rapid Extrication
    - (d) Long Spine Board
      - a) Supine Patient
      - b) Standing Patient
  - (3) Special Considerations
    - (a) Helmets
    - (b) Long-Term Care of Spine Injury
- e) Transport
- f) Conclusion

LECTURE OUTLINE

I. Overview
    A. 13,000 spinal cord injuries a year
    B. Impact
        1. Financial
        2. Familial
II. Anatomy Review
    A. Spinal Column
        1. Protection of Spinal Cord
III. Types of Spine Injuries
    A. Without Neurologic Injury
        1. Ligament Injury
            a) Whiplash
            b) Unstable Column
    B. With Neurologic Injury
        1. Impairments
    C. Region of Spine
        1. Cervical
            a) High Percentage of Fractures
                (1) Result of Motor Vehicle
                    Collisions
        2. Thoracic
            a) Direct Blow
                (1) Great Deal of Force
        3. Lumbar
            a) Pain in Low Back Area
            b) Comon
        4. Sacrococcygeal
            a) Part of Pelvis
            b) Injury Due to Direct Blow
IV. Patient Presentation
    A. Mechanism of Injury
        1. Motor Vehicle Crash
            a) Flexion/Extension/Rotation
        2. Falls
            a) Compression
            b) Axial Loading
        3. Firearms
            a) "Center of Mass"
                (1) Neck
                (2) Chest
                    (a) Abdomen
        4. Recreation
            a) Football
            b) Diving
        5. Associated Injuries
            a) Head
                (1) Loss of Consciousness
            b) Face

                (1) 20 percent with Facial
                    also Spinal
            c) Chest
                (1) More Rare
                (2) Direct Blow
            d) Abdomen
                (1) Low Back Pain
                    (a) Lumbar
    B. Signs and Symptoms
        1. Limitations
            a) Intoxication
                (1) Inability to Feel Pain
            b) Distracting Injury
                (1) Overwhelming Pain
                    Masks Spine Injury
            c) Altered Mental Status
                (1) Associated with Mecha-
                    nism of Injury
        2. Neck or Back Pain
        3. Neurologic Abnormality
            a) Respiratory Failure
                (1) Phrenic Nerve at Cervical
                    3-4-5
                    (a) 3-4-5 keeps you
                        alive
            b) Neurogenic Shock
                (1) Normal Vasoconstriction
                (2) Injury
                    (a) Massive Vasodilation
                        (i) Signs of
                            Hypoperfu-
                            sion
                      (ii) Cool above,
                            warm below
            c) Paralysis
                (1) Loss of movement
            d) Paresthesias
                (1) Loss of sensation
                    (a) Pins and Needles
                      Sensation
            e) Other
                (1) Incontinence
                    (a) Loss of Bladder
                      Control
                (2) Priapism
                    (a) Painful Erection
                        (i) Loss of Spinal
                          Cord Control

C. Assessment
    1. Initial Assessment
    2. Focused History and Physical Examination
    3. Vital Signs
        a) Evaluation for Hypoperfusion
    4. History
        a) Preexisting Neurological Conditions
D. Management
    1. Save the Patient
        a) A comes before B before C
    2. Protect the Cord
        a) Manual Stabilization
            (1) Neutral Inline Position
        b) Cervical Spine Immobilization Device
            (1) Sized to Fit
            (2) 90 Degree Eyes to Ears to Shoulder
            (3) Continous Manual Stabilization
        c) Short Immobilization Device
            (1) Temporary Movement Device
                (a) Transfer to Long Board
        d) Rapid Extrication
            (1) High-Priority Patients
                (a) Life Before Limb
        e) Long Spine Board
            (1) Supine Patient
                (a) Four-Person Lift
                (b) Log-Roll
            (2) Standing Patient
                (c) Standing Takedown
    3. Special Considerations
        a) Helmets
            (1) Fitted
                (a) Football
                    (i) Remain in place unless
                      a. Airway uncontrollable
                      b. Breathing needs to be assisted
            (1) Unfitted
                (a) All Others
                    (i). Remove
        b) Long-Term Care of Spine Injury
            (1) Spinal Cord Transection
                (a) Quadriplegia
                (b) Paraplegia
D. Transport
    1. Ongoing Assessment Imperative
E. Conclusion

TEACHING STRATEGIES

1. Emphasis in this chapter should be on the skills. While practice in the warm confines of a classroom is acceptable initially, EMT students should be taken out-of-doors and encouraged to practice in a number of different types of cars, sports utility vehicles, and trucks.

2. Using a series of slides showing various mechanisms of injury, ask the students to predict the injury (flexion, extension, rotation) and the area of the spine most likely to be effected.

CASE STUDY   PARALYSIS

Officer Shulman knew that something was seriously wrong when he approached the scene of an accident that involved a head-on collision and another rear-end collision. One car was a mess, and the driver was still sitting in the front seat. Usually by the time he arrived all the drivers would be out of the cars or at least fumbling through their glove compartments looking for their insurance cards.

Officer Shulman approached the car and said, "Good evening, Ma'am." The driver of the car softly responded, "I can't feel my legs." Immediately recognizing the seriousness of the situation, Officer Shulman advised the driver not to turn or move her head. He clicked his lapel mike and said, "Control Unit Five. Send EMS and a supervisor to my location, probable spinal injury from the MVC, and tell them to expedite." He then climbed into the backseat of the car and manually stabilized the patient's neck, telling her in a calm voice, "More help is on the way."

ADDITIONAL CASE STUDY

"Eagletown Rescue. A call for injuries from a fall, Partridge Run Estates." As he climbed into ambulance, Brent thought to himself, "There is an old watering hole in Partridge Run." When the ambulance pulled up to the scene the crew was waved in by a couple of teenagers in shorts or swim trunks.

The teenagers had managed to pull Scott up on shore. He had apparently been jumping off a rope dangling over the water and went into the water head first. It was a while before he surfaced so a lifeguard, went in after him. The lifeguard was performing mouth-to-mouth. Next to the lifeguard was a deputy sheriff pouring beer onto the ground.

STOP AND THINK

1. What are the priorities in the assessment of this patient?
2. What special assessment considerations should the EMT use?
3. What special transportation considerations should the EMT use?

ANSWERS TO STOP AND THINK

1. The first priority with every trauma patient is to obtain and maintain a neutral inline position of the cervical spine—unless there is pain with movement or the EMT meets resistance.

2. The EMT should carefully assess, and document, the exact extent of paralysis and paresthesia the patient is experiencing as well as perform repeated and ongoing assessments of the spinal cord injury.

3. Due to the mechanism of injury, the EMT should consider transporting this patient to a trauma center without the use of lights and siren. A cautious ride driven at slow speeds, with a minimum of movement, is in order.

FURTHER STUDY

Bilkasley, M., & Ryder, T. (1997). The halo orthosis. *Journal of Emergency Medical Services, 22* (12), 52–58.

Blank-Reid, C. (1999). Strangulation. *RN, 62* (2), 32–36.

Brown, L. H., Gough, J. E., & Simonds, W. B. (1988). Can EMS providers adequately assess trauma patients for cervical spinal injury? *Prehospital Emergency Care, 2* (1), 33–36.

Cone, D. C., Wydro, G. C., & Mininger, C. M. (1999). Current practice in clinical cervical spinal clearance: Implication for EMS. *Prehospital Emergency Care, 3* (1), 42–46.

Meldon, S. W., Brant, T. A., Cydulka, R. K., Collins, T. E., & Shade, B. R. (1998). Out-of-hospital cervical spine clearance: Agreement between emergency medical technicians and emergency physicians. *Journal of Trauma, 45* (6), 1058–1061.

Murphy, P., & Colwell, C. (2000). Prehospital management of neck trauma. *Emergency Medical Services, 29* (5), 53–60.

Sahni R., Menegazzi, J. J., & Mosesso, V. N., Jr. (1997). Paramedic evaluation of clinical indicators of cervical spinal injury. *Prehospital Emergency Care, 1* (1), 16–18.

VanStralen, D. & Goss, J. (1998). Damage control for pediatric spinal injuries. *Journal of Emergency Medical Services, 23* (3), 114.

ANSWERS TO TEST YOUR KNOWLEDGE

1. The spinal column is a long, segmented bone with a central channel where the spinal cord lies. The spinal cord is part of the central nervous system.

2. Extremes of extension, flexion, and rotation can injure the spinal column and therefore the spinal cord.

3. Facial injuries are often seen with cervical spine injuries. Fractures of the ribs may indicate a concurrent fracture of the spinal column as well.

4. Spinal injuries are divided into those with neurological compromise and those without neurological compromise.

5. Complications of spinal cord injury can include difficulties breathing (phrenic nerve), quadriplegia or paraplegia, and neurogenic (spinal) shock.

6. Any significant mechanism of injury, such as a fall, or evidence of trauma to the center of mass (torso and neck).

7. After immediate manual stabilization, the EMT would check peripheral sensation and movement as well as pulses.

8. When the possibility of spinal injury cannot be ruled out, the EMT must use a jaw-thrust to maintain the airway, avoiding moving the neck.

9. The priorities of care for the spine-injured patient are no different than those of any trauma patient. The EMT would first attend to the ABCs, then proceed to stabilizing the spine with mechanical adjuncts.

10. Spinal immobilization is necessary any time there is significant mechanism of injury, evidence of trauma above the clavicles, neck pain, or paralysis or paresthesia.

11. After the head has been moved to the neutral inline position, the proper-sized cervical immobilization device (CID) should maintain that position without further flexion or extension.

12. The key principles in immobilizing a patient on a short immobilization device is to apply a proper-sized cervical immobilization device, secure the body before the head, and reassess distal pulses, movement, and sensation.

13. A rapid extrication substitutes the short immobilization device with the arms of the rescuers. The patient is still maintained in a neutral position and moved as a unit.

14. After obtaining neutral inline stabilization, the EMTs would lower the patient with the backboard, as a unit, to the ground.

15. A helmet should be removed any time it impedes airway control or ventilation. Unless it is a football helmet, most helmets are removed.

16. All helmet removal follows the same pattern. First, the head and helmet are maintained in a neutral inline position, then straps are removed, then the helmet is backed off the head—all the time maintaining neutral inline stabilization.

Skill 31–1 Application of the Cervical Immobilization Device
Student Name: _____   Date: _____

Purpose: To aid the EMT in stabilization of the cervical spine.

Standard Precautions:
Icon — Handwashing — Gloves

Equipment:
Assortment of Cervical Immobilization Devices (Collars)

Step 1. The EMT first moves the patient's head into neutral alignment. If the patient complains of pain, or resistance is felt, the patient's neck is splinted in position.

YES: _____   RE-TEACH: _____   RETURN: _____   INSTRUCTOR INITIALS _____

Step 2. The EMT assigns a trained assistant to maintain continuous manual stabilization of the patient's head.

YES: _____   RE-TEACH: _____   RETURN: _____   INSTRUCTOR INITIALS _____

Step 3. Next, the EMT checks for distal pulses, movement, and sensation.

YES: _____   RE-TEACH: _____   RETURN: _____   INSTRUCTOR INITIALS _____

Step 4. The EMT measures the patient's neck for a cervical collar, according to manufacturer recommendations.

YES: _____   RE-TEACH: _____   RETURN: _____   INSTRUCTOR INITIALS _____

Step 5. The EMT slides the posterior portion of the collar in the void behind the neck.

YES: _____   RE-TEACH: _____   RETURN: _____   INSTRUCTOR INITIALS _____

Step 6. Cupping the chin piece in one hand, the EMT slides the anterior portion of the collar up the chest until it captures the chin.

YES: _____   RE-TEACH: _____   RETURN: _____   INSTRUCTOR INITIALS _____

Step 7. With collar in place the Velcro® is securely fastened.

YES: _____   RE-TEACH: _____   RETURN: _____   INSTRUCTOR INITIALS _____

Step 8. Checking for a proper collar fit, the EMT mentally draws a line from the opening of the ear to the middle of the shoulder, and from the opening of the ear to the eyes. There should be a 90-degree angle.

YES: _____   RE-TEACH: _____   RETURN: _____   INSTRUCTOR INITIALS _____

Step 9. The EMT finally rechecks for distal pulses, sensation, and movement.

YES: _____   RE-TEACH: _____   RETURN: _____   INSTRUCTOR INITIALS _____

Step 10. Continuous manual stabilization must be maintained, despite the presence of the cervical immobilization device.

YES: _____   RE-TEACH: _____   RETURN: _____   INSTRUCTOR INITIALS _____

Skill 31–2 Application of the Short Immobilization Device

Student Name: _____ Date: _____

Purpose: To further immobilize the injured patient's spine after the application of the cervical collar.

Personal Protective Equipment:
Icon — Handwashing — Gloves

Equipment:
Assortment of Cervical Spine Immobilization Devices
Short Immobilization Device

Step 1. The EMT applies a proper-sized cervical spine immobilization device after manually stabilizing the spine as well as checking distal pulses, movement, and sensation.

YES: _____ RE-TEACH: _____ RETURN: _____ INSTRUCTOR INITIALS _____

Step 2. While a trained assistant maintains continuous manual stabilization, the EMT places his arms along the anterior and posterior thorax. The patient may now be moved forward as a unit, keeping the spine inline.

YES: _____ RE-TEACH: _____ RETURN: _____ INSTRUCTOR INITIALS _____

Step 3. The device is then positioned behind the patient cautiously, then the patient is leaned back against the device.

YES: _____ RE-TEACH: _____ RETURN: _____ INSTRUCTOR INITIALS _____

Step 4. Next the patient's torso, including the legs, is secured to the device.

YES: _____ RE-TEACH: _____ RETURN: _____ INSTRUCTOR INITIALS _____

Step 5. Finally, the patient's head is secured to the device. The EMT pads the void behind the head as needed.

YES: _____ RE-TEACH: _____ RETURN: _____ INSTRUCTOR INITIALS _____

Step 6. The EMT then reassesses distal pulses, movement, and sensory function of the patient before transferring the patient to the backboard.

YES: _____ RE-TEACH: _____ RETURN: _____ INSTRUCTOR INITIALS _____

Skill 31–3 Rapid Extrication

Student Name: _____   Date: _____

Purpose: To manually immobilize the spine of an unstable patient who may have a spinal injury as a result of a motor vehicle collision.

Personal Protective Equipment:
Icon — Handwashing — Gloves — Turnout Gear

Equipment:
Assortment of Cervical Spine Immobilization Devices
Long Spine Board

Step 1. The EMT first checks distal pulses, movement, and sensation. Then the EMT moves the head to a neutral position, and has another EMT apply a proper-sized cervical collar.

YES: _____   RE-TEACH: _____   RETURN: _____   INSTRUCTOR INITIALS _____

Step 2. With an EMT on each side of the patient, the patient is gently lifted a couple of inches so that a longboard may be inserted under the patient's buttocks.

YES: _____   RE-TEACH: _____   RETURN: _____   INSTRUCTOR INITIALS _____

Step 3. One EMT grasps the patient under the arms, while another grasps the patient at the hips. Then, on command, the EMTs rotate patient to the side about 45 degrees. At this point the EMTs may need to switch places if the car's B post becomes an obstruction.

YES: _____   RE-TEACH: _____   RETURN: _____   INSTRUCTOR INITIALS _____

Step 4. Once the patient is parallel to the backboard, the patient is lowered, as a unit, to the longboard while the EMTs maintain inline immobilization.

YES: _____   RE-TEACH: _____   RETURN: _____   INSTRUCTOR INITIALS _____

Step 4. Once the patient is on the longboard, first the body and then the head are fastened securely. The EMT rechecks the patient's distal pulses, movement, and sensation.

YES: _____   RE-TEACH: _____   RETURN: _____   INSTRUCTOR INITIALS _____

Skill 31–4 Long Axis Drag

Student Name: _____   Date: _____

Purpose: To rapidly remove a patient, who is in immediate danger, from a motor vehicle with a minimum of spinal manipulation.

Personal Protective Equipment:
Icon — Handwashing — Gloves — Turnout Gear

Equipment Needed:
None

Step 1. First, the EMT determines that the patient needs immediate extrication for some reason (for example, if the patient is in cardiac arrest).

YES: _____   RE-TEACH: _____   RETURN: _____   INSTRUCTOR INITIALS _____

Step 2. Opening the closest door and entering the passenger compartment, the EMT disentangles any extremities from pedals and other obstructions.

YES: _____   RE-TEACH: _____   RETURN: _____   INSTRUCTOR INITIALS _____

Step 3. Then the EMT reaches behind the patient's back and under both of the patient's arms, and grabs the wrists.

YES: _____   RE-TEACH: _____   RETURN: _____   INSTRUCTOR INITIALS _____

Step 4. The EMT rotates the patient, as a unit, and places the patient into a semi-inclined position.

YES: _____   RE-TEACH: _____   RETURN: _____   INSTRUCTOR INITIALS _____

Step 5. The EMT drags the patient out of the motor vehicle with the patient's head resting on the EMT's forearms.

YES: _____   RE-TEACH: _____   RETURN: _____   INSTRUCTOR INITIALS _____

Step 6. By dropping to her knees, the EMT can lower the patient and crawl backward with the patient, while performing a long axis drag.

YES: _____   RE-TEACH: _____   RETURN: _____   INSTRUCTOR INITIALS _____

Skill 31-5 Modified Log-roll of the Supine Patient

Student Name: _____ Date: _____

Purpose: To immobilize the spine of a supine patient who may have a spinal injury.

Personal Protective Equipment:
Icon — Handwashing — Gloves.

Equipment Needed:
Selection of Cervical Collars
Long Spine Board
Strapping System
Head Immobilization System

Step 1. An EMT checks distal pulses, movement, and sensation of all four extremities while another EMT maintains manual stabilization.

YES: _____ RE-TEACH: _____ RETURN: _____ INSTRUCTOR INITIALS _____

Step 2. While one EMT holds manual stabilization, two more take positions at the patient's shoulders and pelvis, reaching across the patient and grasping the patient's shoulders and hips, respectively.

YES: _____ RE-TEACH: _____ RETURN: _____ INSTRUCTOR INITIALS _____

Step 3. On command, the three EMTs roll the patient on his side. The patient's arms should be at his side.

YES: _____ RE-TEACH: _____ RETURN: _____ INSTRUCTOR INITIALS _____

Step 4. One EMT pulls the longboard under the patient. The longboard should end at the back of the patient's knees. The bottom of the longboard is at the patient's knees.

YES: _____ RE-TEACH: _____ RETURN: _____ INSTRUCTOR INITIALS _____

Step 5. On command, the patient is rolled back onto the longboard, and the patient is pulled up to the center of the board, using a long axis drag.

YES: _____ RE-TEACH: _____ RETURN: _____ INSTRUCTOR INITIALS _____

Step 6. Once the patient is centered on the longboard, the EMT secures the patient to the longboard and reassesses distal pulses, movement, and sensation.

YES: _____ RE-TEACH: _____ RETURN: _____ INSTRUCTOR INITIALS _____

Skill 31–6 Four-Person Lift

Student Name: _____   Date: _____

Purpose: To immobilize the spine of a supine patient who may have a spinal injury.

Personal Protective Equipment:
Icon — Handwashing — Gloves

Equipment Needed:
Assortment of Cervical Collars
Long Spine Board
Strapping System
Head Immobilization System

Step 1. The first EMT kneels at the patient's head and immediately obtains manual stabilization. The second EMT checks the patient's distal pulses, movement, and sensation and applies a cervical collar.

YES: _____   RE-TEACH: _____   RETURN: _____   INSTRUCTOR INITIALS _____

Step 2. The second EMT then straddles the patient and drops one knee to the ground. Placing his hands under the patient's arms, he grasps the shoulder girdle.

YES: _____   RE-TEACH: _____   RETURN: _____   INSTRUCTOR INITIALS _____

Step 3. A third EMT straddles the patient at the hips and drops his opposite knee to the ground. He then grasps the patient around the hips.

YES: _____   RE-TEACH: _____   RETURN: _____   INSTRUCTOR INITIALS _____

Step 4. On command, all three EMTs gently and evenly lift the patient about 2 inches while a fourth EMT slides the longboard under the patient.

YES: _____   RE-TEACH: _____   RETURN: _____   INSTRUCTOR INITIALS _____

Step 5. Once the patient is properly positioned, the EMTs proceed to immobilize the torso and then the head of the patient. Then the EMTs recheck distal pulses, movement, and sensation.

YES: _____   RE-TEACH: _____   RETURN: _____   INSTRUCTOR INITIALS _____

Skill 31–7 Longboard Immobilization of the Standing Patient

Student Name: _____   Date: _____

Purpose: To immobilize the spine of a standing patient who has a potential spine injury.

Personal Protective Equipment:
Icon — Handwashing — Gloves

Equipment:
Assortment of Cervical Collars
Long Spine Board
Strapping System
Head Immobilization System

Step 1. The EMT approaches the patient from the front and takes immediate anterior head stabilization.

YES: _____   RE-TEACH: _____   RETURN: _____   INSTRUCTOR INITIALS _____

Step 2. Another EMT takes head stabilization from the rear, while the first EMT assesses distal pulses, movement, and sensation.

YES: _____   RE-TEACH: _____   RETURN: _____   INSTRUCTOR INITIALS _____

Step 3. An appropriate-sized cervical collar is applied to the patient.

YES: _____   RE-TEACH: _____   RETURN: _____   INSTRUCTOR INITIALS _____

Step 4. Another EMT places the longboard upright behind the patient and between the arms of the EMT holding stabilization.

YES: _____   RE-TEACH: _____   RETURN: _____   INSTRUCTOR INITIALS _____

Step 5. An EMT then stands on either side of the patient. Another EMT holds the board under the patient's arms and stabilizes the bottom of the board with a foot.

YES: _____   RE-TEACH: _____   RETURN: _____   INSTRUCTOR INITIALS _____

Step 6. Slowly, the board and the patient are lowered to the ground, while the EMT at the head stabilizes the head and neck. Another EMT then immobilizes and rechecks distal pulses, movement, and sensation.

YES: _____   RE-TEACH: _____   RETURN: _____   INSTRUCTOR INITIALS _____

Skill 31–8 Helmet Removal

Student Name: _____   Date: _____

Purpose: To immobilize the spine of a patient who is wearing a full-face helmet and may have a spine injury.

Standard Precautions:
Icon — Handwashing — Gloves

Equipment:
Backboard
Scissors
Assortment of Cervical Collars

Step 1. The first EMT manually stabilizes the patient's head in the helmet, while the second EMT assesses distal pulses, movement, and sensation. Any glasses should be removed at this time.

YES: _____   RE-TEACH: _____   RETURN: _____   INSTRUCTOR INITIALS _____

Step 2. The second EMT then cuts the chin strap, slides one hand under the head, stabilizing the head from below, and places her hand on the jaw, stabilizing the head from above.

YES: _____   RE-TEACH: _____   RETURN: _____   INSTRUCTOR INITIALS _____

Step 3. The first EMT then removes the helmet by spreading the helmet apart gently while moving the helmet from the back of the head.

YES: _____   RE-TEACH: _____   RETURN: _____   INSTRUCTOR INITIALS _____

Step 4. Once the helmet is completely removed, the first EMT assumes manual stabilization of the head. It may be necessary to pad under the head.

YES: _____   RE-TEACH: _____   RETURN: _____   INSTRUCTOR INITIALS _____

Step 5. A cervical collar is then fitted to the patient.

YES: _____   RE-TEACH: _____   RETURN: _____   INSTRUCTOR INITIALS _____

Step 6. With the collar in place, and the head in a neutral position, the EMT rechecks distal pulses, movement, and sensation.

YES: _____   RE-TEACH: _____   RETURN: _____   INSTRUCTOR INITIALS _____

CHAPTER 32

Chest and Abdominal Trauma

OBJECTIVES

Upon completion of this chapter, the reader should be able to:

1. Recognize the impact of chest and/or abdominal trauma.
2. Recognize the signs and symptoms of the following chest injuries:
   Simple pneumothorax
   Tension pneumothorax
   Fractured ribs
   Flail segment
   Pulmonary contusion
   Cardiac contusion
   Pericardial tamponade
   Aortic injury
   Traumatic asphyxia
3. Explain the management of an open chest wound.
4. Explain the management of closed chest injuries.
5. Recognize the signs and symptoms of the following open abdominal wounds:
   Evisceration
   Impaled object
6. Explain the management of the open abdominal wound.
7. Recognize the signs and symptoms of the following closed abdominal injuries:
   Liver and spleen injuries
   Pelvic fracture
8. Explain the management of closed abdominal injuries.

GLOSSARY

cardiac contusion   Bruising of the heart.
evisceration   An abdominal wound with abdominal contents protruding through the wound.
flail segment   An unconstrained portion of the chest.
hemoptysis   Spitting up blood.
hemothorax   Bleeding in between the lung and the chest wall.
paradoxical motion   Movement in the opposite direction.
pericardial tamponade   Blood within the sac around the heart.
petechiae   Small spider-like hemorrhages under the skin.
pneumothorax   Air in between the lung and the chest wall.
pulmonary contusion   Bruising of the lungs.
pulse pressure   The difference between systolic and diastolic blood pressures.
subcutaneous emphysema   Air under the skin and above the chest wall.

sucking chest wound   Air passing in and out of an open chest wound.

tension pneumothorax   Increased intrathoracic pressure that compresses the heart and great vessels.

tracheal deviation   Movement of the trachea from the midline.

traumatic asphaxia   A crushing blow that forces air and blood out of the chest.

PREPARATORY

Materials: EMS Equipment: Exam gloves, stethoscope (dual and single head) (1:6), blood pressure cuffs (adult, infant, and child) (1:6), penlights (1:6).

Personnel: Primary Instructor: One EMT-Basic instructor knowledgeable in patient assessment. Assistant Instructor: The instructor-to-student ratio should be 1:6 for psychomotor skill practice. Individuals used as assistant instructors should be knowledgeable in assessing baseline vital signs and SAMPLE histories.

Recommended Minimum Time to Complete: 2 hours

STUDENT OUTLINE

I. Overview

II. Anatomy Review

III. Chest Trauma

   A. Mechanism of Injury
      1. Blunt Chest Trauma
      2. Penetrating Trauma
   B. Signs and Symptoms
   C. Assessment
   D. Management
   E. Transport
   F. Specific Injuries
      1. Open Chest Wounds
         a) Management of the Open Chest Wound
      2. Tension Pneumothorax
      3. Rib Fractures
         a) Management of Fractured Ribs
      4. Flail Segment
         a) Management of the Flail Segment
      5. Pulmonary Contusion
         a) Management of a Pulmonary Contusion
      6. Cardiac Contusion
         a) Management of a Cardiac Contusion
      7. Pericardial Tamponade
         a) Management of Pericardial Tamponade
      8. Aortic Injury
         a) Management of an Aortic Injury
      9. Traumatic Asphyxia
         a) Management of Traumatic Asphyxia

IV. Abdominal Trauma

   A. Mechanism of Injury
      1. Penetrating Abdominal Trauma
      2. Blunt Abdominal Trauma
   B. Signs and Symptoms of Abdominal Injury
   C. Assessment of Abdominal Injuries
   D. Management of Abdominal Injuries
   E. Transport
   F. Specific Conditions
      1. Liver and Spleen Injuries
         a) Management of Liver and Spleen Injuries
      2. Evisceration
         a) Management of Evisceration
   G. Pelvic Fractures
      1. Management of Pelvic Fractures

V. Conclusion

LECTURE OUTLINE

I. Overview
  A. 50 percent of serious trauma involves chest and/or abdomen
  B. EMTs can have positive impact on survival
    1. Two-thirds arrive at emergency department alive

II. Anatomy Review
  A. Thoracic and Abdominal Cavities

III. Chest Trauma
    1. Core organs involved
  A. Mechanism of Injury
    1. Force applied
      a) Blunt
      b) Penetrating
    2. Blunt Chest Trauma
      a) Mechanism of Injury Key
    3. Penetrating Trauma
      a) Gunshot Wound (GSW)
  B. Signs and Symptoms
    1. General
      a) Chest Pain
        (1) Increases with Respiration
      b) Difficulty Breathing
  C. Assessment
    1. DCAP-BTLS
    2. Subcutaneous Emphysema
    3. Crepitus
  D. Management
    1. Oxygenation
    2. Ventilation
  E. Transport
    1. High Priority
      a) Trauma Center
  F. Specific Injuries
    1. Open Chest Wounds
      a) Pneumothorax
    2. Sucking Chest Wound
      a) Collapse of Lung
    3. Hemothorax
      a) Loss of 1,500 cc Blood
  G. Management of the Open Chest Wound
    1. Occlusive Dressing
    2. Oxygenation
    3. Injured Side Down
    4. Tension Pneumothorax
      a) Collapse of Lung Impinges on Heart
        (1) Hypotension
        (2) Difficulty Breathing
        (3) Jugular Venous Distention
        (4) Tracheal Deviation
    5. Rib Fractures
      a) Symptoms
        (1) Painful
        (2) Point Tenderness
      b) Management of Fractured Ribs
        (1) Stabilization
        (2) Self-Splinting
        (3) Position of Comfort
    6. Flail Segment
      a) Defined
        (1) Two or more ribs fractured in two or more places
        (2) Unstable chest wall segment
        (3) Paradoxical motion
      b) Management of the Flail Segment
        (1) Manual Stabilization
        (2) Dressing Taped in Place
        (3) Internal Splinting
          (a) Positive Pressure Ventilation
    7. Pulmonary Contusion
      a) Lung Bruise
      b) Symptoms
        (1) Soft Crackles
        (2) Chest Pain
        (3) Point Tenderness
        (4) Localized Swelling
        (5) Hemoptysis
      c) Management of a Pulmonary Contusion
        (1) Oxygenation
        (2) Ventilation
    8. Cardiac Contusion
      a) Symptoms
        (1) Heart Bruise
        (2) Impaired Pump Action
        (3) Hypotension
        (4) Skipped Beats
      b) Management of a Cardiac Contusion
        (1) Oxygenation
        (2) ALS Intercept

（a) Cardiac Monitor
9. Pericardial Tamponade
 (1) Blood in Sac Around the Heart
 (2) Symptoms—Beck's Triad
  (a) Narrowed Pulse Pressure
  (b) Jugular Venous Distention (JVD)
  (c) Muffled Heart Sounds
 (3) Management of Pericardial Tamponade
  (a) Surgical Emergency
10. Aortic Injury
 a) Rupture of Great Vessel
  (1) Rapid Decompensation
 b) Management of an Aortic Injury
  (1) Surgical Emergency
11. Traumatic Asphyxia
 (1) Massive Chest Compression
 (2) Symptoms
  (a) Jugular Venous Distention
  (b) Facial Cyanosis
  (c) Petechiae
 (2) Management of Traumatic Asphyxia
  (a) Surgical Emergency

IV. Abdominal Trauma
 1. Mechanism of Injury
  a) Penetrating Abdominal Trauma
  b) Blunt Abdominal Trauma
 2. Signs and Symptoms of Abdominal Injury
  a) Abdominal Pain
  b) Signs of Hypoperfusion
  c) Evisceration
 A. Assessment of Abdominal Injuries
  1. DCAP-BTLS
 B. Management of Abdominal Injuries
  1. Control Hemorrhage
  2. Treat Hypoperfusion
  3. Cover Eviscerations
 C. Transport
  1. High Priority
   a) Surgical Emergency
 D. Specific Conditions
  1. Liver and Spleen Injuries
   (1) Management of Liver and Spleen Injuries
 E. Treat Hypoperfusion
  1. Eviseration
   a) Management of Evisceration
    (1) Nonadherent Dressing
    (2) Stabilize Impaled Objects
  2. Pelvic Fractures
   a) Management of Pelvic Fractures
    (1) Use of MAST

V. Conclusion
 A. Treatment of Chest and Abdominal Trauma
  1. Lifesaving

TEACHING STRATEGIES

1. Consider using a model-victim for several scenarios involving a gunshot, a stabbing, an assault with a blunt weapon, and a severe motor vehicle collision. Encourage the students, as a team, to rapidly assess and treat the patient within the "10-minute" rule.

2. Consider inviting a trauma surgeon to class to discuss serious blunt and penetrating thoracic-abdominal trauma and its impact on lives, and the lives of the patient's family.

3. Consider taking the students on a tour of a trauma center. Have the students note the team approach and the integration of many medical disciplines in the care of the patient.

FURTHER STUDY

Hunt, D. (1997). Thoracic park re-visited. *Emergency Medical Services, 26*(7), 47–57.
Keenan, D., & Phrampus, P. (1999). Puncture pathways. *Journal of Emergency Medical Services, 24*(9), 76–79.

Murphy, P. (1997). Gunshot wounds. *Journal of Emergency Medical Services, 22*(6), 74–79.

Phillips, K. (1997). Prehospital evaluation and care of the abdomen. *Emergency Medical Services, 26*(8), 37–40.

Rhodes, M., & Heightman, A. (1999). Retroperitoneal injuries. *Journal of Emergency Medical Services, 24*(4), 58–64.

Sahni, R. (1998). Chest trauma. *Journal of Emergency Medical Services, 23*(10), 86–90.

Stewart, C. (1999). Prehospital management of cardiothoracic trauma. Emergency Medical Services, 28(9), 37–45.

CASE STUDY   ROLL-OVER

The first sheriff's unit on County Highway 11 reported, "Possible Rollover. No Victim Found." The deputy knew someone had to have been driving the car recently, as the engine was still warm, but he could not find the driver. When the state trooper and the county sheriff arrived, they started a search of the roads and local farmhouses while EMS staged on-scene.

Waiting for the order to "return to service," EMT Clayton went down to inspect the car in the ditch. The crushed roof indicated that the car may have rolled, and the windshield was starred, indicating that someone or something had been thrown forward. The top of the steering wheel was bent, and the directional signal was snapped in two midshaft. Drops of blood were visible across the seat and over the backseat. The rear window appeared to have been kicked out, and blood was evident on the trunk and the ground behind the car.

The radio crackled to life. "Police Unit 4, report from the Eveleigh farm, Route 11, possible prowler, man banging on the front door, appears to be bleeding. Says he needs an ambulance because he can't breathe."

ADDITIONAL CASE STUDY

"Shots fired, officer down, units to assist respond code three to corner of South Pearl and Clinton Avenue, meet the Sergeant. Switch to tac 2. Repeat, all units responding switch to tac 2," the message came over the radio's speaker. Immediately, Ahmed's chest tightened. Ahmed's brother was a police officer. "I wonder if he was shot? I wonder if he wore his vest?" Ahmed thought as he turned on the siren.

Ahmed remembered that even if his brother did wear a bulletproof vest, a gunshot can leave a serious injury underneath the vest even if the bullet does not penetrate it.

STOP AND THINK

1. Based on the mechanism of injury, what injuries might an EMT suspect?
2. What are the assessment priorities for this patient?
3. What are the management priorities for this patient?
4. How could this patient deteriorate?

ANSWERS TO STOP AND THINK

1. Based on the mechanism of injury and the evidence on-scene, the EMT should suspect blunt head, neck, and chest trauma.

2. The chief complaint of trouble breathing would lead the EMT to suspect that the patient may have a life-threatening injury. Therefore, the EMT should perform an initial assessment and focus on the patient's breathing.

3. The first management priority is cervical spine stabilization. Following that, the EMT should manage the difficulty breathing with high-flow oxygen, and control any serious bleeding.

4. The patient could deteriorate from any number of serious head, chest, and abdominal wounds due to the serious nature of the collision.

CASE STUDY FALL   FROM A ROOF

"Where's the paramedic?" asked the triage nurse. Kvar, a new EMT for the Village Ambulance, answered, "His vital signs were stable on-scene, so the medic thought we could take it in alone."

The triage nurse interrupted the conversation to alert the staff to the impending arrival of the patient needing trauma resuscitation. Then she told Kvar, "Look, he has barely has a radial pulse, his heart's racing, and his belly is as hard as a rock. Even a rookie EMT could see this was going to happen!"

Kvar stammered as he replied, "We just thought it was the pai . . . but he looked like a rose!"

Just then, as the team passed the patient from the gurney to the stretcher, the ER physician interrupted. "Tell me the story again."

Kvar answered, "He was replacing his roof, slipped, and fell, oh, maybe 15 feet and landed on his side. His only complaint was that his ribs hurt."

ADDITIONAL CASE STUDY

Jillian moaned as she rolled over in her sleep. She had been out drinking the night before, got into an argument with another woman, and was beaten as a result. All she remembered was rolling into a ball as the woman continued to kick her while she was down. Now her back and her legs ached.

Thinking a little cold water on her face would feel good, she sat up in bed. Immediately, she felt dizzy, like she was going to pass out. Lying back down in bed, she picked up the phone and called 9-1-1.

STOP AND THINK

1. Based on the mechanism of injury, what injuries might an EMT suspect?
2. What are the assessment priorities for this patient?
3. What are the management priorities for this patient?
4. How could this patient deteriorate?

ANSWERS TO STOP AND THINK

1. The lower ribs protect vital organs, such as the spleen and liver. A fall onto those ribs, and the organs lying underneath, could result in serious internal bleeding.

2. While completing the entire initial assessment, the EMT might focus on assessing the patient's breathing and circulation.

3. The management priorities for a trauma patient do not change: stabilize the spine, manage the airway, assist breathing, and control bleeding. This patient would be high-priority and needs rapid transportation to definitive care.

4. This patient has already started to deteriorate. Unchecked, the bleeding could eventually cause the patient to experience a cardiac arrest.

ANSWERS TO TEST YOUR KNOWLEDGE

1. Blunt trauma distributes a force across a broader area of the body than does penetrating trauma. Therefore, penetrating trauma is easier to identify, usually by an opening or wound, but injuries from blunt trauma are harder to recognize because blunt trauma leaves fewer signs on-scene.

2. When a lung collapses, whether from trauma or a medical condition, it creates a simple pneumothorax. When the air in the simple pneumothorax collects, it begins to create a pressure, a tension, against the heart and great vessels. This pressure, or tension, can become so great that the heart's functions are compromised and the patient becomes hypotensive.

3. An open chest wound is immediately sealed with an occlusive dressing, often a gloved hand initially. When the EMT has time he should fashion a three-sided occlusive dressing to cover the wound.

4. The signs of a fractured rib are the same as for any other broken bone: pain, crepitus, point tenderness, and deformity. A patient with a fractured rib also exhibits greater pain with inspiration.

5. The key to managing a flail segment is to control the amount of paradoxical motion. Frequently, the EMT obtains that control, initially, by placing her hands over the flail segment. In less severe cases the EMT may choose to tape the flail segment to control the paradoxical motion. In more severe cases, it may be necessary for the EMT to ventilate the patient with positive pressure from a bag-valve mask device.

6. An evisceration is when abdominal contents, typically small bowel, protrude through a wound in the abdomen.

7. To manage an evisceration, the EMT should first control any serious bleeding, then cover the protruding abdominal organs with a dry sterile dressing. Different regions and states have different management techniques for an evisceration. The EMT should follow local protocols.

8. Blunt trauma to the lower ribs typically produces injury to the lower lobes of the lungs (pulmonary contusion), injury to the solid abdominal organs (liver, spleen, and kidneys) leading to hemorrhage, and injury to the hollow organs (stomach and intestine).

9. A closed abdominal injury can lead to life-threatening hemorrhage. The EMT should treat the patient for hypoperfusion, and ensuing hypotension. High-flow oxygen, positioning the patient supine with legs elevated, and preserving warmth are a few of the immediate actions an EMT can take but rapid transportation to an appropriate facility is imperative.

CHAPTER 33

Cuts and Bleeding

OBJECTIVES

Upon completion of this chapter, the reader should be able to:

1. Identify different types of bleeding.
2. Describe the principles of bleeding control.
3. Describe the purpose of a sterile dressing.
4. Describe the major classifications of wounds.
5. Discuss the indications and contraindications for using a tourniquet.
6. Classify the different types of bandages according to their use.
7. Explain why neck wounds are potentially lethal.
8. Explain the field care of an evisceration.
9. Explain the field care of an amputation.
10. Describe the classification of burn injuries.
11. Explain the care and management of a burn injury.
12. Explain how chemical burns are managed.
13. Describe the injuries that can occur from an electrical injury.
14. Explain the management of an electrical injury.

GLOSSARY

abrasion A type of wound in which the uppermost layer of skin is torn away.

amputation The cutting off of an extremity.

avulsion The forceful separation of an extremity.

bandage A strip of cloth applied to hold a dressing in place.

coagulation The process of blood clotting.

cold zone The area where there is no contamination at a hazardous materials spill.

compartment syndrome A buildup of pressure from swelling within muscle cavities.

compress A cotton dressing integrated into a two-tailed bandage.

conductors Materials that easily carry a current.

contusion The medical term for a bruise, a collection of blood under the skin.

cravat A triangular bandage folded into a band.

crush injury Prolonged pressure on the skin and underlying tissues.

current The passage of electricity through an object.

degloving avulsion The forceful separation of skin from an extremity.

direct pressure Constant firm pushing on the bleeding site.

dressing A sterile absorbent cloth used to cover a wound.

ecchymosis   A wider collection of blood under the skin like a contusion.

elevate   Raising the bleeding site above the level of the heart.

embolism   A physical blockage in the bloodstream.

entrance wound   Damage created as electricity enters the body.

evisceration   Intestines protruding through an abdominal wound.

exit wound   Damage created as electricity exits the body.

fasciotomy   A surgical procedure whereby skin is cut to relieve pressure.

figure-of-eight   A roller bandage that turns across itself.

full-thickness burn   A burn that affects all three layers of the skin.

gauze dressing   Sterile cotton weave cloth.

hematoma   An accumulation of blood under the skin caused by rupture of a large blood vessel.

hemorrhage   Medical term for bleeding.

impaled object   An object embedded in the body.

incision   A cutting of the skin.

inflammation   The body's attempt to prevent infection and begin healing.

insulators   Materials that resist the passage of current.

integumentary system   The cells and tissues that make up the skin.

laceration   A type of wound characterized by a full-thickness tear in the skin.

linear   A straight course of broken skin.

material safety data sheet (MSDS)   A sheet that contains information about specific chemicals and how to treat exposures.

necrotic   Dying tissue.

North American Emergency Response Guidebook (NAERG)   A reference book that gives safety information on a wide variety of chemicals.

occlusive dressing   Impenetrable covering that prevents escape of air and moisture from a wound.

Occupational Safety and Health Administration (OSHA)   The federal organization that monitor's industry safety.

palmar method   A method of determining the percentage of burned skin using the patient's palm.

partial-thickness burn   A burn that affects the epidermis and the dermal layer of the skin.

pressure dressing   A dressing that adds another layer of bandage as well as pressure to an underlying wound.

puncture   A hole created in the skin by a sharp object.

recurrent bandage   A bandage that is laid back and forth across the tape of a dressing, then anchored.

reinforce   Brace or strengthen a bandage.

roller bandage   Cotton cloth rolled into a cylinder for easier control when unwrapping.

rule-of-nines   A formula to determine the percentage of burned skin.

spiral bandage   A roller bandage that is wrapped around a limb.

stellate   A starlike pattern of broken skin.

straddle injury   Damage to the perineal area.

stridor   A low-pitched inspiratory sound heard in constricted airways.

sucking chest wound   Wound in which air moves in and out of the chest cavity.

superficial burn   A burn in which only the uppermost layer of skin is affected.

tattooing   A peppering of gun powder on the skin.

tourniquet   A tight constricting band that stops blood flow to a limb.

trauma dressing   A large cotton dressing placed over a major open wound.

triangular bandage   A 36 x 42 triangular piece of muslin cloth.

universal dressing   Large 9 x 36 gauze dressing.

wound   Damage to the skin as a result of trauma.

Equipment: EMS Equipment: Universal dressing, occlusive dressing, 4 x 4 gauze pads, self-adherent bandages, roller bandages, triangular bandage, burn sheets, sterile water or saline.

Personnel: Primary Instructor: One EMT-Basic instructor knowledgeable in soft tissue injuries. Assistant Instructor: The instructor-to-student ratio should be 1:6 for psychomotor skill practice. Individuals used as assistant instructors should be knowledgeable in soft tissue injuries.

Recommended Minimum Time to Complete: 2 hours

STUDENT OUTLINE

I. Chapter Overview
   A. Anatomy Review
   B. Injury to the Skin
   C. Assessment
      1. Scene Size-Up
      2. Initial Assessment
         a) Bleeding
   D. Management
      1. Principles of Bleeding Control
         a) Dressings
            (1) Types of Dressings
         b) Pressure Dressing
         c) Tourniquet
   E. Transportation
II. Wound Bandaging
   A. Assessment
      1. Scene Size-Up
         a) General Impression
      2. Initial Assessment
      3. Rapid Trauma Assessment
         a) Types of Wounds
            (1) Abrasions
            (2) Lacerations
      4. Incisions
      5. Punctures
      6. Avulsions and Amputations
   B. Management
      1. Bandages
            (1) Principles of Wound Bandaging
               (a) Recurrent Bandage
               (b) Spiral Bandage
               (c) Figure-of-Eight
            (2) Special Bandages
               (a) Neck Wounds
               (b) Sucking Chest Wound
               (c) Evisceration
               (d) Straddle Injury
            (3) Impaled Objects
      2. Avulsions and Amputations
         a) Degloving Avulsions
   C. Transportation
      1. Ongoing Assessment
III. Special Wounds
   A. Assessment
         a) Scene Size-Up
         b) Initial Assessment
         c) Rapid Trauma Assessment
      1. Bruising
         a) Hematoma
      2. Assessment of Contusions
   B. Crush Injury
      1. Compartment Syndrome
   C. Management
   D. Transportation
      1. Ongoing Assessment
IV. Thermal Burns
   A. Assessment
      1. Scene Size-Up
         a) General Impression
      2. Initial Assessment
         a) Rapid Trauma Assessment
            (1) Burn Trauma
            (2) Classifications of Burn Injury
            (3) Burn Severity
               (a) Critical Burns
   B. Burn Management
      1. Burn Field Dressing
   C. Transportation
V. Chemical Burns
   A. Assessment
      1. Chemical Burns
      2. Scene Size-Up
      3. Initial Assessment
      4. Treatment
         a) Dry Chemicals
         b) Wet Chemicals
         c) Eye Injury
VI. Electrical Burns
   A. Assessment
      1. Electrical Burns
      2. Scene Size-Up
   B. Assessment
   C. Management of Electrical Burns
   D. Transportation
      1. Ongoing Assessment
VII. Conclusion

LECTURE OUTLINE

I. Chapter Overview
   A. Impressive Blood Loss
      1. Seldom Life-Threatening
         a) Controlled
   B. Anatomy Review
      1. Integumentary System
         a) Functions
            (1) Protection from Infection
            (2) Maintains Shape/Form
   C. Injury to the Skin
      1. Inflammation
         a) Pain
         b) Clotting
         c) Scarring
   D. Assessment
      1. Scene Size-Up
         a) Blood Visible
         b) Personal Safety
            (1) PPE
      2. Initial Assessment
         a) Bleeding
            (1) Secondary to Airway/
                Breathing
            (2) Simple Measures to
                Control
                (a) Uncontrollable
                    Bleeding
                    (i) High Priority
   E. Management
      1. Principles of Bleeding Control
         a) Reinforce Natural Process
            (1) Clotting
                (a) Dressing
            (2) Vasoconstriction
                (a) Direct Pressure
                (b) Elevation
                (c) Regional Pressure
                    (i) Pressure
                        Dressing
                    (ii) Pulse Point
                        Compression
                    (iii) Tourniquet
         b) Dressings
                (a) Sterile
                (b) Clean Application
            (1) Types of Dressings
                (a) Gauze Dressing
                (b) Trauma Dressing
                (c) Occlusive Dressing

                (d) Universal Dressing
            c) Pressure Dressing
                (1) Conforming Bandage
                   over Dressing
                  (a) Military Field (Com-
                     press) Dressing
         d) Tourniquet
            (1) Last Resort
                (a) Seldom Needed
            (2) Constricting Band
            (3) Pressure Device
                (a) Spanish Windlass
            (4) Left in Place
            (5) Time Noted
   F. Transportation
      1. Function of Control
         a) Low Priority
            (1) Controlled
         b) High Priority
            (1) Uncontrolled
            (2) Hypoperfusion
II. Wound Bandaging
   A. Assessment
      1. Scene Size-Up
         a) General Impression
      2. Initial Assessment
      3. Rapid Trauma Assessment
            (1) DCAP-BTLS
         a) Types of Wounds
            (1) Abrasions
                (a) Debrided Epithe-
                   lium
            (2) Lacerations
                (a) Deep Subendothe-
                   lial Injury
            (3) Incisions
                (a) Surgical Lacerations
            (4) Punctures
                (i) Point Incision
            (5) Avulsions and Amputa-
                tions
                (a) Partial or Complete
                   Removal
   B. Management
         a) Control Bleeding
            (1) Apply Dressing
         b) Maintain Control
            (1) Apply Bandage
      1. Bandages

(1) Principles of Wound Bandaging
   (a) Hold Dressing in Place
      (i) Roller Bandage
      (ii) Triangular Bandage
         (1) Cravat
      (iii) Binders
   (b) Apply Pressure to Wound
      (i) Compress
   (c) Recurrent Bandage
      (i) Large Area
   (d) Spiral Bandage
      (i) Extremity
   (e) Figure-of-Eight
      (i) Joints
(2) Special Bandages
   (a) Neck Wounds
      (i) Air-Occlusive
   (b) Sucking Chest Wound
      (i) Three-Sided Dressing
   (c) Evisceration
      (i) Sterile
      (ii) Moist
      (iii) Nonadherent
      (iv) Heat-retaining
   (d) Straddle Injury
      (i) Diaper Dressing
(3) Impaled Objects
   (a) Immobilization
2. Avulsions and Amputations
   a) Principles
      (1) Control Bleeding
      (2) Retrieve Part
         (a) Cool
         (b) Moist
   b) Degloving Avulsions
C. Transportation
   1. Ongoing Assessment
      a) Assess Dressing
         (1) Tourniquet Effect
         (2) Bleed-Through
            (a) Reinforce Dressing

III. Special Wounds
   A. Assessment
      (1) Entrapment

   a) Scene Size-Up
      (1) Scene Safety First
   b) Initial Assessment
      (1) Life-Threats First
   c) Rapid Trauma Assessment
      (1) DCAP-BTLS
1. Bruising
   a) Hematoma
      (1) Significant Blood Loss
2. Assessment of Contusions
   a) Size
   b) Age
      (1) Black and Blue
      (2) Greenish-Brown
B. Crush Injury
   a) Prolonged Entrapment
   1. Compartment Syndrome
      a) Signs
         (1) Paresthesia
         (2) Pulselessness
         (3) Paralysis
   2. Impact
      a) Toxic Washout
      b) Swelling
         (1) Loss of Peripheral Pulses
            (a) Fasciotomy
C. Management
   1. Rapid Transport
   2. ALS Intervention
      a) Intravenous Fluids
      b) Medications
D. Transportation
   1. Ongoing Assessment
IV. Thermal Burns
   A. Assessment
      1. Scene Size-Up
         a) General Impression
            (1) Safety First
      2. Initial Assessment
         a) Airway
      3. Rapid Trauma Assessment
         (1) Burn Trauma
            (a) Loss of Protective Skin Covering
         (2) Classifications of Burn Injury
            (a) Superficial
            (b) Partial-Thickness
            (c) Full-Thickness
         (3) Burn Severity
            (a) Critical Burns
               (i) Rule of Nines

(1) Greater than 20 percent over 10, less than 50
(2) Greater than 10 percent under 10, over 50
    (ii) Face
    (iii) Hands or Feet
    (iv) Genitalia
    (v) Preexisting Medical Condition

B. Burn Management
  1. Burn Field Dressing
    a) Greater than 10 percent
      (1) Dry Sterile Dressing
    b) Less than 10 percent
      (1) Moist Dressing
C. Transportation
  1. Regional Burn Center

V. Chemical Burns
  A. Assessment
    a) Scene Safety
    1. Chemical Burns
      a) Identify the Source
        (1) Material Safety Data Sheets
        (2) North American Emergency Response Guidebook

        (3) Shipping Manifest
  2. Scene Size-Up
  3. Initial Assessment
    a) Remove the Source
  4. Treatment
    a) Dry Chemicals
      (1) Brush Off
    b) Wet Chemicals
      (1) Wash Down
    c) Eye Injury
      (1) Irrigate

VI. Electrical Burns
  A. Assessment
    1. Electrical Burns
    2. Scene Size-Up
      a) Identify the Source
      b) Duration of Contact
  B. Assessment
      a) Remove the Source
      b) Identify Entrance and Exit Wounds
  C. Management of Electrical Burns
    1. External
      a) Treat as Thermal
    2. Internal
      a) Surgical Emergency
  D. Transportation
    1. Ongoing Assessment
      a) ALS Worthy

VII. Conclusion
  A. First—Protect Yourself
  B. Second—Protect the Patient
  C. Prevent Further Injury
  D. Treat and Transport

TEACHING STRATEGIES

1. Consider inviting a local Red Cross first aid instructor to class. The Red Cross did much of the pioneering work in bleeding control and bandaging and have developed a number of techniques for bandaging wounds.

2. Assemble a large quantity of dressings and bandages. Then give the students a list of bleeding injury sites to bandage. When the students are done the patient should look like an Egyptian mummy.

3. Ask an army medic (91-Bravo) to bring a field kit to class. Ask the medic to demonstrate the methods that the army uses to control bleeding wounds on the battlefield.

FURTHER STUDY

Bozinko, G., Lowe, K., & Reigart, C. (1998). Burns. *RN, 61*(11), 37–40.

Carroll, P. (1999). Chest injuries. *RN, 62*(1), 36–42.

Hansen, S., Paul. C. & Voigt. D. (1999). Chemical injuries. *Journal of Emergency Medical Services, 24*(8), 82–88.

Shellenbarger, T. (2000). Nosebleeds: Not just kid's stuff. *RN, 63*(2), 50–54.

Wiebelhaus, P., & Hansen, S. (1999). Burns; Handle with care. *RN, 62*(11), 52–58.

CASE STUDY PROFUSE BLEEDING

"Oh, that was stupid!" thought Janine. "I'm always in too much of a hurry." While dashing out of the house, Janine had reached for the door, missed the handle, and put her arm through the glass. Instinctively, she had pulled her arm back out, which resulted in a long cut down the length of her forearm. Now she is bleeding profusely.

"This ought to be a trick. How am I going to do this?" Janine ponders as she holds a towel with one hand over the other arm and she looks at the phone. "Maybe I can dial 9-1-1 with my nose." Janine drops the towel, dials 9-1-1, and picks up the towel noticing her arm is bleeding again. A voice on the other end of the phone line says, "9-1-1, what is your emergency?"

"EMS?" Janine asks. "Yes, ma'am," replies the communicator. "I'm bleeding," says Janine, "I cut my arm on some glass and now I'm bleeding and I can't stop it. Can you send help?"

STOP AND THINK

1. What are the immediate priorities in this case?
2. How would an EMT control this bleeding?
3. Is there a life-threat here?

ANSWERS TO STOP AND THINK

1. The first and immediate priority is to control the bleeding.

2. First apply a dressing to reinforce the natural clotting process. If this is ineffective, then the EMT should elevate the affected limb above the level of the heart. If this is ineffective, the dressing will need to be reinforced by a pressure dressing and use of a pressure point to control blood flowing into the area. Finally, if all else fails, the EMT would need to consider a tourniquet.

3. Excessive blood loss with or without continued bleeding can lead to hypoperfusion and shock.

CASE STUDY POSSIBLE STABBING

"Hey man, your back is all wet," Jeremy exclaimed. "Yeah, I'm pretty sweaty after wrestling with that guy back there," Harry explained. Jeremy replied, "No man, look at your shirt, it's darker. Hey, you're bleeding!"

Harry quickly lifted his shirt and looked at his front, while Jeremy looked at his back. Jeremy said, "Hey man, you've been cut! Look here, above your belt, you got a cut. That jerk must have had a knife or something and cut you when you were wrestling."

Harry used his cell phone to call the police. When the police arrived, the officer examined the wound. The bleeding had stopped but the wound looked deep so the officer called for EMS.

STOP AND THINK

1. If the bleeding has stopped, why is EMS needed?
2. What should be the EMT's priorities at this scene?
3. Does this patient need transportation to the hospital?

ANSWERS TO STOP AND THINK

1. While external bleeding may appear to be controlled, the more dangerous internal injuries may continue to bleed.
2. The EMT should initially manage the ABCs, assessing for signs of hypoperfusion. This patient would be a high-priority patient.
3. As a high-priority patient this patient needs immediate transportation to a trauma facility where surgeons are immediately available.

CASE STUDY   CONSTRUCTION ACCIDENT

"Help, I'm trapped," yells Fred. Fred had been working in a ditch when the shoring gave way and tons of sand and rock poured over and around him like an angry river. Now Fred can hardly breathe and is yelling for help.

Fortunately, nearby workers call the local emergency services department immediately. The EMTs in the rescue squad that arrives have just received training with confined space rescue. The rescue squad quickly and efficiently frees Fred from his entrapment and delivers him to the waiting ambulance in a Stokes® basket. Aboard the ambulance is Theola, a new EMT, and her field training officer Sam. "Go ahead, Theola, check him out," Sam directs while he prepares to call for a paramedic intercept from the county.

STOP AND THINK

1. What are the potential harms that could have befallen this patient while he was trapped?
2. What assessment findings could the EMT expect to find when examining the patient?
3. What are the EMT's priorities for managing the patient?

ANSWERS TO STOP AND THINK

1. While the rescue was "quick and efficient," the patient's limbs were entrapped for a prolonged period of time. This could lead to crush injuries.
2. If crush injury is present, the EMT should discover pain, pallor, paralysis, paresthesia, and pulselessness due to compartment syndrome.
3. After assessing and treating any problems discovered in the initial assessment, the EMT should proceed to assess and manage the extremities.

CASE STUDY   MAN DOWN

Josh is sitting on a picnic table watching the firefighters do their thing. He has been assigned to an aid post on the far side of the building while the rest of the crew is busy setting up a rehab station. Bored out of his wits, Josh is starting to wonder if he should ask for relief at his post when the radio crackles, "Firefighter down! Exposure B."

"Exposure B?" Josh thinks, "That's around the corner!" Josh grabs his aid bag and the oxygen and runs to the other side of the building.

On the ground is a firefighter. Other firefighters are already busy stripping the turnout gear off the injured firefighter as smoke rolls off his coat. As Josh approaches the patient, it hits him, that smell, the smell one never forgets, the smell of burned flesh.

STOP AND THINK

1. What are the priorities in the assessment of this patient?
2. What special assessment considerations should the EMT think about?
3. What special transportation considerations should the EMT think about?

ANSWERS TO STOP AND THINK

1. In all cases where a patient is burned, the first priority has to be the airway.
2. The patient who is burned is experiencing a great deal of pain. The patient's complaints of pain can distract the EMT.
3. The patient who is burned should be transported to a burn center as soon as possible provided the airway is controlled.

CASE STUDY   CHEMICAL EXPOSURE

Thatcher was checking the valves and gauges in the plant as a part of his regular duties. "High pressure gauge check, steam release valve tight and check, drainage tube valve tight." As soon as he had spoken the words, the valve over his head blew off, and the hot, steamy chemical solution bathed him from above. Screaming out in pain, Thatcher clawed his way on all fours to the wall. Running his hand across the wall, he found the alarm and yelled into the PA system, "I've got something in my eyes!" Then he reached out and pulled the shower handle, and 50 gallons of water began pouring over his head.

STOP AND THINK

1. What are the priorities in the assessment of this patient?
2. What special assessment considerations should the EMT think about?
3. What special transportation considerations should the EMT think about?

ANSWERS TO STOP AND THINK

1. While an eye injury can be very distracting, it is usually not life-threatening. The EMT should remain focused on initial assessment before proceeding to assess and treat the eye injury.
2. The patient with an injured eye is typically in a great deal of pain. The EMT should explain to the patient that the treatment will help alleviate some of the pain.
3. The patient with an eye injury from a chemical or thermal source should be transported immediately to a burn center if possible. ALS should be intercepted as soon as possible.

CASE STUDY   ELECTRIC SHOCK

As the EMS crew disembarks from the ambulance, the power company foreman approaches them, saying, "He's over there. Got blown clean off the pole. He's got a pulse and is breathing, but he looks pretty shook up." The EMT looks in the general direction in which the foreman is pointing. "Boy, I'll bet that tingled," the EMT says. Then the EMT asks the foreman, "Hey, are the lines safe? I mean, is the power shut down?" "Yeah," the foreman replies, "we shut it down the moment it happened. I called the main switch and told them to keep it shut down until you boys get out of here."

Picking up the ready bages, the EMS crew approaches the patient. Another lineman is already at the patient's head holding manual stabilization of the patient's neck. The patient looks a little pale but is obviously awake and alert. "What hurts you the most?" asks the EMT.

ADDITIONAL CASE STUDY

"Timber!" yells the foreman. The crews are busy trying to harvest the trees before sunset. Suddenly someone yells out, "Help!" The foreman sprints to the side of a fallen lumberjack. His chainsaw apparently kicked back and struck him in the face. As the foreman hits the kill switch to turn off the chainsaw a flickering gleam of light catches his eye—a nail in the tree's stump.

Turning his attention to the fallen lumberjack, he sees a long jagged gash in his left cheek that is vigorously spurting blood. He immediately realizes that he is going to need more help. Sprinting to the skidder, he grabs the mobile radio and calls. "Suzy, this is Charlie on the Northridge."

STOP AND THINK

1. What are the priorities in the assessment of this patient?
2. What special assessment considerations should the EMT think about?
3. What special transportation considerations should the EMT think about?

ANSWERS TO STOP AND THINK

1. Whenever an electrical injury has occurred the EMT's first priority has to be personal safety. The EMT needs to ask, "Is the power shut off? Is the scene safe?"

2. Burn injuries can be deceiving. The external entrance and exit wounds are not representative of the amount of internal injury present.

3. Burn patients should be transported to a burn center immediately.

ANSWERS TO TEST YOUR KNOWLEDGE

1. All bleeding must be controlled. First, apply a dressing. If that is not effective, then the EMT proceeds with direct pressure, elevation, a pressure dressing, use of a pressure point, and, as a last resort, use of a tourniquet.

2. There are three types of bleeding: arterial, capillary, and venous.

3. Dressings are intended to support the body's clotting function and protect the wound from further injury and/or contamination.

4. A tourniquet should only be used as a last resort when all other bleeding control methods fail. If the tourniquet is to remain on for more than 4 hours, then it should be a life versus limb decision.

5. Most bandages are cotton cravats or cotton gauze packaged in a roller. Occlusive dressings are used for special situations.

6. A wound to a neck vein can allow air to be entrained into the wound when the patient takes a breath in. The result is a bubble of air, called an air embolism, in the patient's circulation.

7. The different wound types are abrasions, lacerations, punctures, incisions, avulsions, and amputations.

8. An evisceration should be covered with a nonadherent dressing and then padded with a bulky dressing to prevent further injury.

9. The first priority with an amputation is to control the bleeding at the stump. Typically a bulky dressing will be sufficient. In extreme cases it may be necessary to apply a tourniquet. The next priority would be to find the amputated part and wrap it in a sterile dressing. The amputated part should then be placed in a plastic bag that is cooled on ice.

10. Burns are either superficial burns of the skin (first degree), partial thickness burns of the skin (second degree) and/or full-thickness burns of the skin (third degree).

11. The field care of a burn starts with stopping the burning. Once the burning has stopped, the EMT needs to determine the extent of the burn. If the burn is minor (i.e. less than 10 percent), then a moist dressing is applied. If the burn is greater than 10 percent, then a dry sterile dressing should be applied.

12. If the chemical is still on the patient (the patient is contaminated), then the chemical contaminate represents a danger to the EMT.

13. Electrical burns create an intensive injury that can be compared to an iceberg. The entrance wound could be compared to the tip of the iceberg while the injury under the surface could be compared to the mass of the iceberg that lies just under the surface and extends deep into the body.

14. The field care of the electrical burn begins with identifying the source, then assessing the patient for entrance and exit wounds. After dressing the external wounds, the patient should be treated as a surgical emergency and transported to a trauma center for further care.

CHAPTER 34

Bony Injuries

OBJECTIVES

Upon completion of this chapter, the reader should be able to:

1. List three mechanisms of force that can cause injury to a bone.
2. Describe a ligament and a tendon.
3. Describe and differentiate between a closed and an open fracture.
4. Define when a dislocation becomes an emergency.
5. Describe the common signs and symptoms of a bone injury.
6. List the principles of splinting.
7. Describe the different techniques of splinting.
8. Describe a splinting technique for the following bone injuries:
   a. Collarbone
   b. Shoulder blade
   c. Acromioclavicular dislocation
   d. Shoulder
   e. Upper arm
   f. Elbow
   g. Forearm
   h. Wrist and hand
   i. Hip
   j. Proximal femur
   k. Midshaft femur
   l. Patella
   m. Knee
   n. Lower leg
   o. Ankle
   p. Foot
9. Discuss the importance of differentiating a knee dislocation from a kneecap dislocation.
10. Describe when an EMT can straighten a fracture or dislocation.

GLOSSARY

acromioclavicular (A/C) dislocation A separation of the shoulder and clavicle.

appendicular skeleton The bones of the shoulders, arms, pelvis, and legs.

axial skeleton The bones of the cranium, spine, and thorax.

bipolar traction splint A traction splint with a double shaft.

calcaneus The heel bone.

closed fracture A broken bone in which the bone ends do not break the skin.

Colles fracture A broken wrist that is shaped like a silver fork.

crepitus The sound of bone ends grinding against one another.

direct force The transfer of energy to a point of impact of violence.

dislocation A bone that slips out of joint, and out of alignment.

dorsiflexion Movement of the toes upward, toward the nose.

false motion Movement in the bone where there is not supposed to be movement.

flexible splint Any material that can be formed to fit any angle and then made rigid.

footdrop A loss of nervous control that results in a flaccid foot.

fracture A sudden breaking of a bone.

guarding When a patient attempts to prevent contact with a painful area.

indirect force The transfer of energy as a result of violence away from the point of impact.

ligament The connective tissue that connects bone to bone.

locked A bone that is unable to return to its natural position.

motor nerves The nervous tissue that carries impulses that initiate muscular contraction.

open fracture A broken bone in which the bone ends erupt through the skin.

osteoporosis A softening of the bones from calcium loss.

paralysis An inability to move a limb.

paresis Muscular weakness.

paresthesia A sensation of numbness or tingling.

patella The kneecap.

pelvic girdle The bones of the pelvis and the attached legs.

pneumatic splint A splint that conforms to the shape of the injury by either inflation or vacuum.

point tenderness A finite area that is painful when pressed.

position of function The natural relaxed position of a hand or foot.

range of motion (ROM) The movement that a bone, or limb, is allowed in a joint.

rigid splint Any firm material that can provide support for a limb.

sciatic nerve The primary sensory and motor nerve of the leg.

self-splint When a patient uses his or her body to protect and stabilize a limb.

sensory nerves The nervous tissue that carries impulses of feelings such as pressure or pain.

shoulder dislocation A separation of the scapula and the humerus.

shoulder girdle The scapulas, the clavicles, and the attached arms.

sling and swathe (S/S) The use of a cravat and a triangular bandage to splint a limb.

spontaneous reduction A bone that returns to its natural position, within a joint, without assistance.

sprain A stretch of a ligament or tendon beyond its range of motion resulting in tissue injury.

symphysis pubis The union of the two halves of the pelvis.

tendon The connective tissue that attaches the muscle to the bone.

traction The application of a steady pull inline with an axis.

traction splint A splint that provides a continuous pull along the axis of the bone.

twisting force A turning force of violence.

unipolar traction splint A traction splint with a single shaft.

PREPARATORY

Equipment: EMS Equipment: splints (padded arm and leg, air, traction, cardboard), ladder, blanket, pillow, pneumatic antishock garment, improvised splinting material (e.g., magazines, etc.).

Personnel: Primary Instructor: One EMT-Basic instructor knowledgeable in musculoskeletal injuries and splinting techniques. Assistant Instructor: The instructor-to-student ratio should be 1:6 for psychomotor skill practice. Individuals used as assistant instructors should be knowledgeable in musculoskeletal care and splinting techniques.

Recommended Minimum Time to Complete: 4 hours

STUDENT OUTLINE

1) Overview
2) Anatomy Review
3) Injury
    a) Muscular Injuries
    b) Joint Injuries
    c) Broken Bones
4) Assessment
    a) Scene Size-Up
        i) General Impression
    b) Initial Assessment
        i) Focused Physical Examination
            (1) Signs and Symptoms
    c) Management
        i) Splinting
            (1) Principles of Splinting
                (a) Distal Pulses
                (b) Realigning Bones
        ii) Splinting Devices
    d) Transportation
        i) Ongoing Assessment
5) Injuries to the Shoulder Girdle
    a) Assessment
    b) Management
        (1) Injury of the Clavicle
        (2) Injury of the Scapula
        (3) Injury of the Acromioclavicular (AC) Joint
        (4) Injury of the Shoulder
        (5) Injury of the Upper Arm
        (6) Injury of the Forearm
        (7) Injury of the Wrist and Hand
6) Injuries to the Pelvic Girdle
    a) Assessment
    b) Management
        i) Injury of the Hip
            (1) MAST/PASG Application
        ii) Injury of the Proximal Femur
        iii) Injury of the Midshaft Femur
        iv) Injury of the Patella
        v) Injury of the Knee
        vi) Injury of the Lower Leg
        vii) Injury of the Ankle
        viii) Injury of the Foot
    c) Transportation
        i) Ongoing Assessment
7) Conclusion

LECTURE OUTLINE

1) Overview
   a) Considerable Pain
   b) Typically Non-Life-Threatening
   c) Permanent Disability
2) Anatomy Review
   a) Axial Skeleton
      i) Protects core organs
   b) Appendicular Skeleton
      i) Prone to injury
      ii) Divisions
         (1) Shoulder Girdle
         (2) Pelvic Girdle
3) Injury
      i) Force
         (1) Direct
         (2) Indirect
         (3) Twisting
   b) Muscular Injuries
      i) Connective Tissues
         (1) Tendons
         (2) Ligaments
      ii) Impact Range of Motion
         (1) Importance of MOI
      iii) Injuries
         (1) Sprains
   c) Joint Injuries
      i) Range of Motion
         (1) Importance of MOI
      ii) Dislocation
         (1) Subluxation
      iii) Spontaneous Reduction
   d) Broken Bones
      i) Fractures
         (1) Open
            (a) Eruption Through Skin
      ii) Closed
         (1) Painful, Swollen Deformity
4) Assessment
   a) Scene Size-Up
      (1) Mechanism of Injury
         (a) Violence
            (i) Lines of Force
      ii) General Impression
         (1) Patient Posture
   b) Initial Assessment
      (1) Life-Threats First
      ii) Focused Physical Examination
         (a) DCAP-BTLS
         (2) Signs and Symptoms

(a) Swollen
(b) Painful
(c) Deformity
(d) Pulselessness
   (i) Cynanosis
(e) Paresthesia
(f) Paresis
(g) Paralysis
(h) Crepitus
(i) Point Tenderness
(j) Self-Splinting
(k) Guarding
(l) False Motion
   c) Management
      (1) Manual Stabilization
      (2) Exposure of Injury Site
      (3) Assessment of Distal Function
         (a) Pulses
         (b) Movement
         (c) Sensation
      ii) Splinting
         (1) Purpose
            (a) Prevent Movement
            (b) Prevent Further Tissue
                Damage
            (c) Relieve Painful Spasm
            (d) Control Bleeding
         (2) Principles of Splinting
            (a) Function
               (i) External Support
            (b) Actions
               (i) Manual Stabilization
               (ii) Distal Pulses/Move-
                    ment/Sensation
      1. Radial
      2. Posterior Tibial
      3. Dorsalis Pedis
   (iii) Realigning Bones
      1. Purpose
         a. Position of Function
         b. Return of Distal Pulses
      2. Process
         a. Inline Traction
            i. Resistance
            ii. Pain
   iii) Splinting Devices
      (1) Sling and Swathe
      (2) Flexible Splint
      (3) Rigid Splint

(4) Pneumatic Splint
(5) Traction Splint
   (a) Unipolar
   (b) Bipolar
d) Transportation
   i) Ongoing Assessment
5) Injuries to the Shoulder Girdle
   a) Assessment
   b) Management
      (1) Injury of the Clavicle
         (a) Presentation
            (i) Step-Off
            (ii) Handlebar Deformity
         (b) Treatment
            (i) Sling and Swathe
      (2) Injury of the Scapula
         (a) Presentation
            (i) Rare
               1. Severe Forces
            (ii) DCAP-BTLS
               1. Deformity
                 Unusual
         (b) Treatment
            (i) Sling and Swathe
      (3) Injury of the Acromioclavicular
         (AC) Joint
         (a) Presentation
            (i) Downward Force
            (ii) Step-Off
         (b) Treatment
            (i) Sling and Swathe
      (4) Injury of the Shoulder
         (a) Presentation
            (i) Dislocation
               a. Common
                 Joint
                 Injury
               b. Squared-
                 Off
                 Appear-
                 ance
             2. Anterior
               a. More
                 Common
               b. History of
                 Previous
                 Injury
         (b) Treatment
            (i) Bedroll/Pillow
               Under Arm
            (ii) Sling and Swathe

(5) Injury of the Upper Arm
   (a) Presentation
      (i) Classic Presentation
         1. Swollen,
            Painful
            Deformity
   (b) Treatment
      (i) Padded Board Splints
         Along Axis
      (ii) Sling and Swathe
(6) Injury of the Forearm
   (a) Presentation
      (i) Classic Presentation
   (b) Treatment
      (i) Splint in Position
         Found
(7) Injury of the Wrist and Hand
   (a) Presentation
      (i) Colles Fracture
         1. Silver Fork-Shaped
            Deformity
      (ii) Clavicular Bone Frac-
         ture
         1. Pain in Auto-
            nomic Sniff
            Box
   (b) Treatment
      (i) Splint in Position of
         Function
         1. Holding Bar
            Can
      (ii) Board Splint Along
         Axis
      (iii) Sling and Swathe
6) Injuries to the Pelvic Girdle
   a) Assessment
      i) Severe Force
         (1) Mechanism of Injury
      ii) Point Tenderness
      iii) Inability to Ambulate
   b) Management
      i) Injury of the Hip
         (1) MAST/PASG Application
      ii) Injury of the Proximal Femur
         (a) Presentation
            (i) Foot Drop
            (ii) Pain Upon Compres-
               sion of Insertion
         (b) Treatment
            (i) Maintain Position
               1. Pillows

Between Legs
2. Secure to Long Backboard
iii) Injury of the Midshaft Femur
  (a) Presentation
    (i) Painful
    (ii) Swollen
      1. Significant Blood Loss
  (b) Treatment
    (i) Application of Traction
      1. External Skeleton
        a. Unipolar Device
        b. Bipolar Device
iv) Injury of the Patella
  (a) Presentation
    (i) Mechanism
      1. Twisting Action
    (ii) Lump Lateral
    (iii) Painful
  (b) Treatment
    (i) Stabilization
    (ii) Immobilization
    (iii) Ice to Reduce Swelling
v) Injury of the Knee
  (a) Presentation
    (i) Step-Off
    (ii) Surgical Emergency
      1. Location of Veins, Arteries, and Nerves
  (b) Treatment

(i) Pulses
  1. Immobilize and Transport
(ii) No Pulses
  1. Straighten Position of Function
    a. Immobilize and Transport
vi) Injury of the Lower Leg
  (a) Presentation
    (i) Classic
  (b) Treatment
    (i) Splint Along Axis
vii) Injury of the Ankle
  (a) Presentation
  (b) Treatment
viii) Injury of the Foot
  (a) Presentation
    (i) Deformity
  (b) Treatment
    (i) Pillow Splint
c) Transportation
  (1) Typical Low Priority
  (2) High Priority
    (a) Loss of Distal Function
    (b) Loss of Distal Pulses
      (i) Knee Dislocation
ii) Ongoing Assessment
  (1) Reassess Distal Functions
    (a) Splints Acting as Tourniquets
7) Conclusion
  a) Stick to the Principles

TEACHING STRATEGIES

1. Practice makes perfect and nothing drives the techniques of splinting like drill. A pile of splinting supplies should be placed in the middle of the floor, but only one of each. Assembling all the student teams together, give them all the same bone injury. After each team has finished splinting, check for immobilization of joints above and below. Then have each team present its unique solution to the splinting problem. Several rounds of splinting will reinforce splinting principles as well as encourage problem-solving skills.

CASE STUDY   FOOTBALL INJURY

It was fourth down and a yard to go. There was the snap and the run and another snap, only this time the second snap came from the quarterback's leg. The referees ran to the downed player, then waved EMS onto the field.

The two EMTs followed the athletic trainer, who pulled a stretcher loaded with gear and a backboard. Once they were at the patient's side, an EMT maintained manual stabilization of the player's helmet while the trainer asked, "Roger, where do you hurt?"

"It's my leg," the patient replied. "I think I broke my leg." After a few more questions, both the EMT and the trainer were satisfied that the patient's only injury was in his left leg. The second EMT immediately started to cut the pant leg off the injured leg using a trainer's angel. There was blood at the site of the deformity.

ADDITIONAL CASE STUDY

The Harley™ was on its side and the driver was pinned under it when the ambulance arrived. The pinned biker, Billy-Joe, was cursing and pounding on his leg and yelling that his leg hurt. "Hold on, the fire department's on its way and we'll get that thing off your leg," explained Hunter.

"O.K., lady but you'd better not cut the colors," replied the biker. The bike was stable, so Hunter performed her initial assessment and then tried to do as much of rapid trauma assessment as she could under the circumstances.

STOP AND THINK

1. Based on the mechanism of injury, what injuries might an EMT suspect?
2. What are the assessment priorities for this patient?
3. What are the management priorities for this patient?
4. How could this patient deteriorate?

ANSWERS TO STOP AND THINK

1. Based on the mechanism of injury, the player could have a broken femur, hip injury, or knee injury.

2. The first priority, after the initial assessment, is to stabilize the injured leg. Following stabilization, the EMT should check distal pulses, motion, and sensation.

3. The patient's injured limb should be splinted on-scene after a dry sterile dressing is applied to the wound.

4. If the bone ends cut an adjacent artery, then the patient could potentially lose a significant amount of blood into the thigh. If the bone ends are near a nerve, they could potentially cause direct injury, or swelling could cause indirect injury, resulting in paresis, paresthesia, or paralysis.

CASE STUDY   CLIMBING ACCIDENT

It was Ranger Fish's last winter on the job before he retired. He had seen it all. Campers mauled by bears, campers burned by campfires, campers infected with "beaver fever," but what made him nervous were the ice climbers.

Recently, the Trap Dike, next to Mount Colden, had become a new sensation for ice climbers and it seemed like busloads of them were trekking in for a weekend and a shot at glory. There had already been three major rescues this season and Ranger Fish was carefully watching the newest group of climbers ascend over the waterfalls.

Then it happened. A misstep or a lost point, it did not matter. The climber made a short slide, then fell backward for what seemed like forever. Finally an ice screw grabbed hold and the climber hung in midair, upside down, yelling.

As Ranger Fish made his way across the frozen lake, he could not help but think, "Darn fool kids." The other climbers had already managed to get the injured climber off the ice and onto the ground as Ranger Fish approached. "Hi, what's your name? Where do you hurt?" he asked.

"Steve, and I think I hurt my shoulder," replied the climber. "Do you think you can walk?" asked the ranger. "Sure," Steve replied. "Well, let me check you out," the ranger said, "and then we'll get back to the station." The ranger unslung his backpack and removed the necessary first aid gear.

ADDITIONAL CASE STUDY

"Last one, got to make this last one," Bill grunted as he pulled the dumbbell over his head and let it fall back over his head. At that moment something shifted, there was a sudden pain, and Bill dropped the dumbbell. Letting out a yelp as the weight fell, Bill sat straight up.

Sean, hearing the noise of the crashing dumbbell and Bill's yelp, came running over. "What happened?" he asked. "I think I've screwed up my shoulder again," Bill said as he got up from the bench. Clutching his forearm to his side, Bill proceeded to the locker room. "Look," Sean said, " I'll call EMS."

STOP AND THINK

1. Based on the mechanism of injury, what injuries might an EMT suspect?
2. What are the assessment priorities for this patient?
3. What are the management priorities for this patient?
4. How could this patient deteriorate?

ANSWERS TO STOP AND THINK

1. Based on the mechanism of injury, it would appear that the patient may have a shoulder injury.

2. Ensuring that this patient's only injury is his shoulder. A shoulder injury can produce a significant amount of pain, pain that may distract the patient's attention away from seemingly more minor, but potentially more dangerous, injuries.

3. After ensuring that the patient has no other significant injuries, the EMT should proceed with assessing and stabilizing the injured shoulder.

4. A large bundle of veins, arteries, and nerves run close to the shoulder. An injury to the shoulder could potentially injure these important structures.

CASE STUDY   FALL FROM A HORSE

The horse was galloping along when suddenly its front leg when into a hole. The horse fell sideways, right on top of its young rider, Carolyn.

Realizing immediately what had happened, Katie, the trainer at Three Pines Stables, ran to Carolyn and immediately pulled her from underneath the horse. Carolyn, not comprehending what had happened, tried to stand up but could not. So she remained on her back while Katie ran to the barn to call 9-1-1.

The engine company arrived quickly, and the officer-in-charge ordered two men to get the basket, while the EMT on the crew, Stanley, went to the patient's side.

"Please don't move," Stanley advised his young patient. "My name is Stanley and I am with the fire department. The ambulance is coming from the city but it might be a few minutes. Can you tell me what hurts?"

Carolyn, who was starting to feel the pain, said, "My hip hurts." Stanley started to take a set of vital signs. He looked at the horse and then decided he had better have a paramedic-pumper respond to the scene.

ADDITIONAL CASE STUDY

The cardboard boxes toppled, like dominos, on top of Mona. Mona cried out for help from underneath the heap. The warehouse supervisor, hearing her pained cries, picked up the house phone and told the operator to call out the plant's quick response squad. Marshaling the other workers, the plant supervisor started organizing a detail to unbury Mona.

"Mona, Mona, it's Chris. I'm an EMT. Where does it hurt?" asked Chris, who crawled on his belly to be near Mona's head as the heavy boxes were removed. "Chris, It's my hips. And I can't feel my legs either."

STOP AND THINK

1. Based on the mechanism of injury, what injuries might an EMT suspect?
2. What are the assessment priorities for this patient?
3. What are the management priorities for this patient?
4. How could this patient deteriorate?

ANSWERS TO STOP AND THINK

1. The EMT should immediately suspect a hip and pelvis injury. However, other injuries cannot be dismissed without a physical examination.

2. The first priority with this, and every patient, is to perform an initial assessment. After an initial assessment and a rapid trauma exam, the EMT may want to perform a focused examination of the affected limb.

3. A large number of organs (the bladder, the uterus, the intestine, to name a few) lie in close proximity to and are protected by the pelvis. The pelvis, and the spine, should be stabilized on a long backboard to prevent further injury.

4. A pelvic injury could lead to serious internal injury as well as life-threatening hemorrhage. The patient should be packaged, preferably with a backboard, for rapid transport to a trauma center.

FURTHER STUDY

Payne, B. (1997). Knee trauma. *Journal of Emergency Medical Services, 22*(10), 72–78.

Schultz, C., & Koenig, K. (1997). Preventing crush syndrome. *Journal of Emergency Medical Services, 22*(2), 30–38.

Stewart, C. (1999). Lower extremity trauma part I. *Emergency Medical Services, 28*(4), 43–46.

Stewart, C. (1999). Lower extremity trauma part II. *Emergency Medical Services, 28*(5), 57–59.

Stewart, C. (1999). Prehospital management of crushing injuries. *Emergency Medical Services, 28*(7), 51–55.

Suter, R. (1997). Nontraumatic extremity complaints. *Journal of Emergency Medical Services, 22*(2), 52–58.

Ward, B., & Godbout, B. (1999). Foul play. *Journal of Emergency Medical Services, 24*(7), 66–69.

Wood, S. (1998). Hip fractures and dislocations. *Journal of Emergency Medical Services, 23*(11), 154–158.

ANSWERS TO TEST YOUR KNOWLEDGE

1. The three mechanisms of force are direct force, indirect force, and twisting force.

2. Ligaments attach bone to bone, whereas tendons attach muscles to bone.

3. When a dislocation disrupts either peripheral circulation or neuromuscular function it is considered an emergency.

4. A closed fracture means that the bone ends remain within the limb, whereas an open fracture means that the bone ends have erupted through the skin.

5. The common signs and symptoms of a bone injury include deformity, point tenderness, crepitus, swelling, and pain. Serious bone injuries have muscular weakness (paresis), numbness (paresthesia), and even loss of movement (paralysis) as well as pulselessness.

6. The twelve principles of splinting are:
    1. Always consider life before limb.
    2. Manually stabilize a suspected fracture.
    3. Expose the injury.
    4. Control bleeding.*
    5. Check for pulses, movement, and sensation distal to the injury.
    6. Never allow the patient to bear weight on the injured limb.
    7. Splint in the position found.
    8. Immobilize the joints above and below the injury (if a joint, then the bones above and below).
    9. Elevate the injury above the level of the heart.
    10. Pad the voids between the splint and the limb.
    11. Avoid placing straps directly over the injured area.
    12. Recheck distal pulses, movement, and sensation after the splint is applied.
    *Life-threatening bleeding would have been dealt with during the initial assessment.

7. Splinting techniques include use of a rigid splint, a flexible splint, a pneumatic splint, a sling and swathe, and a traction splint.

8. The following bones can be splinted with the following techniques:

a. Collarbone	Sling and Swathe
b. Shoulder blade	Sling and Swathe
c. Acromioclavicular dislocation	Sling and Swathe
d. Shoulder	Sling and Swathe
e. Upper arm	Rigid Splint
f. Elbow	Flexible Splint
g. Forearm	Rigid Splint
h. Wrist and hand	Flexible Splint
i. Hip	Rigid Splint
j. Proximal femur	Traction Splint
k. Midshaft femur	Traction Splint
l. Patella	Flexible Splint
m. Knee	Flexible Splint
n. Lower leg	Rigid Splint
o. Ankle	Pneumatic Splint
p. Foot	Pneumatic Splint

9. A kneecap (patella) dislocation does not endanger/involve any important adjacent structures. A true knee dislocation can potentially disrupt the popliteal artery, nerves, and veins behind the knee, resulting in significant disability for the patient.

10. When a suspected bone injury (fracture/dislocation) to a joint has interrupted blood flow to a distal limb, the EMT may have to attempt a gentle realignment to reestablish pulse. An EMT will frequently realign a midshaft long bone injury in order to splint the limb.

Skill 34–1 Application of a Bipolar Traction Splint

Student Name: _____   Date: _____

Purpose: To apply a traction device to a possible midshaft femur fracture.

Standard Precautions: Icon — Handwashing — Gloves
Equipment:
Bipolar Traction Splint

Step 1. The EMT applies manual stabilization of the limb while instructing another trained assistant to grasp the leg just above the knee and apply manual stabilization of the affected leg.

YES: _____   RE-TEACH: _____   RETURN: _____   INSTRUCTOR INITIALS _____

Step 2. Then the EMT checks distal pulses, movement, and sensation in the affected leg.

YES: _____   RE-TEACH: _____   RETURN: _____   INSTRUCTOR INITIALS _____

Step 3. The EMT prepares the traction device, adjusting it beyond the length of the uninjured leg and moving the straps into place.

YES: _____   RE-TEACH: _____   RETURN: _____   INSTRUCTOR INITIALS _____

Step 4. Next, the EMT applies the ankle hitch to the ankle and assumes traction of the leg.

YES: _____   RE-TEACH: _____   RETURN: _____   INSTRUCTOR INITIALS _____

Step 5. Then the EMT slides the traction splint under the legs and secures the ischial strap across the thigh.

YES: _____   RE-TEACH: _____   RETURN: _____   INSTRUCTOR INITIALS _____

Step 6. In the last step, the EMT applies the ankle hitch to the ratchet and applies mechanical traction. With the straps in place, the EMT rechecks distal pulses, movement, and sensation.

YES: _____   RE-TEACH: _____   RETURN: _____   INSTRUCTOR INITIALS _____

Skill 34–2 Application of a Unipolar Traction Splint

Student Name: _____ Date: _____

Purpose: To apply a traction device to a possible midshaft femur fracture.

Standard Precautions: Icon — Handwashing — Gloves
Equipment:
Scissors
Unipolar Traction Device

Step 1. The EMT applies manual stabilization of the limb, while instructing another trained assistant to grasp the leg just above the knee and apply manual stabilization of the affected leg.

YES: _____ RE-TEACH: _____ RETURN: _____ INSTRUCTOR INITIALS _____

Step 2. Then the EMT checks distal pulses, movement, and sensation in the affected leg.

YES: _____ RE-TEACH: _____ RETURN: _____ INSTRUCTOR INITIALS _____

Step 3. The EMT prepares the traction device, adjusting it about 3 to 4 inches past the leg.

YES: _____ RE-TEACH: _____ RETURN: _____ INSTRUCTOR INITIALS _____

Step 4. Then the EMT slides the traction splint between the legs, and secures the ischial strap across the thigh.

YES: _____ RE-TEACH: _____ RETURN: _____ INSTRUCTOR INITIALS _____

Step 5. Next, the EMT applies the ankle hitch to the ankle and applies traction of the leg.

YES: _____ RE-TEACH: _____ RETURN: _____ INSTRUCTOR INITIALS _____

Step 6. In the last step, the EMT places the straps in place, and the EMT rechecks distal pulses, movement, and sensation.

YES: _____ RE-TEACH: _____ RETURN: _____ INSTRUCTOR INITIALS _____

CHAPTER 35

Prenatal Problems

OBJECTIVES

Upon completion of this chapter, the reader should be able to:

1. Identify the components of the female reproductive system.
2. Explain how the body changes during pregnancy.
3. Describe the care of the pregnant patient with abdominal pain.
4. Explain how to care for a victim of a sexual assault.
5. Review the risk factors that contribute to complications of pregnancy.
6. Describe the care of the pregnant patient with vaginal bleeding.
7. Explain the care of the woman who is suffering from preeclampsia and eclampsia.
8. Explain what protective mechanisms the fetus has against blunt trauma.

GLOSSARY

abortion   The premature termination of a pregnancy.

cervix   The opening to the uterus at the bottom.

childbirth   The act of delivering a child.

eclampsia   A convulsive disorder seen only during pregnancy.

ectopic pregnancy   A pregnancy that develops outside the uterus.

fallopian tube   The passage between the ovary and the uterus.

fetus   The ovum after it is implanted in the uterine wall.

fundus   The top of the uterus.

miscarriage   A spontaneous termination of a pregnancy.

ovary   The receptacle for a woman's eggs.

ovulation   The release of an egg from the ovary.

ovum   The fertilized egg.

placenta   The interface between the uterus and the fetus.

placenta previa   A condition in which the placenta grows over the cervix opening.

placental abruption   A condition in which the placenta prematurely detaches from the uterine wall.

preeclampsia   A condition of pregnancy that may lead to eclampsia.

quickening   The first movements of the fetus that a mother senses.

sexual assault   A physical and psychological trauma of a sexual nature.

spontaneous abortion Loss of a pregnancy.

supine hypotensive syndrome Compression of the vena cava when a pregnant woman lies flat, resulting in a loss of blood pressure.

uterus A muscular chamber that holds the products of conception; also known as the womb.

PREPARATORY

Materials: EMS Equipment:Childbirth kit, airway management equipment, eye protection, gloves.

Personnel: Primary Instructor: One EMT-Basic instructor familiar with childbirth who has either delivered a child in the out-of-hospital setting or has seen or assisted with a vaginal delivery within the hospital. Assistant Instructor: The instructor-to-student ratio should be 1:6 for psychomotor skill practice. Individuals used as assistant instructors should be knowledgeable in obstetric/gynecological emergencies.

Recommended Minimum Time to Complete: 2 hours

STUDENT OUTLINE

1) Overview
2) Anatomy Review
3) Conception and Pregnancy
   a) The Changes of Pregnancy
4) Abdominal Pain in Women of Childbearing Age
   a) Ectopic Pregnancy
   b) Assessment
   c) Management
   d) Transportation
5) Sexual Assault
   a) Assessment
   b) Management
   c) Transporation
6) Complications in Early Pregnancy
   a) Bleeding During Early Pregnancy
      i) Spontaneous Abortion
   b) Assessment of the Pregnant Woman
   c) Signs and Symptoms
   d) Management
7) Complications of Pregnancy
   a) Bleeding Late in Pregnancy
      i) Placental Abruption
      ii) Placenta Previa
   b) Toxemia of Pregnancy
      i) Preeclampsia
      ii) Eclampsia
   c) Management
8) Blunt Abdominal Trauma
   a) Assessment
      i) Scene Size-Up
         (1) Falls
         (2) Intentional Trauma
         (3) Motor Vehicle Collisions
   b) Assessment
   c) Management
   d) Hypoperfusion in Pregnancy
      i) Transportation
9) Conclusion

LECTURE OUTLINE

1) Overview
   a) Risk
      i) Bodily Changes
   b) Benefits
      i) Newborn
2) Anatomy Review
   a) Uterus
      i) Womb
      ii) Fundus
      iii) Cervix
   b) Vagina
      i) Birth Canal
3) Conception and Pregnancy
      i) Ovulation
         (1) Ovum
      ii) Fertilization
         (1) Fetus
   b) The Changes of Pregnancy
      i) Placenta
         (1) Fetal Circulation
            (a) Hypoperfusion
4) Abdominal Pain in Women of Childbearing Age
   a) Etiology
      i) Pregnancy
         (1) Potentially Life-Threatening
   b) Ectopic Pregnancy
      i) Pregnancy Outside Uterus
   c) Assessment
      i) Lower Abdominal Pain
      ii) Scant Vaginal Bleeding (Possible)
      iii) Signs of Hypoperfusion
   d) Management
      i) Abdominal Pain in Woman of Childbearing Age is Ectopic Until Proven Otherwise
      ii) Treat Hypoperfusion
   e) Transportation
      i) High Priority
      ii) ALS Intercept
         (1) Intravenous Fluids
5) Sexual Assault
      i) Violence
         (1) Physical Trauma
         (2) Psychological Trauma
   b) Assessment
      i) Life-Threats First
      ii) Limited Exam

         (1) Same-Sex EMT
         (2) Confidential Discussion
   c) Management
      i) Criminal Complaint
         (1) Voluntary
      ii) Evidence
         (1) Brown Paper Bag
         (2) Chain of Evidence
      iii) Cleansing
         (1) Avoid Showers, Urination, Douche, etc.
   d) Transporation
      i) Low Priority
6) Complications in Early Pregnancy
   a) Bleeding During Early Pregnancy
      i) Spontaneous Abortion
         (1) Miscarriage
            (a) Loss of Pregnancy
   b) Assessment of the Pregnant Woman
   c) Signs and Symptoms
      i) History
         (1) Expected Date of Delivery (EDD)
         (2) Prenatal Care
         (3) Complications
         (4) Past Medical History
            (a) History of Pregnancy
               (i) Live versus miscarrage
   d) Management
      i) Treat Hypoperfusion
      ii) Vaginal Bleeding
         (1) Sanitary Napkin
      iii) Save Tissue/Clots
7) Complications of Pregnancy
      i) Infant Survival Likely
   b) Bleeding Late in Pregnancy
      i) Placental Abruption
         (1) Detachment of Placenta from Uterine Wall
         (2) Abdominal Pain
      ii) Placenta Previa
         (1) Low Attachment of Placenta
            (a) Leakage
               (i) Cervical Opening (Os)
   c) Toxemia of Pregnancy
         (1) Poisoned Pregnancy

(2) Fluid and Electrolyte Imbalances
  ii) Preeclampsia
    (1) Hypertension
    (2) Fluid Retention
    (3) Headaches
  iii) Eclampsia
    (1) Seizures
  d) Management
    i) No Bright Lights
    ii) No Vaginal Examinations
    iii) Left Lateral Recumbent
    iv) Treat Hypoperfusion
8) Blunt Abdominal Trauma
  a) Assessment
    i) Scene Size-Up
      (1) Falls
        (a) Center of Balance
      (2) Intentional Trauma
        (a) Domestic Violence

(3) Motor Vehicle Collisions
    (a) Improperly Worn Seatbelt
  b) Assessment
    i) Late Pregancy
      (1) Post Quickening
      (2) DCAP-BTLS
  c) Management
    i) Treat Hypoperfusion
      (1) Pecking Order
        (a) First Fetus
  d) Hypoperfusion in Pregnancy
    i) Transportation
      (1) Left Lateral Recumbent
        (a) Supine Hypotensive Syndrome
      (2) Destination
        (a) Consider Surgical Capabilities
9) Conclusion

TEACHING STRATEGIES

1. Consider having a sexual assault nurse examiner (SANE) or sexual assault victims examiner (SAVE) come to class and explain the manner and methods that they use when they are called into the hospital for a patient.

2. Consider asking a woman in advanced pregnancy to come to class to discuss the changes that have occurred in her body, some of the difficulties that she has experienced, and what her experience has been with other health care providers.

CASE STUDY   ABDOMINAL PAIN

"Mom, I'm going to stay home! I don't feel so well," Erin yelled down the stairs. "OK, Honey, but you'll miss your senior picture. Call me at the office if you get worse," her mother yelled back as she went out the front door.

Her mother had been at work less than an hour when the phone rang. "Mom, I really hurt," Erin cried. Her mother said, "Look, I'm coming home and I'll call the ambulance as soon as I hang up." Mrs. Ward then called the local emergency number and explained to the operator how to locate the house, where the emergency house key was, and that she would be home in about 30 minutes.

"Hello! It's Officer McCall, Cherry Valley Police. Hello!" cried out the police officer as he entered the house. "Here!" Erin replied. Led by Officer McCall, the ambulance crew walked toward the low sounds of sobbing and into the living room. The girl was curled in fetal position on the sofa, with the phone on the floor, and obviously had been crying for some time. "My belly hurts, it really hurts!" she said.

ADDITIONAL CASE STUDY

The middle school nurse met the ambulance crew at the front door and escorted them to the office. As she walked with the crew she explained, "I thought it was the stomach flu, it's been going around you know, then she started to get really uncomfortable. She was tachycardic before but when her blood pressure started to drop I decided to call EMS. By the way, her mother is on her way."

"Hi, Mary, my name is Jennifer and I'm an EMT," said Jennifer as she closed the curtain behind her, "What's bothering you today?" Mary winced as she straightened from her fetal position to point at her left lower quadrant.

STOP AND THINK

1. Based on the patient presentation, what medical conditions might an EMT suspect?
2. What are the assessment priorities for this patient?
3. What are the management priorities for this patient?
4. How could this patient deteriorate?

ANSWERS TO STOP AND THINK

1. Any female of childbearing age with lower abdominal pain should be suspected of having an ectopic pregnancy until proven otherwise. While other possibilities exist, including appendicitis, for example, the most life-threatening possibility is an ectopic pregnancy.

2. After the initial assessment demonstrates that the patient is not hypotensive and going into shock, the EMT should focus the examination on her abdomen. Some women also experience scant vaginal bleeding. The EMT should inquire about the use of vaginal pads, and if affirmative, start a pad count.

3. The management priorities for this patient include administering high-flow oxygen, treating the patient for hypoperfusion, and transporting to a hospital with surgical capabilities.

4. If an ectopic pregnancy ruptures, the patient will suffer massive hemorrhage that could lead to severe shock and death.

CASE STUDY   RAPE

Officer Gould was making her usual rounds on campus, when her radio crackled and a message came across the air. The dispatcher announced, "Units in the vicinity of the soccer field, acknowledge and respond to the south end for a panic alarm activation."

Officer Gould, who was near the soccer field, responded to the dispatcher with "on-scene" as the first arriving unit. As she looked she saw a young woman, maybe in her late teens, standing behind a tree.

As she moved closer, Gould could see that the young woman was partially clothed and that she was valiantly trying to hold up the remains of her shirt to cover her chest. The words the young woman spoke cut through the cold night air like a knife. "I've been raped," the woman told the officer.

ADDITIONAL CASE STUDY

Feeling a little more groggy then usual from the night before celebration, Yolanda braced herself and stood up. Only then did she notice that she was wet. Confused, because her period ended a week ago, she went into the bathroom. Taking her pants down she discovered that she didn't have on any underwear. She always wore underwear. Then her foggy memory of the night before started to clear up. She had been drinking, felt like she was going to pass out, and someone offered to carry her to her dorm room. "Who was he?" she thought to herself. Well, it didn't matter. "I think I've been raped."

STOP AND THINK

1. Based on the patient presentation, what injuries might an EMT suspect?
2. What are the assessment priorities for this patient?
3. What are the management priorities for this patient?
4. How could this patient deteriorate?

ANSWERS TO STOP AND THINK

1. Rape victims may suffer tears to the vagina and rectum; however most are not life-threatening.

2. If at all possible, a same-sex EMT should be performing the assessments. Without minimizing the impact of the rape, the EMT must remember that rape is about control and often battering occurs along with the rape. The EMT should assess the patient, to the degree possible, for signs of a beating, such as abrasions and contusions to the torso, lacerations of the scalp, fractures of the face, and the like. If possible, a rapid trauma assessment may be in order.

3. Barring life-threatening injuries, the EMT should focus his or her management on meeting the psychological needs of the patient and transporting her to the emergency department. While rape is a crime, the patient has the right to not report the crime and the EMT must respect that right. If any clothing, particularly underclothing, is removed, it should be placed in a brown paper bag. Finally, the patient should be discouraged from cleansing the area immediately.

4. If the patient suffered a battering during the rape, it is possible that she could hemorrhage from internal wounds.

CASE STUDY   EXCESSIVE BLEEDING

The EMT team and sheriff's deputy were met at the door by a middle-aged woman who reeked of cigarette smoke. "It's my daughter, she's in the bathroom." With those words, the woman turned around, sat down in her chair, and continued to watch the soap opera on television.

Walking in single file down the narrow hallway, the team came to a closed bathroom door. From behind the closed door came a muffled "I'll be right there." In about a minute, the door opened and a teenaged girl motioned Shelley, one of the EMTs, inside, and indicated that the men should stay out.

"Look," the girl started, "I'm pregnant, but my momma don't know. I'm bleeding down there," she pointed at her crotch. "More than usual. I told Momma I had the diarrhea so she'd call EMS." While listening to the girl's story, Shelley peered into the toilet. It was full of blood.

ADDITIONAL CASE STUDY

"Not again," thought Samantha. Samantha had already lost two babies early in pregnancy and she was hopeful, with the new medicine, that she would not lose this one. But here she was lying on the floor, bleeding heavily. Her husband frantically called 9–1-1 and was waiting at the door for the ambulance.

Fortunately, the ambulance was literally around the corner and arrived in moments. When the first EMT, David, entered the room, he saw the patient lying on the floor. She was ghostly pale and covered in sweat. Wasting no time he called out to his driver, "Call for the paramedics!" then knelt next to his patient.

STOP AND THINK

1. Based on the patient presentation, what medical conditions might an EMT suspect?
2. What are the assessment priorities for this patient?
3. What are the management priorities for this patient?
4. How could this patient deteriorate?

ANSWERS TO STOP AND THINK

1. A woman who is bleeding, after a confirmed pregnancy, may be suffering a spontaneous abortion (miscarriage).

2. This patient needs to be assessed for signs of hypoperfusion during the initial assessment. The EMT is going to need to know if the patient has had any prenatal care, if she knows her expected date of delivery (EDD), if she has been pregnant in the past, and if there were any complications.

3. The EMT should focus on treating the hypoperfusion and transporting the patient to the emergency department. Sanitary napkins will help collect the blood. Any tissue or clots should be preserved.

4. While the likelihood of a spontaneous abortion is high, other life-threatening possibilities do exist, particularly placenta previa.

CASE STUDY   VAGINAL BLEEDING

"Dr. Fitz's office," the receptionist announced. "Did someone there call EMS, Ma'am?" asked EMT Waite. "Yes, please come in," replied the receptionist. "Down to the end of the hall, last door on the left. The nurse will meet you there."

Pulling the stretcher behind them, the two EMTs went down the narrow hall to the last door on the left and knocked on the door. "Come in," shouted a voice from within.

The EMTs were then led to the cramped examining room, where they met their obviously pregnant patient.

"Hello," EMT Waite said to the patient. Immediately the nurse provided a long patient history that included 26 weeks of pregnancy and heavy painless vaginal bleeding for the past 2 hours.

The last remark was like a slap in the face for the EMTs. Heavy, painless vaginal bleeding for 2 hours! The two EMTs immediately leapt into action.

ADDITIONAL CASE STUDY

"Please come on in," said the gentleman at the door. "My name is Peter and this is my wife Naomi." Peter explained that his wife, who was in her last month of pregnancy, was bleeding and how they called the doctor and he told them to call an ambulance.

"Listen, the doctor was very specific. He said this was no emergency and to tell you guys to take her to the hospital without lights and siren so that he could examine her. Can you do that?"

"Well, sir, let's talk to your wife first and let me get her vital signs before we make any decisions," said the EMT.

STOP AND THINK

1. Based on the patient presentation, what medical conditions might an EMT suspect?
2. What are the assessment priorities for this patient?
3. What are the management priorities for this patient?
4. How could this patient deteriorate?

ANSWERS TO STOP AND THINK

1. Bleeding late in pregnancy would make the EMT suspect a problem with the placenta's placement—perhaps placenta previa.

2. The EMT should focus assessment on signs of hypoperfusion. It is inappropriate for an EMT to perform a vaginal exam; instead ask the patient if she is bleeding or leaking.

3. The first priority would be high-flow oxygen, followed by other supportive treatments intended to hold off the hypoperfusion.

4. Continued bleeding could threaten the fetus and even possibly induce premature labor.

CASE STUDY   SPOUSAL ABUSE

As the EMTs parked the ambulance, they could see a police officer leading a man away from the house in handcuffs. Puzzled by what they were seeing, EMT Nabinger approached the police supervisor, Sargent McNally and inquired, "What's going on? We got a call for a woman who had fallen."

"More like pushed, down a flight of stairs," Sergeant McNally replied. "She's over there, in the patrol car. Look, I've got to take a statement, so do you mind if I listen in while you guys get your history?"

"It's entirely up to her but as far as I'm concerned, you're welcome to come," replied Nabinger. As McNally turned to wave down a passing patrol car with its red lights flashing, he added, "Oh, by the way, she's six months pregnant. I'll be right with you in a minute."

"Six months pregnant," Nabinger thought. He felt his stomach begin to knot.

ADDITIONAL CASE STUDY

"I swear. I fell down the stairs and hit my belly," said the woman, who appeared to be cowering a little from the man behind her who was standing with his arms crossed over his chest, glaring down on the EMT.

"Look, buddy, just take her to the hospital and stop asking your fool questions," demanded the man. Sensing the hostility, the EMT elected to package the patient and perform the rest of the assessment in the back of the ambulance.

"Sir, I take it you will be following the ambulance in your car?" asked the EMT hopefully.

STOP AND THINK

1. Based on the patient presentation, what injuries might an EMT suspect?
2. What are the assessment priorities for this patient?
3. What are the management priorities for this patient?
4. How could this patient deteriorate?

ANSWERS TO STOP AND THINK

1. Unfortunately, the focus of many domestic violence attacks are upon pregnant women. The pregnant woman who has been assaulted should be suspected to have sustained injuries to the uterus, possibly leading to placenta abruptio.

2. After an initial assessment has been made for signs of hypoperfusion, the EMT should focus on the abdomen. Is the baby moving? Is the woman bleeding or leaking from the vagina?

3. The patient should be treated for shock, as appropriate, and transported in the left lateral recumbent position, to prevent supine hypotensive disorder. A decision should be made to transport to a hospital with surgical capabilities.

4. If the placenta does detach, the patient may experience premature labor. The EMT should be prepared for a field delivery of a premature infant.

FURTHER STUDY

Cascio, A., & Polk, D. (1997). Trauma in the pregnant patient. *Journal of Emergency Medical Services*, *22*(8), 90–97.

Gregoire, A. (1997). When the trauma patient is pregnant. *RN*, *60*(2), 44–50.

Mattera, C. (1999). Obstetrical complications. *Journal of Emergency Medical Services*, *24*(3), 124–128.

Phillips, K. (1996). Teen abortion. *Emergency Medical Services*, *25*(5), 41–43.

ANSWERS TO TEST YOUR KNOWLEDGE

1. Starting from the outside: vagina, cervix (also called Os), uterus, fallopian tubes, and ovaries.

2. As the pregnant uterus enlarges, it starts to crowd other pelvic organs, including the bladder and the intestines. The blood volume of the pregnant woman starts to increase as well, to accommodate the demands of the uterus.

3. As the uterus grows it leaves the protective confines of the pelvis, making it more susceptible to injury from trauma. The pregnant, or gravid, uterus also moves a woman's center of gravity, making her more susceptible to falls.

4. A sexual assault victim should be treated by a same-sex EMT whenever possible. The EMT should make the discussion as private and confidential as possible, permitting the patient control over the situation and questions.

5. The early sign of placenta previa is leakage of uterine contents, such as blood and amniotic fluid—what is commonly referred to as *spotting*.

6. The fetus is somewhat protected by the uterus during pregnancy. During early pregnancy, the uterus lies within the protective confines of the bony pelvis. As the pregnancy develops, the fetus is bathed in and protected by a pool of amniotic fluid that acts like a hydraulic cushion.

7. The patient with preeclampsia should not be exposed to bright lights or excessive stimulation, like the type that lights and sirens produce. The EMT should not perform a vaginal examination; rather, the patient should be placed in the left lateral recumbent position and transported quietly.

CHAPTER 36

Childbirth

OBJECTIVES

Upon completion of this chapter, the reader should be able to:

1. Describe the normal female anatomy during pregnancy.
2. Describe the components of the three stages of labor.
3. Identify signs and symptoms of impending delivery.
4. Recognize the importance of a brief predelivery history.
5. Describe how to assist with a normal delivery in the field.
6. Identify the presentation and the prehospital management of a prolapsed umbilical cord.
7. Describe how to manage a breech or a limb presentation.
8. Describe special considerations with the passage of meconium-stained amniotic fluid.
9. Identify special considerations associated with multiple gestations or premature delivery.
10. Describe the proper care of the mother postdelivery.

GLOSSARY

amniotic sac   The membranous sac that surrounds the fetus and placenta within the uterus.

bloody show   The expulsion of a small amount of bloody mucus from the cervix as the cervix begins to thin.

braxton hicks contractions   Random contractions that occur in the third trimester that are not associated with cervical effacement or dilation; also known as "false labor."

breech presentation   The presentation of a foot or buttocks instead of the fetal head.

cardinal movements of labor   The series of natural movements the infant makes upon descent through the birth canal.

cervical dilation   Progressive opening of the cervix that occurs as the fetal head descends into the pelvis.

cesarean section   The surgical removal of a newborn from the uterus through an abdominal incision.

crowning   The term used to describe the appearance of the fetal head at the vaginal opening when delivery is imminent.

effacement   Thinning of the cervix that occurs as a pregnancy nears its conclusion.

first stage of labor   The process of cervical effacement and dilation.

gravidy   The total number of pregnancies a woman has had.

labor   The process by which the uterus expels the fetus and placenta.

meconium   Fetal stool.

molding   Movement of the fetal cranial bones as the fetus passes through the birth canal.

multiparous   A term used to describe a woman who has previously had children.

parity   The total number of live children born to a woman.

premature delivery   A delivery that occurs prior to 36 weeks of gestation.

primiparous   A term used to describe a woman who is in her first pregnancy.

prolapsed umbilical cord   The presentation of the umbilical cord prior to the infant, resulting in compression of the cord.

second stage of labor   The phase of childbirth that begins when the cervix is completely dilated and ends with the delivery of the infant.

third stage of labor   The last stage of labor during which the placenta is delivered.

PREPARATORY

Materials: EMS Equipment: Childbirth kit, airway management equipment, eye protection, gloves.

Personnel: Primary Instructor: One EMT-Basic instructor familiar with childbirth who has either delivered a child in the out-of-hospital setting or has seen or assisted with a vaginal delivery within the hospital. Assistant Instructor: The instructor-to-student ratio should be 1:6 for psychomotor skill practice. Individuals used as assistant instructors should be knowledgeable in obstetric/gynecological emergencies.

Recommended Minimum Time to Complete: 2 hours

STUDENT OUTLINE

(1) Chapter Overview

(2) Anatomy Review

(3) Normal Childbirth

    a) Stages of Labor

        i) Stage One

        ii) Stage Two

        iii) Stage Three

4) Emergency Childbirth

    a) History

    b) Assessment

    c) Preparation for Delivery

    d) Normal Delivery

5) Special Delivery Scenarios

    a) Prolapsed Umbilical Cord

        i) Signs and Symptoms

        ii) Management by the EMT

    b) Breech Presentation

        i) Signs and Symptoms

        ii) Management by the EMT

    c) Meconium

        i) Signs and Symptoms

        ii) Management by the EMT

    d) Multiple Gestation

        i) Signs and Symptoms

        ii) Management by the EMT

    e) Premature Delivery

        i) Signs and Symptoms

        ii) Management by the EMT

6) Postdelivery Care

    a) Mother

    b) Infant

7) Conclusion

LECTURE OUTLINE

1) Chapter Overview
    a) Field Birth Uncommon
    b) Frequent In-Service Necessary
2) Anatomy Review
    a) Fetus/Infant
    b) Uterus
        i) Amniotic Sac
    c) Placenta
        i) Umbilical Cord
    d) Vaginal Canal
        i) Cervix
3) Normal Childbirth
        i) Progressive
    b) Stages of Labor
        i) Stage One
            1) Mucous Plug
                a) Bloody Show
            2) Onset of Contractions
        ii) Stage Two
            1) Cervix Dilated
            2) Infant Delivery
                a) Crowning
            3) Birth
        iii) Stage Three
            1) Delivery of Placenta
            2) Uterine Contractions
4) Emergency Childbirth
    a) History
        i) Expected Date of Delivery (EDD)
            1) Due Date
        ii) Complications of Pregnancy
        iii) Number of Babies
        iv) Color of Amniotic Fluid
            1) Green-tinged
        v) Past Pregnancies
        vi) Number of Live Births
    b) Assessment
        i) Membranes Ruptured
        ii) Contractions
        iii) Crowning
    c) Preparation for Delivery
        i) Body Substance Isolation
        ii) Medical Control
        iii) Set-Up
    d) Normal Delivery
        i) Mother Supine
            1) Knees to Chest
            2) Head Elevated
        ii) Drape Vaginal Opening

        iii) Break Amniotic Sac as Needed
        iv) Assist Infant's Head
            1) Unloop or Clamp/Cut Umbilical Cord
        v) Suction Mouth and Nose
        vi) Assist Shoulders Down Then Up
        vii) Support Infant's Body
        viii) Clamp Umbilical Cord
        ix) Infant to Mother's Breast
        x) Deliver Placenta
        xi) Transportation
5) Special Delivery Scenarios
    a) Prolapsed Umbilical Cord
            1) Delivery of Umbilical Cord First
        ii) Signs and Symptoms
            1) Visible Cord
                a) Pulsations Usually Present
        iii) Management by the EMT
            1) 100% Oxygen to Mother
            2) Sims Position (Buttocks Up)
            3) Contact Medical Control
    b) Breech Presentation
            1) Buttock or Limb Presentation
        ii) Signs and Symptoms
            1) Buttocks or Limb(s) Visible
        iii) Management by the EMT
            1) Same as Prolapsed Cord
    c) Meconium
            1) Infant's First Stool
            2) Respiratory Compromise
        ii) Signs and Symptoms
            1) Green-Tinged Amniotic Fluid
                a) Ranges from Green Water to Pea Soup
        iii) Management by the EMT
            1) Suction Oropharnyx
            2) ALS Intercept
    d) Multiple Gestation
            1) Twins/Triplets
        ii) Signs and Symptoms
            1) Mother's Ultrasound
        iii) Management by the EMT
            1) Prepare for Two or More Deliveries
    e) Premature Delivery
            1) Birth Before 36 Weeks
        ii) Signs and Symptoms
            1) Normal Labor
        iii) Management by the EMT

1) Normal Delivery
2) Hypothermia
6) Postdelivery Care
a) Mother
i) Control Bleeding
1) Breast-Feeding
2) Uterine Massage
b) Infant
i) APGAR Scoring
1) One Minute
a) Acrocyanosis
2) Five Minutes
ii) Hypothermia
7) Conclusion
a) Natural Process
i) Little Assistance

TEACHING STRATEGIES

1. Consider borrowing a pregnancy vest from a childbirth class. These vests allow both male and female EMT students to "feel" what it is like to be pregnant. Have a student act in the role of a mother about to deliver and have the other EMTs assess the mother, gathering vital signs as well as a history.

2. Consider having the class view a childbirth tape. There are many excellent childbirth videos on the market. These videos allow the students to see and hear what occurs in an actual delivery.

3. Consider inviting a childbirth educator to the class. Ask the childbirth educator to review natural birthing techniques, like LaMaze, and also review the role of the nurse-midwife during a delivery.

CASE STUDY DELIVERY

"This has got to be the biggest snowstorm on record," said Mike as he stirred his coffee and looked out the window. The words had barely left Mike's lips when the call went out. "Woman in labor, contractions less than 4 minutes apart. 200 Ponderosa."

Fortunately, a county snowplow was standing by for just such an emergency. The snowplow quickly swung onto the ambulance ramp and cleared a wide path, then proceeded, at about 20 miles per hour, toward 200 Ponderosa. The ambulance followed it.

After what seemed like forever, the ambulance finally arrived. Grabbing the obstetrics kit as well as the first-in bag, Mike went to the door and knocked. He was met at the door by a middle-aged man who ushered the crew into a second-floor bedroom.

Sitting up in a knees-to-chest position was a woman in her mid-thirties who was panting. Around the bed were three other children, all playing and seemingly oblivious to their mother's situation.

"Hi, my name is Mike. What's your name?" Mike asked. "Hi, my name is Dawn," the patient replied, "and this isn't what I had planned. The nurse-midwife was supposed to be here by now." Mike was quick to reply. "It's understandable, the snow is about 3 feet deep now. Tell me, how do you feel?"

Dawn stopped panting, and looked at Mike and said, "I feel like pushing!"

ADDITIONAL CASE STUDY

Approaching the farmhouse, the EMT could see and smell the smoke from the woodstove. He was being waved into the house by a burly man who was yelling, "My wife is having a baby!"

Going through the kitchen the EMT noticed that the water was well water from an old-fashioned hand pump and that there were few electric lights. He ducked as he entered the bedroom and on top of an overstuffed quilt was a woman in her early twenties. Using his flashlight to look around the room, he noted that the quilt was soaking wet.

"Look, sir, could you get us some clean sheets, start to boil some water, and please take the dog in another room," asked the EMT.

STOP AND THINK

1. What are the signs of impending delivery?
2. What should be included in the assessment of a woman in labor?
3. What equipment should the EMT prepare if he thinks childbirth is imminent?
4. What should the EMT do if the umbilical cord presents first?
5. What should the EMT do if the infant's buttocks present first?
6. What would the EMT do if the amniotic fluid were green-tinged?
7. What would the EMT do if the patient said "I'm having twins"?
8. What would the EMT do if she is delivering ahead of schedule?
9. What should the EMT do for the mother after the delivery?
10. What should the EMT do for the infant after the delivery?

ANSWERS TO STOP AND THINK

1. The classic sign of an impending childbirth is the urge to push. Other signs include frequent labor pains, crowning, and rupture of the bag of waters.

2. The history of the pregnant woman should include her expected date of delivery (EDD), if she has had any complications during her pregnancy, history of prenatal care, previous pregnancies and how these deliveries went. The physical examination should include timing contractions and then, if the contractions are 2 minutes apart, looking for crowning.

3. The EMT should have equipment for the mother, oxygen and the like, as well as a fully stocked obstetrics kit.

4. If the umbilical cord presents first (a prolapsed cord), the EMT should apply 100% oxygen to the mother, ask her to assume the knee-to-chest position (Sims), and transport immediately while contacting medical control en route.

5. The EMT's management of a breech, footling, or buttock presentation is the same as for a prolapsed cord.

6. Green-tinged amniotic fluid may indicate infant meconium. If the meconium is thin and watery, the EMT should suction the oropharynx. If the meconium is thicker, like pea-soup, the EMT should suction the oropharynx and consider ALS assistance for more invasive procedures.

7. Whenever multiple births are anticipated, the EMT should prepare a similar number of childbirth kits.

8. The EMT should prepare for an imminent childbirth of a premature infant. This may include requesting ALS assistance to the scene as well as contacting medical control. As premature infants are prone to hypothermia, the EMT should warm the room as well as prepare more heated blankets.

9. After delivery of the baby, the EMT should place the infant on the mother's breast. This encourages maternal bonding as well as stimulating hormones that aid in the delivery of the placenta.

10. Immediately after childbirth, the EMT needs to dry, warm, and stimulate the infant's breathing. An APGAR score should also be obtained at the 1-minute and 5-minute mark.

FURTHER STUDY

Mattera, C. (1998). Emergency childbirth. *Journal of Emergency Medical Services, 23*(7), 60–69.

ANSWERS TO TEST YOUR KNOWLEDGE

1. During pregnancy, the woman's body undergoes many changes. Her uterus enlarges as the infant grows, the mother's blood volume increases to reflect new demand, the woman's breasts enlarge in anticipation of breast-feeding, and the hormones circulate throughout the body.

2. During the first stage of labor, the woman's contractions start, preparing for eventual childbirth. During the first stage, the mucous plug stopping the cervix is often discharged and a bloody show alerts the mother to impending delivery. During the second stage of labor the cervix dilates and thins and the infant is born. During the third and final stage of labor the placenta is delivered as the uterus continues contractions and returns to a more normal size.

3. The classic signs of impending delivery include an urge to push and crowning at the vaginal opening. Other signs or symptoms can be the bloody show, rupture of the bag of waters, and, more frequent, labor contractions.

4. The predelivery history alerts the EMT to any potential complications that the mother may experience. This history will help guide the questions that the EMT will ask medical control.

5. After donning personal protective equipment, the EMT can assist the mother with delivery. First, the EMT can help the patient obtain a comfortable position with knees-to-chest and head elevated. Then the

EMT drapes the vaginal opening. As the infant is being born, the EMT breaks the amniotic sac, as needed, then moves the umbilical cord clear of the neck. Next, the EMT suctions the mouth and nose as the head presents. The EMT then supports the infant's head and assists the delivery of the shoulders (down then up). Once the infant is out of the birth canal, the EMT proceeds with drying and warming the infant.

6. After delivery of the baby, the EMT should place the infant on the mother's breast. This encourages maternal bonding as well as stimulating hormones that aid in the delivery of the placenta.

7. If the umbilical cord presents first (a prolapsed cord), the EMT should apply 100% oxygen to the mother, ask her to assume the knee-to-chest position (Sims), and transport immediately while contacting medical control en route.

8. The EMT's management of a breech, footling, or buttock presentation is the same as for a prolapsed cord.

9. Whenever multiple births are anticipated, the EMT should prepare a similar number of childbirth kits.

10. Green-tinged amniotic fluid may indicate infant meconium. If the meconium is thin and watery, the EMT should suction the oropharnyx. If the meconium is thicker, like pea-soup, the EMT should suction the oropharynx and consider ALS assistance for more invasive procedures.

Skill 36–1 Emergency Delivery

Student Name _____ Date_____

Purpose: To assist the mother in the natural delivery of a newborn infant.

Personal Protective Equipment: Icon — Handwashing — Gloves — Gown — Mask - Googles

Equipment:

Surgical Scissors or Cord Clamps	Bulb Suction Device
Towels	Gauze Sponges
Baby	Blanket
Sanitary Napkins	Plastic Bag or Bucket

Step 1. The EMT positions the mother supine with knees drawn up and spread apart and assists the mother by helping her elevate her buttocks on a pillow or blankets.

YES: _____   RE-TEACH: _____   RETURN: _____   INSTRUCTOR INITIALS _____

Step 2. The EMT creates a clean area around the vaginal opening with clean towels or paper barriers.

YES: _____   RE-TEACH: _____   RETURN: _____   INSTRUCTOR INITIALS _____

Step 3. As the infant's head appears, during crowning, the EMT places his fingers gently on the skull and exerts very gentle pressure to prevent explosive delivery.

YES: _____   RE-TEACH: _____   RETURN: _____   INSTRUCTOR INITIALS _____

Step 4. If the amniotic sac has not broken, the EMT uses his thumb and forefinger, or a clamp, to puncture the sac and push it away from the infant's head and face.

YES: _____   RE-TEACH: _____   RETURN: _____   INSTRUCTOR INITIALS _____

Step 5. As the infant's head is delivered, the EMT determines if the umbilical cord is around the neck; if it is, slip it over the infant's head or shoulder. If it is not possible to slip the cord, the EMT should clamp the cord in two places, cut the cord between the clamps, and unwrap the cord from the infant's neck.

YES: _____   RE-TEACH: _____   RETURN: _____   INSTRUCTOR INITIALS _____

Step 6. After the infant's head is born, the EMT supports the head and suctions the newborn's mouth and then the nose several times with the bulb suction device.

YES: _____   RE-TEACH: _____   RETURN: _____   INSTRUCTOR INITIALS _____

Step 7. As the torso and full body are born, the EMT supports the infant with both hands. As the feet are born, the EMT grasps them firmly.

YES: _____   RE-TEACH: _____   RETURN: _____   INSTRUCTOR INITIALS _____

Step 8. After pulsations cease, the EMT clamps the umbilical cord in two places, with the closest clamp about 4 fingers' width away from the infant, and then cuts the cord between the clamps.

YES: _____   RE-TEACH: _____   RETURN: _____   INSTRUCTOR INITIALS _____

Step 9. The EMT gently dries the infant with towels and wraps the infant in a warm blanket. The infant is placed on its side, preferably with the head slightly lower than the trunk.

YES: _____   RE-TEACH: _____   RETURN: _____   INSTRUCTOR INITIALS _____

Step 10. Another EMT should monitor the infant and complete initial care of the newborn.

YES: _____   RE-TEACH: _____   RETURN: _____   INSTRUCTOR INITIALS _____

Step 11. The EMT places a sterile sanitary napkin between the mother's legs and asks her to close her legs. The EMT also comforts the mother and monitors vital signs.

YES: _____   RE-TEACH: _____   RETURN: _____   INSTRUCTOR INITIALS _____

Step 12. While preparing the mother and infant for transport, the EMT watches for delivery of the placenta. When the placenta is delivered, the EMT wraps the placenta in a towel and places it in a plastic bag or container, and transports it to the hospital with the mother.

YES: _____   RE-TEACH: _____   RETURN: _____   INSTRUCTOR INITIALS _____

CHAPTER 37

Newborn Care

OBJECTIVES

Upon completion of this chapter, the reader should be able to:

1. Demonstrate how to obtain an APGAR score on a newborn.
2. Discuss the implications of the APGAR score for the newborn.
3. Identify the treatment priorities for a newborn.
4. Describe the care of a newborn with respiratory distress.
5. Demonstrate a focused physical examination for a newborn.
6. Identify which pregnancies may have complications.
7. Demonstrate the resuscitation of a newborn in cardiac or respiratory arrest.

GLOSSARY

acrocyanosis   Cyanosis of the extremities.
APGAR   A predictive score for measuring the health of newborns.
fontanelles   The soft spots on an infant's skull.
molding   The shaping of a newborn's head to pass through the birth canal.
neonate   A newborn infant up to one month old.
vernix caseosa   A cheesy white substance found on a newborn.

PREPARATORY

Materials: Childbirth kit, airway management equipment, eye protection, gloves.
Personnel: Primary Instructor: One EMT-Basic instructor familiar with childbirth who has either delivered a child in the out-of-hospital setting or has seen or assisted with a vaginal delivery within the hospital. Assistant Instructor: The instructor-to-student ratio should be 1:6 for psychomotor skill practice. Individuals used as assistant instructors should be knowledgeable in obstetric/gynecological emergencies.
Recommended Minimum Time to Complete: 2 hours (shared with childbirth)

STUDENT OUTLINE

1) Overview
2) The Newborn Infant
3) Initial Assessment of the Newborn
    a) Management of the Newborn
4) Focused Assessment of the Neonate
    a) General Appearance
    b) Birth Trauma
        i) Birth Defects
5) Infant Resuscitation
    a) Meconium Aspiration
6) Conclusion

LECTURE OUTLINE

1) Overview
2) First Hour of Life
3) High Risk
4) The Newborn Infant
5) Neonate
6) Supportive Care
7) Initial Assessment of the Newborn
    a) APGAR Score 0–2
        i) Appearance
        ii) Pulse
        iii) Grimace
        iv) Activity
        v) Respiration
    b) Assessment
        i) Straighten Legs
            1) Activity
        ii) Airway
            1) Suction
                a) Protective Reflexes
        iii) Breathing
            1) Strong Cry
        iv) Circulation
            1) Rapid
    c) APGAR Scoring
        i) Acrocyanosis
    d) Management of the Newborn
8) Airway
9) Head Dependent
10) Bulb Suction
11) French Catheter
12) Breathing
13) Blow-by Oxygen
14) Assisted Ventilation
15) Circulation
16) Assisted Ventilation
17) Heart Rate Less Than 60 bpm
18) External Cardiac Compressions
19) Focused Assessment of the Neonate
    a) General Appearance
        1) Fetal Position
        2) Vernix Caseosa
    b) Birth Trauma
        1) Molding
    c) Birth Defects
20) Factual
21) Nonjudgmental
22) Infant Resuscitation
    i) Stimulate Breathing
        1) Suction Airway
    ii) Stimulate Breathing
        1) Positive Pressure Ventilation
    iii) Stimulate Breathing
        1) External Compressions
            a) Heart Rate Less Than
                60 bpm
    b) Meconium Aspiration
        i) Clear the Airway
23) Conclusion
    a) Application of Previous Knowledge to
      New Situation

TEACHING STRATEGIES

1. Using an infant CPR mannequin, ask the students to follow the inverted triangle of resuscitation, step by step.

2. Consider having a pediatric advanced life support (PALS) instructor or a neonatal advanced life support (NALS) instructor come and discuss pediatric resuscitation.

CASE STUDY   ASSESSING THE NEWBORN

"Wow, this is really cool!" thought Jose as he wiped the newborn infant with a dry towel. Jose had just seen a live birth for the first time.

The baby was perfect. She had little tiny hands, a little blue, but perfect. The fingernails are so small, Jose thought. She had a hearty wail that indicated she was moving good air, and she was just kicking, kicking, kicking. So much life in this little one, he thought to himself.

Returning to reality Jose told himself, "Back to work, time for an APGAR score to see how this little one is doing." Looking at the laminated card that he had taken out of the birth kit, he called out, "The APGAR is 9!"

ADDITIONAL CASE STUDY

"Push" were the words of the EMT as the birth partner held the patient's hands. "That's it. Keep pushing, almost there. Great job, Mom," said Fred as he quickly suctioned the newborn's mouth and nose. Assisting the infant's shoulders downward then upward the rest of the body seemed to slip right out of the birth canal.

"It's a girl!" Fred proudly announced as he went about drying and stimulating the child. In his mind Fred was reminding himself he needed to remain calm and to proceed methodically with the assessment of the infant using the APGAR score.

STOP AND THINK

1. What is the importance of obtaining an infant APGAR score?

2. What signs would the EMT observe that might indicate the newborn is having difficulty adjusting to life?

3. What actions would the EMT take to try to support the infant who is having difficulty?

4. What would be the EMT's response to the mother of an infant with a birth defect when the mother asks, "Is my baby alright?"

ANSWERS TO STOP AND THINK

1. The APGAR score helps to establish a baseline commonly accepted by all health care providers.

2. All of the points of the APGAR score indicate an infant's ability to adopt to extrauterine life. These include the appearance of the child (cyanosis) as well as pulse, grimace, activity, and respiration.

3. Typically only minimal effort is needed to stimulate a full-term infant—actions such as warming and drying.

4. The EMT should remain nonjudgmental and state, matter-of-factly, the newborn's condition.

CASE STUDY   INFANT IN DISTRESS

"Infant not breathing at 34 Indian River Boulevard." As this announcement came over the loudspeaker, for a moment, it seemed like nobody was breathing. You could have heard a pin drop. Then a flurry of activity began as people ran to the ambulance bays.

The infant alarm people had called the fire department and left a message that an "apnea" monitor had been installed at 34 Indian River Boulevard for a "high-risk infant."

As the ambulance proceeded down Liberty Street, the wail of the siren blocked out everything. Daphne sat on the bench, looking at the action wall and thinking to herself. "OK, be calm. What am I going to need? What am I going to do?

The ride seemed to take an eternity.

ADDITIONAL CASE STUDY

"Why is my baby blue?" asked the new mother. "He just needs a little oxygen, give us a minute," Paul said as he turned to his side and laid the baby on the bedside table he had set up. The drill ran through his head. First suction the airway. If no success, then stimulate the infant.

As Paul placed the bulb-syringe in the infant's oropharynx, he saw the thick goop of meconium blocking the airway. He suctioned vigorously while turning to his driver and saying, "Go to the rig. Call for ALS. Expedite. Clear." With those words spoken, he turned back to the infant and tried to feel an apical heartrate.

STOP AND THINK

1. Which infants are at "high-risk" for cardiac arrest?
2. What are the treatment priorities?
3. When does an EMT start compressions?
4. What does it mean when an infant has green goop in the mouth immediately following childbirth?

ANSWERS TO STOP AND THINK

1. Premature infants are at high-risk for cardiac arrest as well as infants with birth anomalies, such as cardiac disorders.

2. The treatment priorities revolve around the initial assessment. First, stimulate the infant by vigorously rubbing the infant's back (this can be compared to checking for level of consciousness). Then the EMT should proceed with suctioning the airway. If the infant remains depressed (relatively bradycardic), the EMT should administer oxygen, first by blow-by then by positive pressure ventilation. If all else fails, and the child remains relatively bradycardic, the EMT should proceed with external chest compressions.

3. The EMT should start compressions when the newborn is pulseless, or remains bradycardic (apical heartrate less than 60 beats per minute) after suctioning and ventilation fail.

4. Green goop is an indication of meconium. The EMT should immediately assess the airway, then listen to the lungs, at the armpits, for clear air exchange.

FURTHER STUDY

Hamilton, S. (1999). Prehospital newborn resuscitation. *Emergency Medical Services, 28*(5), 39–45.
Suslowitz, B. (1998). The empty crib. *Journal of Emergency Medical Services, 23*(3), 86–88.

ANSWERS TO TEST YOUR KNOWLEDGE

1. Signs of infant respiratory distress include cyanosis, sternal retractions, seesaw breathing, and bradycardia.

2. The APGAR score is obtained, at 1 and 5 minutes postbirth, by assessing the newborn.

3. The APGAR score includes the appearance, grimace, respiration, pulse, and activity.

4. The APGAR score is fairly predictive of a child's health, or the need for health care providers, including EMTs, to intercede and assist the child.

5. The EMT should focus on assessing the infant for signs of birth trauma, such as limp extremities, as well as any birth defects.

6. Included in the list of high-risk pregnancies are teen-aged women and middle-aged women as well as those who smoke or use illicit drugs.

7. Infant resuscitation starts with the suctioning the airway and follows through with assisted ventilation and external chest compressions as needed.

8. An infant's heart beats much faster than an adult's. Therefore, an EMT should perform external chest compressions at a rate of approximately 120 beats per minute, or 2 a second.

CHAPTER 38

Pediatric Medical Emergencies

OBJECTIVES

Upon completion of this chapter, the reader should be able to:

1. Identify the developmental considerations for infants, toddlers, preschool children, schoolage children, and adolescents.
2. Recall the differences in anatomy and physiology of the infant, child, and adult patient and describe how they affect emergency care.
3. Describe some general techniques that are useful in taking a history and performing a physical examination on a pediatric patient.
4. Describe the typical response to illness of the infant or child.
5. Describe several causes of pediatric airway emergencies and the emergency management of them.
6. Describe several causes of pediatric respiratory emergencies and the emergency management of them.
7. Identify the signs and symptoms of hypoperfusion in the infant and child.
8. State the most common causes of cardiac arrest in infants and children and how they impact emergency management of this condition.
9. Describe several causes of pediatric altered mental status and the emergency management of them.
10. Recognize the need for EMT debriefing following a difficult pediatric transport.

GLOSSARY

abdominal thrusts Forceful application of pressure to the upper abdomen, toward the chest, in an attempt to expel a foreign body from the airway.

asthma A condition consisting of bronchospasm and inflammation in response to multiple stimuli.

back blows Firm blows administered to an infant's upper back in an attempt to expel a foreign body from the airway.

chest thrusts Firm compressions delivered to an infant's midchest in an attempt to expel a foreign body from the airway.

croup A viral illness that can cause upper airway swelling in a child.

debriefing An organized discussion among personnel involved in a difficult situation in an attempt to prevent unnecessary buildup of stress.

epiglottitis A bacterial infection that can cause upper airway obstruction.

febrile seizure A seizure that results from a rapid rise in body temperature.

intercostal retraction   A retraction of skin and muscle between the ribs with each breath seen in a child with respiratory distress.

meningitis   An infection and inflammation of the lining around the brain and spinal cord.

sternal retraction   Sternal depression with each breath seen in a child with severe respiratory distress.

sudden infant death syndrome (SIDS)   The sudden, unexplained death of an infant in the first year of life.

PREPARATORY

Materials: EMS Equipment: Exam gloves, stethoscope, blood pressure cuff, penlight.

Personnel: Primary Instructor: One EMT-Basic instructor, knowledgeable with infants and children. Assistant Instructor: The instructor-to-student ratio should be 1:6 for psychomotor skill practice. Individuals used as assistant instructors should be knowledgeable in infant and child emergencies.

Recommended Minimum Time to Complete: 3 hours

STUDENT OUTLINE

1) Overview
2) Normal Childhood Development
   a) Neonate
   b) Young Infant
   c) Older Infant
   d) Toddler
   e) Preschooler
   f) Schoolage Child
   g) Adolescent
3) General Considerations
   a) Initial Approach
   b) Gathering a History
   c) Performing a Physical Exam
4) Common Pediatric Illnesses
5) Airway Problems
   a) Foreign Body Obstruction
   b) Assessment
      i) Incomplete Obstruction
   c) Management
      i) Infant
      ii) Child
   d) Transportation
6) Trouble Breathing
      i) Croup
      ii) Epiglottitis

   b) Assessment
   c) Management
   d) Transportation
7) Pediatric Asthma
      i) Respiratory Infections
   b) Assessment
   c) Management
8) Hypoperfusion
   a) Assessment
   b) Management
      i) Cardiac Arrest
         (1) SIDS
9) Altered Mental Status
      i) Seizures
      ii) Diabetes
      iii) Behavioral
      iv) Poisoning
      v) Infections
   b) Assessment
   c) Management
10) Stress in Caring for Children
   a) Child
   b) Family
   c) Provider
11) Conclusion

LECTURE OUTLINE

1) Overview
   a) Age-Dependent Care
   b) Application of Previous Training to New Situation
2) Normal Childhood Development
   a) Neonate
      i) Strong Sense of Smell/Hearing
      ii) Maternal Bond
   b) Young Infant
      i) Rapid Growth
      ii) Sense of Sight Developed
   c) Older Infant
      i) Increased Activity
      ii) Stranger Anxiety
   d) Toddler
      i) Mobile
      ii) Independence
      iii) Injury as Punishment
   e) Preschooler
      i) Curious
   f) Schoolage Child
      i) Adult Proportions
      ii) Self-Expression
   g) Adolescent
      i) Adult-like
      ii) Risk-Taking Behaviors
3) General Considerations
   a) Initial Approach
      i) Age-Specific
   b) Gathering a History
      i) Young
         (1) Parent as Historian
      ii) Older
         (1) Child as Historian
   c) Performing a Physical Exam
      i) Young
         (1) Toe-to-Head Approach
      ii) Older
         (1) Standard Approach
         (2) Modesty Issues
4) Common Pediatric Illnesses
5) Airway Problems
   a) Foreign Body Obstruction
      i) Toddler Exploration
   b) Assessment
      i) Incomplete Obstruction
      ii) Cry, Cough, or Speak
   c) Management
      (1) Follow AHA/ARC Guidelines

ii) Infant
   (1) Backblows
   (2) Chest Blows
iii) Child
   (1) Abdominal Thrusts
d) Transportation
   i) ALS Intercept
6) Trouble Breathing
   i) Croup
      (1) Viral Infection
         (a) Self-Limiting
         (b) Ages six months to four years
   ii) Epiglottitis
      (1) Bacterial Infection
         (a) Vaccines available
   b) Assessment
      i) Croup
         (1) Seal-Like Barking Cough
         (2) Worse at Night
      ii) Epiglottitis
         (1) Brassy Cough
         (2) High Fever
         (3) Drooling
   c) Management
      i) Differentiation Not Important
      ii) Humidification of Oxygen
      iii) Nothing in Mouth
   d) Transportation
      i) ALS Intercept
      ii) High Priority
7) Pediatric Asthma
   i) Narrowed Airways
   ii) Increasing Incidence
   iii) Sources of Shortness of Breath
      (1) Upper Respiratory Infections
      (2) Asthma
   b) Assessment
      i) Triggers
      ii) Wheezing
      iii) Evidence of Difficulty Breathing
   c) Management
      i) Assist with Inhaler (Protocols Permitting)
      ii) Oxygen Therapy
      iii) Small-Volume Nebulizer (SVN) (Protocols Permitting)
      iv) ALS Intercept
8) Hypoperfusion

a) Assessment
    i) Source of Fluid Loss
    ii) Shunting
       (1) Sudden Decompensation
b) Management
    (1) Oxgyen Therapy
    (2) Elevation
    (3) Warmth
    (4) ALS Intercept
    ii) Cardiac Arrest
       (1) SIDS
          (a) Unknown Cause
       (2) Resuscitate Unless Hopeless
          (a) Family Care

9) Altered Mental Status
    (1) Number of Causes
    ii) Seizures
       (1) Fever
    iii) Diabetes
       (1) Hypoglycemia Previously Diagnosed
    iv) Behavioral

       (1) Rule Out Medical Causes First
    v) Poisoning
       (1) Identification
       (2) Toxin-Specific Treatment
    vi) Infections
       (1) Meningitis
b) Assessment
    i) Focus on ABCs
c) Management
    i) Supportive Care
10) Stress in Caring for Children
    a) Child
       i) Stranger Anxiety
    b) Family
       i) Parental Concern
          (1) Parental Interference
    c) Provider
       i) Fear of Errors
       ii) CSID
11) Conclusion
    a) Application of Previous Knowledge to Unique Situation

TEACHING STRATEGIES

1. Consider asking a child-development expert/instructor or a local child-care center operator to speak to the class about the developmental milestones of young children. Using the information provided, ask the students to formulate strategies on how to approach different age groups.

2. Consider taking the students on a trip to a local day-care center and have them attempt to obtain some rudimentary demographic information (age, date of birth, address, and telephone number) from the children.

3. Consider asking a pediatrician to speak to the class. Encourage the physician to reveal his or her techniques for getting children of different ages to cooperate with an assessment.

CASE STUDY CHILD CHOKING

The 9-1-1 communicator picked up the phone to hear a man yelling, "He is choking!" Calmly, she proceeded to give the distraught parent step-by-step instructions while she turned the address over to another communicator. As an ambulance responded to the address, the communicator explained each step.

By following carefully scripted instructions, the communicator was able to talk the man through the appropriate maneuvers to remove the marble from his son's airway. By the time the EMTs arrived at the house, she could hear the child crying loudly in the background. The communicator told the parent, "Sir, the ambulance is there; you're in good hands. Let them do their job, and, sir, good luck."

ADDITIONAL CASE STUDY

Jimmy was racing around the house while his watchful mother went about her daily chores. Jimmy was climbing behind the stove, then suddenly started to flail his legs about. When his mother pulled him out from behind the stove, she was shocked to find that he was blue. At the same moment, his body went limp in her arms.

In a panic, she grabbed the telephone and called EMS. Fortunately, the ambulance was posted just down the street at the quickie-mart. EMTs arrived on-scene within minutes and rushed into the house.

STOP AND THINK

1. What makes a child's airway different from an adult's?
2. How can the EMT differentiate between a partial and a complete airway obstruction?
3. What should be done for the child with a complete airway obstruction due to a foreign body?
4. What are the potential causes of pediatric airway obstruction?
5. What should be done after the airway has been cleared?

ANSWERS TO STOP AND THINK

1. The tongue in a pediatric airway is relatively larger than an adult's and the airway is shorter and straighter.

2. A child with a partial airway may be able to speak in short phrases or may exhibit a stridor. The child with a complete obstruction will not be able to talk and because he is unable to exchange air, will fatigue quickly, become cyanotic, and lose consciousness.

3. Standard American Heart Association (AHA) airway maneuvers should be attempted by the EMT until successful or until the child loses consciousness, at which time the EMT should consider beginning transport and intercepting with ALS. If the EMT is trained in endotracheal intubation, the EMT could attempt direct visualization via larygoscopy.

4. Potential causes of pediatric airway obstruction include foreign objects, such as food or toys, as well as infection, including epiglottis.

5. Once the airway is cleared, the patient's ventilation should be observed. If the child is moving adequate air, then high-flow oxygen should be administered and the child transported. If the child is not moving sufficient amounts of air, as evidenced by cyanosis, poor oxygen saturation readings, or a decreased level of conscious, then the child should be ventilated with a bag-valve mask.

CASE STUDY   ASTHMA ATTACK

"You're out!" yelled the umpire as the boy slid into home plate. "All that effort for nothing," thought Jose, as he watched from the bleachers. Jose had been standing by at the Little League game for an hour when one of the coaches brought one of his players over to be "checked out."

The eight-year-old boy was complaining that he was having trouble breathing. The boy stated that he had a history of asthma but did not like to use his puffer because it made him "nervous." Jose started his initial assessment, noting that an anxious father was jogging toward them.

ADDITIONAL CASE STUDY

The school bus was sitting on the side of the road with its flashers on. One of the children on the bus complained that she could not breathe. The temperature had dropped last night and it was a cold 20 degrees outside and the cold had triggered her trouble breathing.

So the bus driver, thinking quickly, called his dispatcher on the cell phone, advised her what was going on, and asked for instructions. He was told to drive to the corner of West Street and State Street and await the arrival of EMS.

STOP AND THINK

1. What is asthma?
2. What can trigger an asthma attack?
3. What are the signs and symptoms of asthma?
4. What is the treatment for asthma?

ANSWERS TO STOP AND THINK

1. Asthma is a reactive airway disease that causes bronchospasm and bronchoconstriction.

2. Allergens, such as dust or mold, can trigger an asthma attack. The trigger for some patients is exercise or cold air.

3. The typical complaint of a patient with asthma is "I can't breathe." Often this shortness of breath is accompanied by tripod positioning, pursed-lip breathing, and auditory wheezes.

4. Bronchodilators, administered in metered dose inhalers (MDIs) or small-volume-nebulizers (SVNs), are used in emergencies. These "rescue inhalers" provide immediate relief in most cases.

CASE STUDY ILL CHILD

Dana, the EMT-in-charge, is led down the hall to the bedroom. Charity, the boy's mother, says, "He's not acting right. He sleeps all the time and he isn't keeping anything down." Dana finds out that the mother called the pediatrician's office, who directed her to call 9-1-1.

The child had diarrhea for the past three days and just started vomiting this morning. Other than that the boy has not had any complaints. Dana finds a pale, listless child lying in bed. He is awake but his eyes are lackluster and his lips are cracked. "Hi," he says. "My name is Dana, and I am an EMT."

ADDITIONAL CASE STUDY

At first the EMT was struck by how limp the baby was in the crib, like a rag-doll. And the child's cry was pitiful, a low screech that was barely audible. But what stuck him the most were the eyes, sunken and dry despite the fact the child was crying. The mother related a night of frequent diaper changes and vomiting. The pediatrician's office said they could not see the infant until 10:00 a.m. but the mother decided she could not wait.

STOP AND THINK

1. Can vomiting and diarrhea lead to hypoperfusion?
2. What are signs of hypoperfusion?
3. What should the EMT do to treat the hypoperfusion?

ANSWERS TO STOP AND THINK

1. Severe vomiting and diarrhea leads to dehyration, and hypoperfusion. If left untreated, this can be life-threatening.

2. Signs of hypoperfusion in a child include tachycardia, pallor, poor capillary refill, and a decreased level of consciousness. Hypotension is a relatively late sign of hypoperfusion in a child.

3. Field treatments for pediatric hypoperfusion are largely supportive. The child should receive high-flow oxygen, be placed supine with legs elevated, and a blanket should be provided to maintain warmth.

CASE STUDY   CHILDHOOD SEIZURE

The fourteen-year-old babysitter met EMS at the door. "Thank God you guys got here so fast!" she blurted out. "He's in here. I've called his mother. I didn't know what to do. This is my first job. Did I do the right thing?" "Miss, slow down, relax," George responded as he carried his pediatric bag into the living room.

On the couch, a small boy, maybe three years old, was lying on his side covered with a blanket. He was talking gibberish and responded slowly when the babysitter Irene called his name. Irene explained that the boy had not been feeling well and he had been running a fever. Suddenly, the boy had gone into convulsions, which prompted her to call 9-1-1.

Irene could not offer much history, except that she was sure that the boy had never seized before and now he was not acting right. Just then the boy's mother came running into the room, and Irene exclaimed, "He was shaking all over!"

ADDITIONAL CASE STUDY

Tepid baths weren't working and the grandmother started to wash him down with isopropyl alcohol in hopes of reducing his fever. While she was washing him down he started to convulse. The startled grandmother called her son-in-law at work and asked what she should do. He told her, "Call 9-1-1, Nana, and I will meet you at the emergency department." And then he hung up.

Grandma, doing as she was instructed, called EMS. She was becoming increasingly concerned because the child didn't seem to be waking up. When the doorbell rang, she let out an audible sigh of relief.

STOP AND THINK

1. What are some causes of altered mental status in a child?
2. What is a febrile seizure?
3. What should the EMT do for the child who may have had a seizure?
4. Are there potential causes other than seizures for altered mental status?
5. What questions should the EMT ask the mother?

ANSWERS TO STOP AND THINK

1. The mnemonic AEIOU-TIPS is useful in children as well as adults. The emphasis should be on causes of hypoxia (lack of oxygen), fever (infection), and toxic ingestion (overdose).

2. A febrile seizure occurs when a child's temperature rises quickly and the irritated brain seizes.

3. The EMT should treat the postictal child the same way as an adult. It is not usually necessary to cool the child, for example, if he had a febrile seizure.

4. Causes of altered mental status, other than seizure, include hypoxia, hypoglycemia, and toxic ingestion.

5. Beyond the SAMPLE history, the EMT should ask the mother about the child's recent activities and illnesses.

FURTHER STUDY

Ball, R. (1999). Seize the moment—Assessment and management of febrile seizures. *Journal of Emergency Medical Services, 24*(3), 78.

Deschamp, C., & Sneed, R. (1997). EMS for children with special healthcare needs. *Emergency Medical Services, 26*(11), 57–62.

Ojanen-Thomas, D. (1996). Assessing children—It's different. *RN, 59*(4), 38–45.

Perkin, M., & VanStralen, D. (1999). My child can't breathe. *Journal of Emergency Medical Services, 24*(9), 42–48.

Perkin, R., & Van Stralen, D. (2000). Pediatric passages. *Journal of Emergency Medical Services, 25*(3), 50–58.

Raidow, S. (1998). Meeting the emotional needs of the pediatric patient. *Emergency Medical Services, 27*(4), 28.

Shaner, K., & Bechtal, N. (1997). Bridging the gap. *Emergency Medical Services, 26*(3), 46–50.

Werfel, P. (1998). The gentle art of pediatric assessment. *Journal of Emergency Medical Services, 23*(3), 58–64.

ANSWERS TO TEST YOUR KNOWLEDGE

1. Generally, the EMT should approach the child to be assessed slowly, first making contact with the mother or other caregiver. Then the EMT should proceed with a toe-to-head approach to assessment. This allows the child to become comfortable with the EMT.

2. The EMT should integrate knowledge of pediatric development into the assessment. The neonate is relatively helpless and depends on mother for protection. The EMT will not have any difficulty assessing the neonate provided he or she has obtained permission from the mother or caregiver. The infant eventually develops stranger anxiety and the EMT will need more assistance from the mother to complete the assessment.

The toddler has become increasingly more mobile and independent. While this child may agree to an examination, his or her propensity will be to say "No" to questions asked.

The schoolage child is quickly becoming an adult, and should be questioned directly. Finally, the adolescent may be more concerned about appearances than health. This pediatric patient needs to be given decision-making ability within the restrictions of her or his limited experience.

3. The infant's and child's airway is relatively smaller and the tongue is relatively larger, making airway control more difficult. Airway difficulty, and compromise, are more common in children than adults.

Infants and children have weaker chest muscles than adults and therefore are more prone to respiratory distress and exhaustion. However, the heart of a child is free of most cardiovascular disease. Therefore, the most likely etiology of pediatric arrest is respiratory, not cardiac, in nature.

Finally, the cardiovascular system of a child is capable of compensating well. Indications of decompensated shock, like hypotension, do not occur until late in the patient's illness.

4. Typically, a child turns to the mother during times of illness. Toddlers may believe that their illness is a punishment for something that they did wrong.

5. The most common pediatric airway emergency is a foreign body airway obstruction (FBAO). FBAOs are dealt with using the standard AHA or ARC FBAO manuevers.

Other causes of pediatric airway problems include infections such as croup and epiglottitis. The EMT can only offer supportive care while transporting the patient for definitive care in the emergency department.

6. The most common pediatric respiratory disease is asthma. The EMT should provide supportive care and consider assisting the patient with the prescribed meter dose inhaler (MDI).

7. Signs and symptoms of hypoperfusion in a child include tachycardia, pallor, poor capillary refill, decreased level of consciousness, and hypotension.

8. The most common cause of pediatric cardiac arrest is respiratory arrest. Therefore, the EMT should focus attention on maintaining an airway, ventilating the patient, and providing high-flow oxygen.

9. Common causes of pediatric altered mental status include hypoxia (administer high-flow oxygen or ventilate), hypoglycemia (administer glucose to the conscious patient), fever (reduce fever with cool washclothes), and toxic ingestion (identify causative agent and call medical control).

10. Adults tend to link hopes, dreams, and aspirations to children. When a child dies it tends to have a greater impact on the health care provider. Therefore, to lessen the psychological impact, EMTs should be routinely debriefed after a pediatric death.

CHAPTER 39

Pediatric Trauma

OBJECTIVES

Upon completion of this chapter, the reader should be able to:

1. Recognize trauma as the leading cause of pediatric mortality.
2. Explain how pediatric anatomy alters patient assessment.
3. Explain how pediatric anatomy relates to chest trauma.
4. Explain how pediatric anatomy relates to abdominal trauma.
5. Explain how pediatric anatomy relates to head injuries.
6. Discuss the causes of pediatric spinal trauma.
7. Explain the treatment of pediatric spinal trauma.
8. Explain how pediatric anatomy relates to bone injury.
9. Identify pediatric trauma cases that are high-priority.
10. Discuss pediatric burn care.
11. Define and recognize examples of child abuse.
12. Discuss the emergency care of the child with special needs.

GLOSSARY

central venous catheter   An intravenous tube that may be left in for long periods of time and may be used for intravenous medication administration or blood sampling.

cerebrospinal fluid (CSF) shunt   A special catheter that is used to drain excess CSF off the brain and into the abdomen, where it can be easily absorbed.

child abuse   An emotional, physical, or sexual injury inflicted upon a child.

feeding tube   A soft, flexible tube that is placed into the stomach, either through the nose or through the anterior abdominal wall, to allow nutritional supplementation.

mandated reporter   A person who is required by law to report suspicions of child abuse.

mechanical ventilator   A machine that provides artificial ventilation for a patient who cannot breathe effectively on his or her own.

tracheostomy   A surgically created hole in the front of the neck that extends into the trachea.

tracheostomy tube   A rigid tube that is placed into a tracheostomy to maintain a patent airway.

PREPARATORY

Materials: EMS Equipment: Exam gloves, stethoscope, blood pressure cuff, penlight.

Personnel: Primary Instructor: One EMT-Basic instructor knowledgeable in care of infants and children. Assistant Instructor: The instructor-to-student ratio should be 1:6 for psychomotor skill practice. Individuals used as assistant instructors should be knowledgeable in infant and child emergencies.

Recommended Minimum Time to Complete: 3 hours (all pediatric sections)

STUDENT OUTLINE

1) Overview
2) Pediatric Trauma Assessment
    a) Mechanism of Injury
    b) Anatomic Differences
    c) Pediatric Trauma Initial Assessment
        i) General Impression
        ii) Mental Status
        iii) Airway
        iv) Breathing
        v) Circulation
    d) Focused Trauma History and Physical
3) Blunt Trauma
    a) Hypoperfusion
        i) Management
    b) Chest Injury
        i) Management
    c) Abdominal Injury
        i) Management
    d) Head Injuries
        i) Management
    e) Spinal Injury
        i) Management
            (1) Immobilization in Car Seat
            (2) Removing a Child from a Car Seat
    f) Bony Injuries
        i) Management
    g) Burn Injuries
        i) Management
    h) Child Abuse
4) Children with Special Needs
    a) Tracheostomies
        i) Management Considerations
    b) Mechanical Ventilators
        i) Management Considerations
    c) Central Venous Catheters
        i) Management
    d) Feeding Tubes
        i) Management Considerations
    e) Cerebrospinal Fluid (CSF) Shunts
        i) Management Considerations
5) Conclusion

LECTURE OUTLINE

1) Overview
   a) Number One Cause of Pediatric Death
   b) Preventable Deaths
   c) Lifelong Impact
2) Pediatric Trauma Assessment
     i) Children Are Not Small Adults
     ii) Match Mechanism to Size
   b) Mechanism of Injury
     i) Curiousity Leads to Trouble
     ii) Boundary Testing
     iii) Risk-Taking Behaviors
   c) Anatomic Differences
     i) Proportionally Larger Heads
       (1) Top Heavy
     ii) Larger Body to Mass Ratio
   d) Pediatric Trauma Initial Assessment
     i) General Impression
       (1) 90 Percent of Assessment from the Door
     ii) Mental Status
       (1) Ill-Appearing
       (2) Lackluster
       (3) Tearless
     iii) Airway
       (1) Open-Mouth Breather
       (2) Air Hunger
         (a) Pain
         (b) Hypoxia
     iv) Breathing
       (1) Limited Tolerances
       (2) Seesaw Respiration
       (3) Retractions
         (a) Sternal
         (b) Intercostal
     v) Circulation
       (1) Capillary Refill
       (2) Small Volume Is Life-Threatening
   e) Focused Trauma History and Physical
3) Blunt Trauma
   a) Hypoperfusion
     i) Compensation
       (1) Shunting
     ii) Assessment
       (1) Capillary Refill
       (2) Comparative Pulses
         (a) Central versus Peripheral
       (3) Rapid Decompensation
         (a) Hypotension—Premorbid

         (b) Bradycardia—Premorbid
     iii) Management
       (1) High Index of Suspicion
   b) Chest Injury
     i) Assessment
       (1) Soft Cartilage
       (2) Rib Fractures = Severe Force
     ii) Management
       (1) Oxygenation
       (2) Ventilation
       (3) Stabilization of Injuries
   c) Abdominal Injury
     i) Assessment
       (1) Liver/Spleen Unprotected
         (a) Hypoperfusion
     ii) Management
       (1) Hypoperfusion
       (2) Rapid Transport
   d) Head Injuries
     i) Assessment
       (1) Loss of Consciousness
         (i) Nausea/Vomiting Frequent
       (2) Seizure Post-Trauma
     ii) Management
       (1) ABCs
       (2) High Priority
   e) Spinal Injury
     i) Assessment
       (1) Head-Heavy
     ii) Management
       (1) Immobilization in Car Seat
         (a) Pediatric Cervical Collar
           (i) Horseshoe Collar
         (b) Modification Required
       (2) Removing a Child from a Car Seat
         (a) Unable to Maintain Airway
   f) Bony Injuries
     i) Assessment
       (1) Flexible
       (2) Seldom Break
     ii) Management
       (1) Manual Stabilization
       (2) Immobilization
   g) Burn Injuries
     i) Assessment
       (1) Nonintentional
         (a) Curious Behavior

(2) Intentional
  ii) Management
    (1) Airway First
    (2) Large Body Surface Area
      (a) Modified Rule-of-Nines
  h) Child Abuse
   i) Intentional Trauma
   ii) Mandated Reporters
    (1) Patient Care Comes First
4) Children with Special Needs
  a) Children with Disabilities
   i) Congential
   ii) Acquired
  b) Tracheostomies
   i) Airway
   ii) Management Considerations
    (1) Suctioning
    (2) Assisted Ventilation
  c) Mechanical Ventilators
   i) Management Considerations
    (1) Remove Child from Machine

(2) Manually Ventilate
  d) Central Venous Catheters
   i) Management
    (1) Routine Bleeding Control
    (2) Transportation
  e) Feeding Tubes
   i) Soft Tubes in Abdomen
   ii) Management Considerations
    (1) Supportive Care
    (2) Transport
  f) Cerebrospinal Fluid (CSF) Shunts
   i) Assessment
    (1) Presence of Fever
      (a) Meningitis
   ii) Management Considerations
    (1) Maintain Supportive Care
    (2) Moniter ABCs
      (a) Prepared for Seizures
5) Conclusion
  a) Application of prior knowledge to unique situation

TEACHING STRATEGIES

1. Consider a visit to the pediatric trauma center. Nurses and physicians on staff are usually willing to describe the typical types of pediatric trauma patients that are seen at the trauma center.

2. Consider having the local aeromedical transport service send representatives to discuss pediatric trauma. Frequently, pediatric trauma patients are seen at a local hospital, especially in rural areas, then transported to a regional trauma center.

3. Consider a visit to a local disabled citizens center to meet children with special needs. A few hours spent with these children is invaluable to an EMT when he or she has an EMS call in the future.

CASE STUDY   BICYCLE ACCIDENT

The siren screamed as the pumper raced through the streets. The report was "child hit by a car on Highway 66." An engine, an ambulance, and a paramedic-rescue had all been dispatched to the scene.

Emotions were running high when the crew left the station. Just four days before, the crew had worked a pediatric arrest that was caused by a fall from a third-story window. The child did not survive.

Now, they were faced with another pediatric trauma, and this one was on the interstate. Cars would be speeding along the highway at speeds of over 70 miles per hour. "Where the heck was the mother?" Mario thought angrily, "Why wasn't she watching the kid?"

Refocusing his thoughts, Mario the EMT on the engine, started to consider his priorities once he was on the scene, "C-spine first," he reminded himself.

ADDITIONAL CASE STUDY

The police arrived at the motor vehicle collision (MVC) first and had already shut down the closest lane to traffic. The first ambulance crew chief was carefully inspecting the vehicle for damage and counting the number of patients. The vehicle was involved in a low-speed rear-end collision on an entrance ramp to a local mall. Despite the fact that the posted speed was 20 miles per hour, the crew chief suspected that the other driver was going much faster.

As the crew chief looked in the front windshield, he noted that the airbags had been deployed, both driver's side and passenger side, and that there was a forward-facing infant's carseat. Both the driver/mother and the infant appeared unconscious.

STOP AND THINK

1. What are the typical causes of pediatric trauma?
2. What are the anatomic differences between a child and an adult?
3. What are the indications for transporting a child to a trauma center?
4. How would an EMT manage a chest injury? An abdominal injury? A spinal cord injury? A long bone fracture?
5. How should an EMT respond to child abuse?

ANSWERS TO STOP AND THINK

1. Typical causes of pediatric trauma include motor vehicle collisions, child-versus-vehicle collisions, falls, and gunshot wounds.

2. Starting from the top, the autonomic differences between a child and an adult are: a child has a larger head, a child has a larger tongue, a child's bones are softer, a child's respiratory muscles are undeveloped, a child's abdominal muscles are weak, and a child's body-surface area to mass-ratio is larger than an adult's.

3. Any child who is struck by a motor vehicle, who is involved in a high-speed motor vehicle collision, who is ejected from a motor vehicle, or has sustained a fall greater than three times his or her height should be transported to a trauma center.

4. An EMT should manage any pediatric trauma in the same manner as an adult with special consideration to the following: any suspected rib fractures should raise suspicions of serious trauma; any signs of abdominal injury should lead the EMT to suspect serious internal injury; any motor vehicle collision or fall should lead the EMT to suspect spinal trauma; and any long-bone fracture should lead the EMT to suspect serious trauma from a significant force.

5. When an EMT suspects child abuse he should not approach the parents; rather he should concentrate his attentions on the child and report his suspicions to a mandated reporter at a later time.

FURTHER STUDY

Ladebauche, P. (1997). Childhood trauma: When to suspect abuse. *RN, 60*(9), 38–40.

Liebesfeld, M. (1997). When love hurts. *Emergency Medical Services, 26*(3), 29–39.

Quirk, P., & Adelson, P. (1997). Shaken-baby syndrome and the EMS provider. *Emergency Medical Services, 27*(9), 32–38.

Santamaria, J. (1999). Pediatric diving injuries for the pre-hospital care provider. *NAEMT News*, 10–14.

Ventura, M. (1997). Airbag safety alert. *RN, 60*(4), 43.

ANSWERS TO TEST YOUR KNOWLEDGE

1. Trauma, specifically accidental death, is the leading cause of pediatric mortality.

2. First, children have a relatively larger head and therefore are prone to falling head-first and sustaining head injuries. Children also have a larger body surface area to mass-ratio making them more prone to hypothermia.

3. The ribcage of a child is largely cartilage and therefore very flexible. The presence of a painful, swollen deformity along a rib (suggesting a rib fracture) would indicate that the child's chest must have sustained a great deal of force.

4. The internal abdominal organs of a pediatric patient are relatively unprotected. The immature ribcage does not cover the liver and spleen and the undeveloped abdominal musculature does not provide substantial protection.

5. A child's head is relatively heavier and larger than the body when compared to an adult's. This makes the child prone to head injury. A head-injured child has a higher incidence of post-traumatic seizures as well as vomiting.

6. The most common cause of spinal injuries in children are motor vehicle collisions and falls, in that order. The child's heavy head is thrown forward, injuring the neck in the process.

7. The treatment for a suspected pediatric spinal injury is the same as for an adult. However, it takes ingenuity for an EMT to modify equipment to fit the child's smaller size.

8. The skeleton of a child is immature, with plates on each end that permit growth. Children's bones are also more flexible and seldom break. When a child does break a bone, the bone has a tendency to fracture along these growth plates, with serious implications for later development if the fracture is not dealt with immediately.

9. The following injuries, signs, or symptoms make a child "high-priority": signs of severe hypoperfusion, uncontrollable airway, severe difficulty breathing, uncontrollable bleeding, paralysis or paresthesia, open fracture, penetrating trauma, head injury, severe facial trauma, child struck at speed greater than 20 mph, fall three times or greater than child's height, unrestrained passenger in a rollover, ejected from motor vehicle, restrained passenger in high-speed crash (> 50 mph).

10. Care of the pediatric burn patient is the same as for an adult, with several very important caveats. Children are prone to respiratory distress and failure; therefore, the EMT should pay special attention the pediatric airway. Children also have larger body-mass to surface-area ratios, so that the standard rule-of-nines does not apply. Instead, the EMT should utilize a pediatric burn chart to estimate the percentage burns. For the same reason, children are prone to hypothermia following a burn injury.

11. Child abuse is the purposeful infliction of harm, either psychological or physical, on a child. Child abuse can also be child neglect—a failure of the caregiver to provide the minimal comfort and care a child needs to grow.

12. Examples of nonaccidental trauma that could be the result of child abuse include cigarette burns, scald burns, multiple bruises in various stages of healing, and a history of falls, with resultant bone injury.

13. Children with special needs can expect to survive, but they become technologically dependent. Examples include tracheotomy tubes and ventilators, CSF shunts, feeding tubes, and central venous catheters.

CHAPTER 40

Geriatric Medical Emergencies

OBJECTIVES

Upon completion of this chapter, the reader should be able to:

1. Identify the neurologic changes characteristic of aging.
2. Identify the cardiovascular changes characteristic of aging.
3. Identify the respiratory changes characteristic of aging.
4. Identify the gastrointestinal changes characteristic of aging.
5. Identify the genitourinary changes characteristic of aging.
6. Identify the musculoskeletal changes characteristic of aging.
7. Identify the integumentary changes characteristic of aging.
8. Describe the problems that can occur with polypharmacy.
9. Describe the pathophysiology and classic physical findings of a stroke.
10. Discuss the treatment priorities for the patient suffering from a stroke.
11. Define the term *dementia*.

GLOSSARY

arthritis   A decrease in the flexibility of joints along with an inflammation within those joints.

cerebrovascular accident   *See* stroke.

delirium   An alteration in the level of consciousness usually caused by an acute medical problem.

dementia   A syndrome that is characterized by a progressive decline in intellectual function that usually leads to deterioration of occupational, social, and interpersonal functions.

dysarthria   Difficulty speaking resulting in garbled or slurred speech.

elder abuse   Mistreatment of an elder person.

facial droop   One-sided facial muscle weakness that indicates focal brain or nerve injury.

hemorrhagic stroke   An injury to brain tissue as a result of rupture of a vessel that supplies it with blood.

ischemic stroke   An injury to brain tissue as a result of blockage of the vessel that supplies it with blood.

osteoporosis   A progressive loss in the calcium content of the bones seen commonly in elderly women.

polypharmacy   The use of multiple medications by a single patient.

pronator drift   A test of neurologic function that involves raising both arms straight out in front of the body, palms up, eyes closed; a positive test involves one arm drifting and indicates weakness in that arm.

silent myocardial infarction   Death of heart tissue that occurs without the patient experiencing classic cardiac symptoms such as chest pain.

Instructor's Manual to *Emergency Medical Care* | 441

stroke An injury to brain tissue that occurs as a result of disruption of blood flow to part of the brain; also known as a cerebrovascular accident.

transient ischemic attack A temporary disruption of blood flow to part of the brain that results in signs and symptoms of a stroke, yet resolve within minutes to hours.

PREPARATORY

Materials: EMS Equipment: Exam gloves, stethoscope, blood pressure cuff, penlight.

Personnel: Primary Instructor: One EMT-Basic instructor, knowledgeable about geriatrics. Assistant Instructor: The instructor-to-student ratio should be 1:6 for psychomotor skill practice. Individuals used as assistant instructors should be knowledgeable about geriatrics.

Recommended Minimum Time to Complete: 1.5 hours.

STUDENT OUTLINE

1) Overview
2) The Aging of Society
3) Physiologic Changes Associated with Aging
    a) Neurologic
    b) Cardiovascular
    c) Respiratory
    d) Gastrointestinal
    e) Genitourinary
    f) Integumentary
4) Assessment of the Elderly Patient
    a) Scene Size-Up
    b) Initial Assessment
    c) Focused History and Physical Examination
    d) Transport
    e) Ongoing Assessment
5) General Medical Considerations in the Elderly
    a) Medication Use by the Elderly
    b) Susceptibility to Disease
    c) Altered Presentation of Disease
    d) Mistreatment of the Elderly
6) Common Illnesses in the Elderly
    a) Stroke
        i) Presentation
            (1) Signs and Symptoms
        ii) Assessment
        iii) Management
    b) Dementia
        i) Alzheimer's Disease
7) Conclusion

LECTURE OUTLINE

1) Overview
   a) Increased Life Expectancy
2) The Aging of Society
   a) Most Rapidly Growing Demographic Group
   b) Advances in Medical Science
3) Physiologic Changes Associated with Aging
   a) Neurologic
      i) Visual Acuity Decreases
      ii) Loss of Hearing
   b) Cardiovascular
      i) Coronary Artery Disease
   c) Respiratory
      i) Decreased Elasticity
   d) Gastrointestinal
      i) Decreased Motility
   e) Genitourinary
      i) Loss of Kidney Function
   f) Musculoskeletal
      i) Osteoporosis
   g) Integumentary
      i) Thinner Skin
         (1) Hypothermia-Prone
4) Assessment of the Elderly Patient
   a) Scene Size-Up
      i) Activities of Daily Living
   b) Initial Assessment
      i) ABCs
   c) Focused History and Physical Examination
      i) Modified for Changes in Aging
   d) Transport
   e) Ongoing Assessment
5) General Medical Considerations in the Elderly
   a) Medication Use by the Elderly
      i) Polypharmacology
   b) Susceptibility to Disease
   c) Altered Presentation of Disease

   i) Altered Pain Perception
   d) Mistreatment of the Elderly
      i) Dependency
      ii) Elder Abuse
6) Common Illnesses in the Elderly
   a) Stroke
      i) Brain Attack
         (1) Loss of Neurological Function
      ii) Presentation
         (1) Signs and Symptoms
            (a) Signs of Increased Intracranial Pressure (See Head Injury)
            (b) One-Sided Paralysis
            (c) Difficulty with Speech
            (d) Visual Changes
      iii) Assessment
         (1) AVPU
         (2) PERRL
         (3) Pronator Drift
         (4) Speech
      iv) Management
         (1) Time-Restricted
            (a) Less Than 3 Hours
               (i) High Priority
   b) Dementia
      (1) Dementia
         (a) Gradual Onset
      (2) Delirium
         (a) Sudden Onset
      (i) Acute Medical Cause
      ii) Alzheimer's Disease
         (1) Most Common Cause of Dementia
            (a) Degrees of Impairment
7) Conclusion
   a) Application of prior knowledge to new situation

TEACHING STRATEGIES

1. Consider a visit to a nursing home. Have the students interview the patients. Often it is interesting to compare the patient's memory of medications and the ones that are given by the nursing staff.

2. Consider using the many resources available from the American Stroke Association. Their "brain attack" educational program is excellent and includes training on the Cincinnati stroke scale.

CASE STUDY VARIED COMPLAINTS

"A2, respond priority two, the Rockenstire residence, 2401 North Main Street. Elderly woman, complains of a fever," the speaker boomed.

The crew, Ivan and Caitlyn, were greeted by an elderly woman, probably in her late seventies, who ushered them through the doorway and into her living room. "Would you like some tea?" was her first response. "No, thank you, ma'am," said Ivan. "Why did you call EMS today, ma'am?"

Mrs. Rockenstire proceeded to list about half a dozen complaints, including trouble breathing when she walked to the mailbox, a sore hip from a fall several days ago, and a general allover ache she thought was from her arthritis.

"Mrs. Rockenstire, what specifically is bothering you today, something that you want checked out at the hospital?" implored Caitlyn as she sought the one answer to the question that would mean the patient needed medical attention.

ADDITIONAL CASE STUDY

"Listen, I've fallen and I can't get up," Mrs. Bugbee explained to the EMT. The patient was apparently standing at the sink washing dishes, as she normally did after dinner, and turned to answer the telephone. She heard a crack and then fell to the ground, with the phone still in her hand. She asked the caller to hang up and call the emergency squad because she couldn't get up.

STOP AND THINK

1. What physiologic changes are common as a person ages?
2. How does this impact a person's health?
3. How might this impact the EMT's care?

ANSWERS TO STOP AND THINK

1. Some of the common physiologic changes that occur with aging include loss of visual acuity and hearing, brittle bones, decreased exercise tolerance due to decreased lung capacity and cardiac function, and decreased kidney function.

2. The physiologic changes of aging can result in age-specific injury. For example, osteoporosis can lead to bone fractures without trauma. Decreased visual acuity can lead to more frequent falls.

3. An EMT must have a higher index of suspicion for injuries in the elderly, despite the apparent minor mechanism of injury. Furthermore, the EMT must supplement routine care with extra efforts to accommodate issues like a decreased tolerance for cold.

CASE STUDY   POSSIBLE STROKE

Carla entered the apartment first. She was led down the hall to the master bedroom, where an elderly man was lying in bed. "Good morning, sir. My name is Carla, and I am an EMT. What seems to be the problem today?" Carla inquired. "Well," the patient tried to say, "I feel very weak and I can't seem to move my left arm." His speech was somewhat slurred and difficult to understand.

Carla proceeded to obtain further history while her partner, Ruscan, started to assess the patient and check his vital signs. "160 over 120," reported Ruscan. "I wonder what his baseline pressure is?"

Carla turned to the patient's daughter and asked, "When did all this start?" The daughter explained that the patient's weakness started during breakfast. With the help of a neighbor, she was able to help get him back to bed, maybe an hour ago. When he did not get better, she called 9-1-1.

"Let's get him packaged," Carla ordered Ruscan while she put the oxygen mask in place, "and get him to the Stroke Center at Memorial."

ADDITIONAL CASE STUDY

"Listen, my grandfather has been getting very short with the kids and today he actually yelled at them," explained Seth, "and it's not normal for Pops to even raise his voice." Jon, the EMT, listened carefully as he observed the older man sitting in his chair. Interestingly, the patient was leaning to one side as he sat in the chair and his face appeared to have a droop.

STOP AND THINK

1. What are the signs and symptoms of a stroke?
2. What are factors that put someone at-risk for a stroke?
3. What should an EMT do to treat the patient who is possibly suffering from a stroke?

ANSWERS TO STOP AND THINK

1. The signs and symptoms of a stroke can be as subtle as a change in behavior to as dramatic as hemiplegia. One-sided weakness (hemiparesia), slurred speech, loss of vision, facial droop, and irregular pupils.

2. Common risk factors for stroke include hypertension, diabetes, and a history of heart disease.

3. After assuring that the airway is patent, the EMT should apply oxygen to a suspected stroke patient and transport immediately. If the stroke is recent, the patient would be considered high-priority.

CASE STUDY   DISORIENTATION

"Ma'am, you can't shop here dressed like that," the store manager pleaded with the elderly woman, then turned to address the EMT. "Thank goodness you're here, officer."

"Sir, I'm an EMT, not a police officer," Mario said. Then he asked, "What's going on here?" "I need more cat food!" Mario turned in the direction of the voice. In front of him stood an elderly woman, probably in her mid-eighties, dressed in a nightgown and slippers. "Ma'am, how did you get here? There's 3 feet of snow outside, and it's still coming down!" The words had scarcely left his lips when he realized that the patient was not paying attention.

Just then Mario heard someone yelling, "Mother, Mother!" and he saw a middle-aged woman rushing toward them. "I'm sorry, officer, sometimes Mother gets confused and wanders off. I'll take her home immediately." Mario waved his hand to stop her. "Please, let me check her out," Mario said to the daughter. "She's been outside in the freezing cold. I want to make sure she's all right."

ADDITIONAL CASE STUDY

Sitting in a wheelchair, the elderly woman was reaching out and grabbing anybody that walked by her. When she got hold of someone, she would dig her fingernails into the person's flesh until the person cried out. Nursing home staff was becoming increasingly alarmed by this change in behavior and called the patient's physician for instruction. He advised the staff to call the ambulance and have her transported to the hospital for testing.

STOP AND THINK

1. What is the difference between delirium and dementia?
2. What are a few causes of dementia?
3. How should the EMT treat the patient with dementia?

ANSWERS TO STOP AND THINK

1. Dementia is a gradual and progressive loss of cognitive function, whereas delirium is a sudden change in behavior that may be the result of many diseases, including stroke and poisoning.

2. Dementia is often the result of either advanced age (senility) or Alzheimer's disease.

3. The EMT should treat the demented patient with kindness and firm direction. The patient cannot be trusted to make even simple decisions without risking personal injury.

FURTHER STUDY

Andresen, G. (1998). As America ages: Assessing the older patient. *RN*, *61*(3), 46–56.

Andresen, G. (1998). Dx: dementia. *RN*, *61*(6), 26–30.

Ball, R. (1997). Geriatric assessment: The patient over 65. *Journal of Emergency Medical Services*, *22*(3), 96–100.

Gerard, D., & Maniscalco. P. (2000). Brain attack: New perspectives on stroke. *Emergency Medical Services*, *29*(1), 51–55.

Keller, V., & Baker, L. (2000). Communicate with care. *RN*, *63*(1), 32–33.

Kothari R. U., Pancioli, A., Liu, T., Brott, T., & Broderick, J. (1999). Cincinnati prehospital stroke scale: Reproducibility and validity. *Annals of Emergency Medicine*, *33*(4), 373–378.

Morris, M. R. (1998). Elder abuse: What the law requires. *RN*, *61*(8), 52–53.

Werfel, P. (1998). Geriatric assessment and specialized pathology. *Journal of Emergency Medical Services*, *23*(11), 63–71.

ANSWERS TO TEST YOUR KNOWLEDGE

1. The human brain physically shrinks as it ages, making it more vulnerable to injury from blows. The elderly person's cognitive function also becomes diminished.

2. As a person ages the heart has less reserve and therefore a limited ability to respond in times of stress. The heart may also be troubled with narrowed arteries, leading to angina.

3. The total lung capacity of the elderly patient is diminished, leading to exercise intolerance and more frequent bouts of shortness of breath.

4. The gastrointestinal tract of the elderly person works more slowly and has a tendency to become obstructed more easily.

5. The kidneys of the elderly patient have lost some of their filtering capacity, often due to lifelong hypertension. This decreased renal function impacts on drug clearance leaving drugs to build up in the bloodstream.

6. The skeletal system of the elderly patient is often more brittle, as a result of osteoporosis, and therefore the elderly person is more prone to injury and fractures of the bones.

7. The skin of the elderly patient is literally thinner. The thinner skin does not conserve heat as well and the patient may feel cold.

8. Commonly, elderly patients see more than one physician, each of whom may prescribe multiple medications. These multiple medications may interact with one another in unpredictable ways.

9. Strokes are caused by either a blockage of a cerebral artery (embolic) or by the rupture of a blood vessel (hemorrhagic). Regardless of the cause, strokes may present with hemiparesis, hemiplegia, slurred speech, and facial drooping.

10. After assuring that the airway of a patient with a suspected stroke is open, the EMT should administer high-flow oxygen and prepare the patient for immediate transport. If the stroke may have occurred in the recent past, then the EMT should consider transporting the patient to a stroke center.

11. Dementia is a gradual loss of cognitive function.

CHAPTER 41

Advance Directives

OBJECTIVES

Upon completion of this chapter, the reader should be able to:

1. Describe an advance directive.
2. Differentiate the different types of advance directives.
3. Explain how the Patient Self-Determination Act affected EMS.
4. Distinguish comfort measures from resuscitation.
5. Discuss treatment decisions in the field when:
   a. A patient does not have an advance directive
   b. The patient's advance directive is insufficient per local protocols

GLOSSARY

advance directive   A method to make a patient's wishes about resuscitation known to family and health care providers before a patient becomes incapacitated.

do not resuscitate (DNR) order   A physician's order to not start CPR or revive a patient in cardiac arrest.

health care proxy   A person chosen to make medical decisions on behalf of another.

hospice   A team of health care professionals who care for dying patients.

living wills   Legal documents directing a patient's care if the patient becomes unable to do so.

out-of-hospital DNR   A DNR that is binding in the prehospital setting that specifies lifesaving measures should not be started.

Patient Self-Determination Act   The federal law that provides protections to a patient's right to decide on matters of life and death.

power of attorney (POA)   A designated person who makes decisions on behalf of another who is incapacitated.

standard comfort measures   Treatments that are provided to ease suffering but which do not include resuscitation of a patient.

terminal   A patient who is at the end of a disease that will result in the patient's death.

PREPARATORY

Materials: EMS Equipment: Exam gloves, stethoscope, blood pressure cuff, penlight.
Personnel: Primary Instructor: One EMT-Basic instructor, knowledgeable about geriatrics. Assistant Instructor: The instructor-to-student ratio should be 1:6 for psychomotor skill practice. Individuals used as assistant instructors should be knowledgeable about geriatrics.
Recommended Minimum Time to Complete: 1.5 hours.

STUDENT OUTLINE

1) Overview
2) Advance Directives
    a) General Principles of Consent and Refusal
    b) Patients Impacted by Advance Directives
    c) Types of Advance Directives
        i) Living Wills
        ii) Durable Power of Attorney
        iii) Do Not Resuscitate Orders
    d) The Patient Self-Determination Act
        i) Health Care Proxy
    e) Out-of-Hospital DNR Orders
        i) Problems with Out-of-Hospital DNRs
    f) Standard Comfort Measures
        i) Hospice
    g) Resuscitation Decision-Making
3) Conclusion
4) Read On

LECTURE OUTLINE

1) Overview
    a) Right to Die
    b) Incurables
2) Advance Directives
        i) Role Conflict
        ii) Lifesaver versus Caregiver
    b) General Principles of Consent and Refusal
        i) Right to Control Body
        ii) Implied Consent When Unconscious
    c) Patients Impacted by Advance Directives
        i) Negate Implied Consent
        ii) Directs Others to Act on Patient Behalf
    d) Types of Advance Directives
        i) Living Wills
            (1) Attorney Created
            (2) Dependent on Physician Good-will
        ii) Durable Power of Attorney
            (1) Attorney Created

            (a) Delegates Authority
        iii) Do Not Resuscitate Orders
            (1) Physician Created
                (a) Binding in Hospital
    e) The Patient Self-Determination Act
        i) Health Care Proxy
            (1) Patient-Physician Created
                (a) Delegated Authority
    f) Out-of-Hospital DNR Orders
        i) Binding on EMT
        ii) Problems with Out-of-Hospital DNRs
            (1) Ambiguity
    g) Standard Comfort Measures
        i) Hospice
            (1) Supportive Care for Dying Patients
    h) Resuscitation Decision-Making
        i) In Doubt—Contact Medical Control
3) Conclusion
    a) Preplanning prevents poor performance

TEACHING STRATEGIES

1. Consider having a health care attorney discuss powers of attorney, living wills, and health care proxies with the students.

2. Have the students research and report on the policy regarding resuscitation in their jurisdiction.

CASE STUDY   A NATURAL DEATH

"9-1-1, what is your emergency?" Taking a deep breath, the patient's daughter Ruby, started to explain, "I think my father is dead. Could you please send someone over here to check on him?"

The patient, an elderly man, is pulseless. The man's wife, Doreen, is standing next to him. She keeps asking that nothing be done and that he be left alone to "die in peace; that's what he would have wanted."

Ruby tells the EMT that her father was gasping for breath and she got scared, so she called 9-1-1. Her father had a long history of Alzheimer's disease and heart failure, and the doctors have told Ruby that nothing can be done for him.

Looking down at the old man, a man who has obviously fought his disease for a long time, the EMT notes that the patient looks oddly at peace.

ADDITIONAL CASE STUDY

"Stop, stop CPR," yelled the woman. The crew looked up to see a middle-aged woman running toward them waving a piece of paper in her hand. The woman explained, "I am his daughter and he made me his health care proxy. So, I order you to stop CPR, now!" The crew, confused by the sudden change in affairs, pauses to wait for the lieutenant's reaction.

STOP AND THINK

1. Is the EMT obligated to start CPR?
2. Is there any order or directive that could have an impact in this case?
3. Would medical control help in this situation?

ANSWERS TO STOP AND THINK

1. In most situations an EMT is obligated to start CPR unless there is a valid DNR present.
2. An out-of-hospital DNR order would instruct the EMT to withhold lifesaving measures.
3. Without a directive, the EMT could contact medical control for instruction.

FURTHER STUDY

Heckerson, E. (1997). Termination of field resuscitation. *Emergency Medical Services, 26*(8), 51–56.

ANSWERS TO TEST YOUR KNOWLEDGE

1. An advance directive is intended to give health care professionals instruction on how to proceed with a patient when the patient is unable to express his or her wishes due to incapacity.
2. Advance directives include living wills, durable power of attorney, and assignment of a health care proxy.
3. A comfort measure is intended to ease the patient's suffering without providing a lifesaving treatment.
4. EMTs are generally obligated to perform CPR and to pursue other lifesaving treatments unless the patient has a recognized advance directive.
5. If an advance directive is incomplete, the EMT should proceed under implied consent and contact medical control for further instruction.

CHAPTER 42

Emergency Vehicle Operations

OBJECTIVES

Upon completion of this chapter, the reader should be able to:

1. Explain the importance of adequate preparation prior to an emergency call.
2. Describe personnel considerations in daily EMS operations.
3. Describe equipment considerations in daily EMS operations.
4. List the phases of an emergency call and the important considerations in each phase.
5. Explain the emergency vehicle operator's considerations during an emergency response.
6. Describe proper emergency vehicle positioning at the scene.
7. List the two general indications for air medical transport from an emergency scene.
8. Describe the factors that go into landing zone preparation.
9. Discuss the importance of safety when operating around a helicopter.
10. List activities that should be completed on the emergency crew's return to the station.

GLOSSARY

approach path An obstacle-free area adjacent to the touchdown area through which a helicopter can approach and depart.

controlled intersection An intersection with a traffic control device.

covering the brake Placing one foot over the brake pedal in anticipation of stopping.

due regard Respect and consideration for others.

emergency ambulance service vehicle (EASV) A vehicle used in service to EMS and staffed by EMS personnel.

emergency ambulance A vehicle specifically designed for patient transportation in an emergency.

emergency services vehicle (ESV) A vehicle used by an emergency service, including law enforcement, fire service, or EMS.

emergency vehicle operator (EVO) A driver of a vehicle used for emergency service.

emergency vehicle operators course (EVOC) A training course for drivers of vehicles used for emergency service.

flashback The strobe of the emergency lights bouncing back into the EVO's eyes.

four-second rule Determining the amount of time between when the vehicle in front of the emergency vehicle passes a landmark and when the emergency vehicle passes it. This time should be greater than 4 seconds.

hot-load   Placing a patient aboard a running helicopter.

landing zone (LZ)   An area intended for the purpose of landing and taking off in a helicopter.

LZ officer   A designated person on the scene of an incident who will be responsible for choosing a landing zone and ensuring its safety.

panic stop   An emergency stop for an unexpected obstacle.

right-of-way   The privilege of proceeding ahead of others on the roadway.

rotor wash   The wind created by the cycling of a helicopter's rotors.

sharps container   A receptacle for needles.

shoreline   An electrical extension linking an ambulance with a building's electricity.

siren mode   Characteristic patterns of sound designed to alert motorists of the vehicle's presence.

spotter   A person who assists the driver with backing up the vehicle.

surrounding area   The space above and around the touchdown site where a helicopter will land.

touchdown area   The area within a landing zone in which a helicopter will actually land.

wail   A long and steady sound that ascends and descends.

wave-off   The vigorous crossing and uncrossing of the LZ officer's hands alerting the pilot that it has become unsafe to land.

wig-wags   Alternating headlights on an emergency vehicle.

wire strikes   The impact of a helicopter's rotors against overhead wires.

yelp   A sharp, quick, fast-paced, almost chirping sound.

PREPARATORY

Materials: EMS Equipment: An ambulance, properly stocked.

Personnel: Primary Instructor: One EMT-Basic instructor, knowledgeable in ambulance and equipment operations. Assistant Instructor: Not required.

Recommended Minimum Time to Complete: 1 hour

STUDENT OUTLINE

1) Overview
2) Readiness
    a) Emergency Vehicle Classifications
    b) Medical Supplies
        i) Portable Medical Supplies
        ii) Emergency Ambulance Supplies
    c) Nonmedical Supplies
        i) Safety Equipment
        ii) Maps
        iii) Protocols/Procedures Manual
        iv) Communications Devices
3) Daily Preparation
    a) Personnel
    b) Equipment Preparedness
        i) Equipment Failure
    c) Vehicle Preparedness
4) Response
    a) Alarm and Alert
        i) Initial Information
        ii) Departure
        iii) Driving
            (1) Emergency Vehicle Operator
            (2) Driving Safety
            (3) Warning Devices
                (a) Markings
                (b) Emergency Warning Lights
            (4) Light Patterns
            (5) Audible Warning Devices
            (6) Priority Response
                (a) Laws and Regulations
            (7) Driving to Conditions
                (a) Adverse Weather

                (b) Heavy Traffic
                (c) Controlled Intersections
                (d) Braking
                (e) Crew
5) Arrival
    a) Emergency Lights
    b) Positioning
        i) Backing and Parking
    c) Scene Size-Up
    d) On-Scene Actions
        i) On-Scene Stabilization
        ii) Transportation
            (1) Helicopter Transport
                (a) Utilization
                (b) Landing Zone
                    (i) Approach
                    (ii) Landing Zone Safety
                    (iii) Hand Signals
                    (iv) Touchdown
                    (v) Lift-Off
            (2) Ambulance Transport
    e) Transport to Facility
    f) Arrival at Facility
    g) Transfer of Care
        i) Charting
        ii) Cleaning
        iii) Restocking
    h) Return to Station
        i) Restock and Refuel
        ii) Reports
        iii) Debriefing
6) Conclusion

LECTURE OUTLINE

1) Overview
   a) Essential Mission
      i) Transportation to Definitive Care
2) Readiness
   a) Emergency Vehicle Classifications
      i) Emergency Service Vehicle (ESV)
         (1) Snow and Ice
         (2) Off-Road
         (3) Water
         (4) Mass Gathering
         (5) Wilderness
   b) Medical Supplies
      i) Portable Medical Supplies
         (1) Care On-Scene
         (2) Secured in Vehicle
      ii) Emergency Ambulance Supplies
         (1) Regulatory Mandates
   c) Nonmedical Supplies
      i) Safety Equipment
         (1) Simple Extrication Tools
      ii) Maps
      iii) Protocols/Procedures Manual
         (1) Standardized Approaches
      iv) Communications Devices
         (1) Radio
         (2) Cellular Phones
3) Daily Preparation
   a) Personnel
      i) Well-Rested
      ii) Dressed for Conditions
   b) Equipment Preparedness
      (1) Equipment Checklist
      ii) Equipment Failure
         (1) Standard Reporting Procedure
   c) Vehicle Preparedness
      i) Fueled
      ii) Mechanically Sound
4) Response
   a) Alarm and Alert
      i) Initial Information
         (1) Initial Impression
         (2) Scene Safety Concerns
      ii) Departure
         (1) Seatbelts
      iii) Driving
         (1) Emergency Vehicle Operator
            (a) Controlled
               (i) Road Rage
            (b) Safety-Conscious

         (2) Driving Safety
            (a) Emergency Vehicle Operators Courses
         (3) Warning Devices
               (i) Request Right of Way
               (ii) Practice Due Regard
            (b) Markings
               (i) ecnalubma
               (ii) Reflective Striping
            (c) Emergency Warning Lights
               (i) Night Visibility
         (4) Light Patterns
            (a) Wig-Wags
            (b) Yellow Rear-Facing Warning
         (5) Audible Warning Devices
            (a) Sirens
               (i) Wail
                  1. Distance
               (ii) Yelp
                  1. Closing Distance
         (6) Priority Response
            (a) Dispatch Mandated
            (b) Laws and Regulations
            (c) No Immunity from Failure to Observe Due Regard
         (7) Driving to Conditions
            (a) Adverse Weather
               (i) Speed Adjusted Accordingly
            (b) Heavy Traffic
               (i) Avoid Squeeze Play
               (ii) Cover the Brake
            (c) Controlled Intersections
               (i) Come to Stop on Red
            (d) Braking
               (i) Four-Second Rule
               (ii) Panic Warning
            (e) Crew
               (i) Seatbelt
5) Arrival
   a) Emergency Lights
      i) House Calls
         (1) Attract Attention
      ii) Roadside
         (1) Wig-Wag Blind Oncoming Drivers
   b) Positioning
      (1) First On-Scene

                    (a) Protect Scene
            (2) Second Responder
                    (a) Path of Exit
        ii) Backing and Parking
            (1) Spotter
                    (a) Clearly Visible in Rearview
                        Mirrors
                    (b) Standard Hand Signals
                    (c) Use of Two Flashlights
    c) Scene Size Up
        i) Initial Size-Up
            (1) First-In Report
            (2) Logistical Support
    d) On-Scene Actions
        i) On-Scene Stabilization
            (1) According to Priority
        ii) Transportation
            (1) Helicopter Transport
                    (a) Utilization
                            (i) High-Priority Patients
                            (ii) Special Skills/
                                Procedures
                    (b) Landing Zone (LZ)
                            1. LZ Officer
                            (ii) Touchdown Area
                                    a. 100-foot-square
                            (iii) Surrounding Area
                                    a. Free of Haz-
                                        ards
                                        i. Wire
                                            Strikes

            2. Communications
            3. Location
        (iv) Landing Zone Safety
            1. Approach Path
                Clearance
        (v) Hand Signals
            1. Wave-Off
        (vi) Touchdown
            1. Rotor Wash
            2. Leading Edges
        (vii) Lift-Off
            1. Hot Load
            2. Rotor Wash
    (2) Ambulance Transport
        (a) Loading
    e) Transport to Facility
        i) Low Priority = Low Risk
    f) Arrival at Facility
        i) Position
        ii) Discharge
            (1) Patient
            (2) Family
    g) Transfer of Care
        i) Charting
        ii) Cleaning
        iii) Restocking
    h) Return to Station
        i) Restock and Refuel
        ii) Reports
        iii) Debriefing
6) Conclusion

TEACHING STRATEGIES

1. Consider having the students perform a literature search of the local newspapers for reports of ambulance accidents. Every major city has emergency vehicle collisions that are frequently reported by the press.

2. Consider having the local aeromedical service provide a safety program to the class. Most services have a program prepared for emergency services workers and many even prepare a landing zone and bring the ship to the class.

3. Consider having the class visit and inspect a number of emergency vehicles. Discuss the advantages and disadvantages of each type of vehicle to emergency service.

CASE STUDY   SHIFT CHANGE

It is 8 o'clock in the morning and shift change time at the 13th Street station. The oncoming EMTs put on the coffee and head for the equipment bay to begin their daily equipment check. Tru, the new EMT on crew, says, "I hear that these new turbo diesels can really fly!" Her partner Barney replies, "We aren't going to test that theory today. The roads are wet from last night, and the temperature is supposed to stay around 30 degrees. Too much chance of icing up."

Tru looks a little dejected when Barney says, "Look, why don't you ride in the back today, and I'll drive." Picking up the vehicle checklist, Barney starts to perform a routine vehicle inspection while Tru inspects the equipment in the rear of the ambulance.

ADDITIONAL CASE STUDY

Drew hated Monday mornings. The weekend crews usually left the rigs a mess. He trudged over to the equipment storeroom and pulled down the clipboard with the detailed equipment ambulance inventory. Typically, it would take Drew an hour to do a complete rig check. That meant he could not meet with the other crews for coffee for at least an hour. But that was his job, and so he went about it cheerfully.

STOP AND THINK

1. What is necessary preparation for duty as an EMT?
2. Why is it necessary to perform an equipment check at the beginning of every shift?
3. Why is it necessary to perform a vehicle inspection at the beginning of every shift?

ANSWERS TO STOP AND THINK

1. Minimally, an EMT needs to check the equipment and the vehicle in preparation for duty.

2. Faulty or missing equipment can impair an EMT's ability to perform. Faulty or missing equipment should be replaced at the beginning of the shift, before the EMT calls in-service.

3. EMS depends on its vehicles to transport EMTs to the scene of an emergency. A vehicle that breaks down delays that response.

CASE STUDY   EN ROUTE

As the emergency call is dispatched, Marc checks the wall map to be sure he is thinking of the most appropriate route to the scene. Nigel unplugs the ambulance, opens the bay door, and starts to climb into the driver's seat. "Not yet, Nigel, you can drive after the course. Until then, it's still me," barks Marc. "Back into your seat!"

With seatbelt fastened, Nigel picks up the radio and advises the communications center that "Rescue 2 is en route." "A rollover with possible entrapment." Nigel asks, "What do you think we'll find when we get there, Marc?"

ADDITIONAL CASE STUDY

Looking over, Le Duc could see the driver's knuckles turn white as he gripped the steering wheel. The roads were slick with black ice and the ambulance seemed like it was barely making progress. Le Duc reached down and gave his seatbelt a reassuring tug. "Let's take our time," Le Duc cautioned.

Sam looked over at Le Duc and nodded his head in affirmation, then turned his eyes back on the road.

STOP AND THINK

1. What are the responsibilities for each crew member prior to and during an emergency response?

2. What are some of the EVO's considerations during an emergency response and upon arrival at the scene?

3. What do your local traffic laws require of emergency vehicles during an emergency response?

ANSWERS TO STOP AND THINK

1. The crew, especially the emergency vehicle operator, is responsible for his or her own safety, the safety of the crew, and the safety of the public. For everyone's protection, the crew should ensure that the vehicle is mechanically sound, and that the crew understands the nature of the emergency and the level of response to that emergency. Finally, the crew should confirm the address and the directions to that address.

2. While operating the emergency vehicle in emergency mode, the emergency vehicle operator is responsible for the safety of self, the crew, and the public. The emergency vehicle operator must therefore show a due regard to the rights of other drivers on the road. Once on-scene, the emergency vehicle operator should place the vehicle in a safe position. Scene safety is also part of the responsibilities of the emergency vehicle operator.

3. In most states, the emergency vehicle does not have an automatic right to the road. That right must be granted to the emergency vehicle operator (EVO) by other drivers on the road. Until the other drivers give the road to the EVO, the EVO must practice caution and show due regard.

FURTHER STUDY

Anderson, R. (1998). Touchdown! Establishing a helicopter landing zone. *EMS Rescue Technology, 1*(2), 64–66.

Burns, L. (1999). So you want to drive an ambulance? *Emergency Medical Services, 28*(11), 53–59.

Meade, D., & Dernocoeur, K. (1998). Street smarts: Principles of vehicle placement. *Emergency Medical Services, 27*(11), 34–36.

Spivak, M. (1998) Learning to driveellipsisall over again. *Emergency Medical Services, 27*(11), 41–43.

ANSWERS TO TEST YOUR KNOWLEDGE

1. Proper preparation before a call ensures that the EMT will have a roadworthy vehicle that will transport him or her to the scene safely.

2. The emergency vehicle operator should be awake and alert, and not under the influence of any drug, prescribed, illicit, or over-the-counter, that would impair her or his ability to safely operate the emergency vehicle.

3. The emergency vehicle operator should ensure the mechanical soundness of the emergency vehicle as well as its readiness to respond.

4. The phases of an emergency call include the alert, the response, arrival or staging, the departure, and the arrival at the destination hospital. The EVO is responsible for knowing the nature of the call and the appropriate level of response. Leaving the station or post, during the response, the EVO is operating the emergency vehicle with due regard to the rights of other drivers. Upon arrival on-scene, the EVO should place, or stage, the vehicle in a safe location and assist the crew. Once the patient is loaded, the EVO operates the emergency vehicle in a safe manner toward the destination hospital. Once at the hospital, the EVO will position the vehicle and assist with the discharge of the patient and crew.

5. The EVO should always be wary of other drivers on the road, prepared to react to the unexpected actions of the other drivers. Using the emergency lights and siren responsibly, the EVO must make his or her way through traffic, asking for the right of way. Additionally, the EVO must make note of and compensate for the road conditions, never exceeding a safe speed.

6. If the emergency vehicle is first on-scene, the EVO must position the vehicle in such a manner as to protect crew-members on-scene from oncoming traffic. If law enforcement officers are on-scene, and have diverted traffic, the EVO may position the emergency vehicle beyond the scene, preferably in the direction of the destination hospital.

7. Once the emergency vehicle has returned to the station, it should be restocked in preparation for the next emergency response. After the vehicle is readied, the crew should complete any necessary reports.

8. There are two general indications for use of helicopter service while on the scene of an emergency. In the first case, the patient, due to the nature of his or her illness or injury, would benefit from the time saved flying the patient to definitive care. In the second case, the patient would benefit from the skills and training that the helicopter crew can bring to help stabilize the patient.

9. The first priority when establishing a landing zone (LZ) is to find a large (100 x 100) flat area clear of any obstacles such as overhead wires and the like. The next priority would be to mark, or illuminate, the area for the helicopter.

10. Whirling helicopter rotors can cause serious personal injury. The EMT should always approach the helicopter from the front and then only after the pilot waves the EMT forward.

CHAPTER 43

Public Safety Incident Management

OBJECTIVES

Upon completion of this chapter, the reader should be able to:

1. Recognize the presence of hazardous materials.
2. Discuss the role of an EMT on the scene of a hazardous materials incident.
3. Explain how to use the *North American Emergency Response Guidebook*.
4. Classify what areas would be in the hot zone, cold zone, and warm zone.
5. Explain the different hazardous materials identification systems in use for fixed facilities and transportation.
6. Explain the initial role of an EMT on the scene of a multiple-casualty incident.
7. Describe the public safety incident management system.
8. Explain the concept of chain of command.
9. Describe the roles of the following officers:
   — Safety
   — Research
   — Public Information
   — Staging
   — Triage
   — Treatment
   — Transportation
10. Describe the START triage system.

GLOSSARY

briefing   A commander provides the most up-to-date information about the current state of affairs at the incident.

chain of command   Assignment of roles and duties to individuals involved in an MCI with a specific order of reporting to superiors.

chemical emergency transportation center (chemtrec)   A 24-hour technical assistance number for carriers of hazardous materials.

cold zone   The area without any risk of contamination to rescue personnel.

command post   A centralized location, often off-site, where the heads of public safety agencies gather and regulate on-scene operations.

decontamination corridor   The area where the hazardous materials are cleaned off the rescuers and patients; also referred to as the warm zone.

emergency response team A group of people who arrive and rescue contaminated persons, and control, confine, contain, and decontaminate the area.

EMS commander An EMT who is in charge of the first arriving unit, the person in charge of EMS.

field hospital A temporary on-site treatment facility.

first responder awareness level A person trained to identify and report a hazardous materials incident.

guides Instructions for evacuation distance, perimeter boundaries, and potential hazards found in the *North American Emergency Response Guidebook (NAERG)*.

hazardous material Any substance that can cause injury or death to exposed persons.

hot zone The immediate vicinity of the hazardous material spill that is considered contaminated and a risk to rescue personnel.

incident commander (IC) A person in command who has overall responsibility for the entire incident.

incident management system Organization and administration involving all emergency services providers that focuses on the three critical components of large incident management, namely, command, control, and communications.

limited-victim incident (LVI) A smaller number of patients than a multiple-casualty incident (MCI).

material safety data sheet (MSDS) A listing of the health and safety information for a chemical substance.

morgue An area set aside for the collection of the deceased.

multiple-casualty incident (MCI) An incident in which there are "more patients that EMTs."

NFPA 704 symbol A diamond-shaped warning sign with four more diamonds inside.

North American Emergency Response Guidebook (NAERG) A guidebook that provides responders instructions and information on how to handle the first 30 minutes of a hazmat spill.

operations level responder A person expected to act and minimize the spread of a hazardous materials spill as well as to prevent further injuries.

placards A sign established by the United States Department of Transportation (USDOT) to identify the presence of a hazardous material.

public information officer (PIO) An individual who is designated by the incident commander to meet with the media and report the state of affairs at the incident.

research officer A person familiar with the computer and reference resources that are available for chemical exposures.

safety officer (SO) An individual designated by the incident commander who is responsible for the safety of all personnel.

shipping papers Paperwork that accompanies hazardous material while in transit; it contains the chemical name of the materials, as well as the UN designation.

staging area An off-scene location where personnel and vehicles assemble and await assignment.

staging officer A manager of an area that assembles and assigns equipment and personnel to specific duties or tasks.

START triage system A standardized system for triage; START stands for *simple triage and rapid treatment*.

tactical command sheet A document that provides specific instructions for how to proceed with managing a specific incident.

transportation officer The individual responsible for the overall movement of patients from the scene to the appropriate hospitals.

trauma intervention program (TIP) A team of people who operate in the field, during an incident, identifying providers who are at-risk and attempting to remove or reduce the stress on those individuals.

treatment officer The person responsible for setting up the field hospital.

triage A system of distribution of patients into treatment classifications according to their injury severity.

triage officer The individual responsible for the distribution of patients into treatment classification according to their injury severity.

triage tag A shortened patient care document utilized during times of mass disaster.

Materials: EMS Equipment: Triage tags.

Personnel: Primary Instructor: One EMT-Basic instructor knowledgeable in hazardous materials, triage, and disaster operations. Assistant Instructor: Not required.

Recommended Minimum Time to Complete: 2 hours

STUDENT OUTLINE

1) Overview
2) Safety and Hazardous Materials
   a) Federal Regulation
   b) Assessment
      i) Scene Size-Up
         (1) Hazmat Identification
            (a) Hazardous Materials Placards
         (2) Fixed Facility Hazardous Materials
            (a) Pre-plans and MSDS
      ii) Incident Response Plan
         (1) Initial Actions
            (a) Evacuation Distances
            (b) Perimeters
   c) Management
      i) Decontamination
      ii) Treatment
   d) Transportation
      i) Ongoing Assessment
3) The Multiple-Casualty Incident
   a) Public Safety Incident Management System
      i) Incident Command
      ii) Chain of Command
      iii) Command Personnel
         (1) Safety Officer
         (2) Public Information Officer
   b) Role of the EMT in Incident Management
4) EMS Operation Sector
   a) EMS Commander
      i) Transfer of Command
   b) Staging Officer
      i) Equipment Staging
   c) Triage Officer
      i) Personnel
      ii) Equipment
      iii) Triage Systems
         (1) START Triage System
         (2) Triage Tags
   d) Treatment Officer
      i) Personnel
      ii) Equipment
         (1) Morgue
   e) Transportation Sector
      i) Equipment
5) Conclusion

LECTURE OUTLINE

1) Overview
   a) Unknown Emergencies
      i) Stressfull
      ii) Safety Hazards
         (1) Hazardous Materials
2) Safety and Hazardous Materials
   a) Federal Regualtion
      i) Emergency Services Training
         (1) Awareness Level
         (2) Operations Level
         (3) Technician Level
   b) Assessment
      i) Scene Size-Up
         (1) Signs or Clues
            (a) Vapor Clouds
            (b) Dead Wildlife
         (2) Hazmat Identification
            (a) Hazardous Materials Placards
               (i) Transportation Regulation
         (3) Fixed Facility Hazardous Material
            (a) National Fire Protection Association (NFPA) Standard 704
               (i) Standardized Symbols
            (b) Material Safety Data Sheet (MSDS)
               (i) Known Dangerous Material
                  1. Health and Safety Information
            (c) Pre-plans and MSDS
               (i) Known Hazards
               (ii) Action Plans
      ii) Incident Response Plan
         (1) Initial Actions
            (i) Shipping Papers
               1. Chemical Emergency Transportation Center (CHEMTREC)
               2. Health and Safety Information
            (ii) *North American Emergency Response Guidebook* (*NAERG*)
               1. Guides—Groupings of Common Hazards
               2. Health and Safety Information
                  a. Evacuation Distances
                  b. Perimeters
                    i. Hot Zone
                    ii. Cold Zone
   c) Management
      i) Decontamination
         (1) Decontamination Corridor (Decon)
      ii) Treatment
         (1) Chemical-Specific
            (a) Research Officer
            (b) Poison Control
   d) Transportation
      (1) Containment
      ii) Ongoing Assessment
3) The Multiple-Casualty Incident
      i) Scale of Incident
         (1) Multiple-Casualty Incident (MCI)
         (2) Limited-Victim Incident (LVI)
   b) Public Safety Incident Management System
      i) Incident Command
         (1) Command Post
      ii) Chain of Command
         (1) Singular versus Unified
      iii) Command Personnel
         (1) Safety Officer
            (a) Incident Safety
         (2) Public Information Officer
            (a) Media Interface
   c) Role of the EMT in Incident Management
4) EMS Operation Sector
   a) EMS Commander
      i) Highest-Ranking EMS Provider First On-Scene
         (1) Tactical Command Sheets
      ii) Transfer of Command
         (1) Briefing
   b) Staging Officer
      i) Resource Control
      ii) Equipment Staging
   c) Triage Officer
      i) Personnel

    ii) Equipment

    iii) Triage Systems

        (1) START Triage System

        (2) Triage Tags

  d) Treatment Officer

    i) Personnel

    ii) Equipment

        (1) Morgue

  e) Transportation Sector

    i) Equipment

5) Conclusion

TEACHING STRATEGIES

1. Consider having the students take a stack of cards and organize them into high and low priorities. Each card would have a list of symptoms consistent with the elements of the START triage system. Students would have about a minute per card to decide. Then each team of students should compare its results to those of other teams.

2. Consider asking the local hazardous materials response team to speak to the class about hazardous materials sites.

3. Consider having the students use incident command vests and organize care at the scene of a nighttime multiple accident response exercise (NightMARE). Using a local scout troop, give each scout a triage card, and then place them in six or more cars.

CASE STUDY   TANKER ROLL-OVER

Traffic was at a standstill, and we were crawling along the shoulder of the road. The fog was so thick you could barely see a hand in front of your face.

The initial dispatch information was for a "possible injury accident near exit 24." As we approached the exit, the fog suddenly changed colors from white to brown, and the air smelled like rotten eggs.

We immediately stopped and started to back up. Grabbing the binoculars, I looked ahead. There it was, a tank trailer on its side. It appeared to be on fire. Brown-black smoke was billowing from its underside.

ADDITIONAL CASE

People were streaming from the building. Many were stopping just outside the door and then vomiting. Most appeared frightened. The initial report was for an odor. Security officers arriving on-scene were reporting that their eyes burned and their throats were scratchy. One officer immediately had an asthma attack.

The entire building was being evacuated when EMS arrived. The source of the odor was the kitchen. Apparently a dishwasher decided to mix some bleach into the green soap-stuff to make it stronger.

STOP AND THINK

1. What are the indications that this is a hazardous materials incident?
2. What other signs should the EMT look for?
3. What would be the EMT's initial priorities?
4. If this was a building, what signs would the EMT look for?
5. Would the EMT's priorities change?

ANSWERS TO STOP AND THINK

1. The change in the color of the fog, the stench of rotten eggs, and the overturned tractor-trailer are all indications of a possible hazardous materials incident.

2. The EMT should be trying to see, using the binoculars, any placards or wording on the side of the tanker as well as the condition of people in the vicinity.

3. The EMT's initial priority would be to alert emergency services that a possible hazardous materials spill may have occurred, then establish a perimeter according to the *North American Emergency Response Guidebook*.

4. If this were a building, the EMT should look for clues of occupancy, perhaps a sign or logo, as well as any NFPA 704 symbols.

5. The priorities are always the same for an EMT regardless of the nature or location of the incident. First, remain safe, then declare the emergency.

CASE STUDY   SCHOOL BUS ACCIDENT

A truck loaded with topsoil was making its way down Route 7, lumbering along at a leisurely 30 miles per hour when it approached Cornish Hill. Easing the truck into low gear, the driver had already started the descent when he realized that he had lost his brakes.

Concerned about what was ahead, the trucker frantically sounded his airhorn and tried to downshift. Glancing ahead, his heart stopped. Crosswise in the middle of the road was a school bus. There was no way to avoid the crash. He just braced for impact.

Siting on the opposite corner was Officer Lee, sipping his coffee and observing the intersection. Suddenly he realized what was going to happen. Dropping his coffee in his lap, he picked up the radio and shouted, "School bus accident, corner of Route 7 and Cornish Hill." He then bounded from the patrol care to the carnage that was before him.

ADDITIONAL CASE STUDY

"Multiple care collisions, entrance ramp to Greenbush Mall, all units responding use caution, reported ice on the roadway," the radio announced. Putting the quick response vehicle into gear, Gergio carefully inched into traffic. This was the third incident of this type since the start of the holiday shopping season.

As Gergio approached the scene, he could see the yellow lights of the mall's security officer as well as the blue lights of the first responding officer. One, two, three, four, five; he could count five vehicles in the line. Without going any farther, Gergio picked up the radio's microphone and declared a level 2 incident.

STOP AND THINK

1. What is the responsibility of the first arriving emergency responder to the scene of a major incident?
2. What are the advantages of the incident management system?
3. What are the various officers in the EMS sector?
4. What are the roles and duties of these officers?
5. How does a major incident compare to a typical EMS call?

ANSWERS TO STOP AND THINK

1. The first arriving unit is responsible for establishing incident command. Then the EMT should determine the type of incident, the potential number of patients, and what resources may be needed. This information is usually transmitted during the first-in report.

2. The incident management system allows the emergency responders to divide tasks into manageable portions while still maintaining centralized control of the incident.

3. The various officers of the EMS sector include triage, staging, transportation, and, if needed, treatment.

4. As the titles imply, each officer is responsible for performing the tasks of the position to which she or he is assigned; for example, the triage officer performs patient triage.

5. All of the activities that occur at a typical EMS call occur at a major incident, just in larger quantities. For example, at a typical call there is a treatment officer; the treatment officer is the EMT.

FURTHER STUDY

Christen, H., & Maniscalco, P. (1998). EMS incident management: The treatment sector in mass casualty events. *Emergency Medical Services, 27*(6), 28–40.

Christen, H., & Maniscalco, P. (1999). EMS incident management: Emergency medical logistics. *Emergency Medical Services, 28*(1), 49–53.

Christen, H., Maniscalco, P., & Rubin, D. (1999). EMS incident management: Traits and characteristics of the incident safety officer. *Emergency Medical Services, 28*(6), 85–90.

Christen, H., Maniscalco, P., & Rubin, D. (2000). EMS incident management: Duties of the incident safety officer. *Emergency Medical Services, 27*(3), 27–33.

Mack, D. (1999). Team EMS. *Journal of Emergency Medical Services, 24*(7), 36–44.

Maniscalco, P., & Rubin, D. (1998). EMS incident management: Personnel roles and responsibilities. *Emergency Medical Services, 28*(4), 64–69.

Maniscalco, P., & Rubin, D. (1998). EMS incident management: The safety sector. *Emergency Medical Services, 27*(11), 59–62.

Maniscalco, P., & Rubin, D. (2000). EMS incident management: Operational communications. *Emergency Medical Services, 29*(5), 93–97.

Streger, M. (1998). Prehospital triage. *Emergency Medical Services, 27*(6), 21–28.

Streger, M. (1999). Mass casualty and disaster. *Emergency Medical Services, 28*(4), 59–63.

ANSWERS TO TEST YOUR KNOWLEDGE

1. Typical signs of the presence of hazardous materials include low-lying vapor clouds, dead wildlife, the occupancy of the building, placards, and NFPA 704 symbols.

2. Minimally, the role of an EMT at a hazardous materials incident is to recognize and report the incident.

3. The *North American Emergency Response Guidebook* (*NAERG*) provides the EMT with initial instructions. First, by using either the placard number, or the chemical's name, the EMT would identify the proper guide, then follow the guide's instruction. If no placard is visible or the chemical is unknown, the EMT should turn to the universal guide 111.

4. The area immediately around the hazardous material is called the *hot zone*. Personnel working within the hot zone must wear protective clothing. The area surrounding the hot zone is called the *warm zone*. Typically the decontamination corridor is within the warm zone. The outermost area, where the public is safe to stand, is called the *cold zone*.

5. The United States Department of Transportation (USDOT) has adopted the United Nations

classification and placard system for hazardous materials in transit, whether by rail, ground, water, or air. The NFPA 704 hazardous materials marking system was developed for fixed hazardous materials storage facilities.

6. Initially, the first EMT on-scene of an multiple-casualty incident would be responsible for identifying the incident, determining the potential number of casualties, and reporting the findings.

7. The public safety incident management system is a method of dealing with emergencies shared by all emergency services.

8. A chain of command is a hierarchy of supervisors, each responsible for a task or mission and who report to an overseer.

9. The following officers have the following responsibilities at a mass casualty: safety: responsible for the overall health and well-being of the responders; public information: acts as a liasion to the press and public; staging: responsible for assembling and distributing supplies, equipment, and personnel; triage: responsible for sorting and classifying patients according to the severity of their injuries; treatment: responsible for caring for injured patients on-scene; transportation: responsible for the movement of patients to definitive care.

10. The START triage system is a simple method of sorting patients into high and low priority based on their initial assessment findings.

CHAPTER 44

Rescue Operations

OBJECTIVES

Upon completion of the chapter, the reader should be able to:

1. Indicate when a technical rescue is needed.
2. Identify the phases common to all rescues.
3. Select the appropriate personal protective equipment for specific hazards of rescue.
4. Recognize situations of confined space rescue.
5. Explain the common hazards encountered in confined space.
6. Restate how the standard of care implies that an EMT must have special training for technical rescue.
7. Recognize the normal hazards at a motor vehicle collision.
8. Explain the importance of stabilizing a motor vehicle before proceeding with a rescue.
9. Differentiate between heavy rescue and rapid extrication.
10. Describe the three most common means of extrication from a vehicle using heavy rescue.
11. Differentiate flat water from swift water rescue.
12. Describe how a shore-based rescue is established for flat water.
13. Describe how a shore-based rescue is established for swift water.
14. Describe what a hasty search is and how to perform one.
15. Explain the importance of searching for clues during a search and rescue operation.

GLOSSARY

clues   Evidence a person was in an area.

confined space   Any area that has limited openings for exit and access and is not designed for worker occupancy.

cribbing   Blocks of wood used to stabilize a vehicle.

flapping the roof   Cutting the uprights or posts to peel back the roof of a motor vehicle.

flat water   A body of water without current.

forcible entry   Using special tools or brute force to overcome an obstacle to gain entrance.

forcing the door   Using a tool to overcome a latching mechanism.

hasty search   A quick search of an area.

heavy rescue   The use of special vehicle extrication equipment.

high life hazards   Known dangerous conditions that could injure or kill someone.

loaded bumpers   Stored energy in a compressed bumper.

nader pin   A case hardened pin designed to prevent the door from springing open in a motor vehicle collision.

personal flotation device (PFD)   A vestlike device or similar affair that has positive buoyancy.

point of contact (POC)   The spot/area where the person was last seen.

pre-planning   An agreed-on response that is planned before an emergency occurs.

redundancy   Having two plans of action in place in case one of them fails.

rescue   Helping another person who is incapable of freeing himself or herself from confinement.

rolling the dash   Pulling back the dashboard off the patient.

safety glass   A piece of glass wedged between two sheets of plastic designed to remain in one piece if damaged.

snag lines   Rescue ropes slung over a stream or river.

stepblocks   A special prefabricated cribbing.

swift water   Rapidly moving body of water.

technical rescue   Complex rescue operations performed by highly trained technicians using specialized equipment.

tempered glass   Special glass designed to shatter into fragments.

throw bag   A length of rope loosely coiled in a sack.

undertow   A powerful downward current in the water.

window punch   A special window glass-breaking tool.

PREPARATORY

Materials: EMS Equipment: Exam gloves, stethoscopes, blood pressure cuffs, penlights.

Personnel: Primary Instructor: One EMT-Basic instructor knowledgeable in gaining access. Assistant Instructor: The instructor-to-student ratio should be 1:6 for psychomotor skill practice. Individuals used as assistant instructors should be knowledgeable in extrication procedures.

Recommended Minimum Time to Complete: 1 hour

STUDENT OUTLINE

1) Overview
    a) Caution
2) Phases of the Rescue
    a) Establishing Command
    b) Scene Size-Up
        i) Confined Space Rescue
    c) Management
        i) Access
            (1) Residence
        ii) Rescue
    d) Treatment
    e) Transport
3) Motor Vehicle Collisions
    a) Preparation
    b) Command
        i) Perimeters
    c) Scene Size-Up
    d) Management
    e) Access
    f) Prioritization
        i) Heavy Rescue
            (1) Patient Safety
    g) Assessment
    h) Transportation
4) Water Rescue
    a) Establishing Command
    b) Scene Size-Up
    c) Management
    d) Access
        i) Shore-based Rescue—Flat Water
        ii) Shore-based Rescue—Swift Water
    e) Treatment and Transport
    f) Transportation
5) Search and Rescue
    a) Establishing Command
    b) Scene Size-Up
    c) Access: Search
        i) Hasty Search
    d) Rescue
    e) Treatment
    f) Transportation
6) Conclusion

LECTURE OUTLINE

1) Overview
    i) Rescue Defined
        (1) Essence is Medical
    b) Caution
        i) Training Needed
        ii) Local Protocols
2) Phases of the Rescue
    a) Establishing Command
        i) Unified versus Singular
    b) Scene Size-Up
        i) Environment Assessment
            (1) Hazard Mitigation
        ii) Confined Space Rescue
            (1) Special High-Risk Rescue
    c) Management
        i) Technical Rescue
            (1) Pre-Plan
            (2) Redundancy
        ii) Access
            (a) Getting an EMT to
                Patient's Side
            (2) Residence
                (a) Caution—Intruder Alert
                (b) Caution—Animals
        iii) Rescue
            (1) Forcible Entry
    d) Treatment
    e) Transport
3) Motor Vehicle Collisions
    i) Heavy Rescue
    b) Preparation
        i) Pre-plan
        ii) Practice
    c) Command
        i) Establish a Command Presence
        ii) Perimeters
            (1) Inner Circle
    d) Scene Size-Up
        i) Walk-Arounds
        ii) Loaded Bumpers
    e) Management
        i) Stabilization
            (1) Cribbing
            (2) Step-Blocks
    f) Access
        i) Windows
            (1) Safety Glass

            (2) Tempered Glass
                (a) Window Punch
    g) Prioritization
        (1) Triage
            (a) Rapid Extrication
            (b) Standard Extrication
        ii) Heavy Rescue
            (1) Techniques
                (a) Forcing the Door
                    (i) Nader Pin
            (2) Flapping the Roof
            (3) Rolling the Dash
            (4) Patient Safety
                (a) Backboards
                (b) Oil-Tarps
    h) Assessment
        i) Focus on ABCs
    i) Transportation
        i) Condition Determines Priority
4) Water Rescue
    i) Community Risk Assessment
    b) Establishing Command
    c) Scene Size-Up
        i) Flat Water versus Swift Water
            (1) Undertows
    d) Management
    e) Access
        i) Point of Contact (POC)
        ii) PPE
            (1) Personal Floatation Device
                (PFD)
        iii) Shore-based Rescue—Flat Water
            (1) Reach, Throw, Row Then Go
                (a) Throw-Bags
        iv) Shore-based Rescue—Swift Water
            (1) Snag Lines
            (2) Upstream and Downstream
                Teams
    f) Treatment
        i) Exposure
    g) Transportation
        i) High Priority
5) Search and Rescue
    a) Establishing Command
        i) Trail Heads
    b) Scene Size-Up
        i) Terrain

ii) High-Life Hazards
c) Access: Search
    i) Hasty Search
        (1) Search for Clues
d) Rescue
    i) Cross-Country Carry

ii) Helicopter Evacuation
    (1) Pre-Planned LZ
e) Treatment
    i) Exposure
f) Transportation
6) Conclusion

TEACHING STRATEGIES

1. Consider having the local fire-rescue company provide a demonstration of the capabilities of the heavy rescue. Encourage the students to ask the firefighters how EMS interacts with rescue on the scene of an extrication.

2. Consider having the local forest ranger or search and rescue team coordinator come to class and discuss search and rescue (SAR) operations and the roles that an EMT can take in such an operation.

3. Consider running a shore-based water rescue drill. Ask the students to assume the roles of incident command, staging, and transportation, as well to form search-based rescue teams.

CASE STUDY   NONACCESS

The caller cried out, "I've fallen, and I can't get up!" Apparently, the elderly woman had fallen during the night and was only able to crawl on her hands to the Lifeline™ to call for help. That effort took her all night. She sounded exhausted as she tried to explain her situation. Lifeline™ had called both 9-1-1 and the neighbor, who was listed as "responder."

The house, a sturdy little brick cottage, was at the end of a winding lane. The neighbor, who was already at the house, explained that the house was completely locked from the inside and that there was no way in.

As the neighbor talked hurriedly to the crew chief, a new EMT, whose name was Trevor, started to look in windows. He called out that he could see the patient lying on the kitchen floor, waving and smiling at him as he peered through the window. The EMT could not hear her through the window but she kept pointing to her hip. Tears were rolling down her cheeks, and Trevor thought to himself, "She's putting up a brave front, but she's obviously in a great deal of pain."

ADDITIONAL CASE STUDY

Karl was walking along the ridge enjoying the fall foliage. A recent light rainfall had the made the trail a little slippery but Karl really loved the colors of the leaves. While gazing upward, Karl made a misstep and slid some 20 feet down a slope. Looking up the hill, Karl prepared to stand up when he realized that his left ankle was painful.

Lying back down on the leaves, Karl pulled his cellular telephone out of his coat pocket and called 9-1-1.

STOP AND THINK

1. What are the phases of a rescue operation?
2. What is the difference between a simple rescue and a technical rescue?
3. What are some common hazards on the scene of a rescue?
4. Why are confined space rescues dangerous?
5. What would be a typical approach to a locked entry call?

ANSWERS TO STOP AND THINK

1. The phases of any rescue operation include establishing command, performing a scene size-up, and managing the rescue.

2. To perform a simple rescue the EMT does not need special training or special equipment, whereas a technical rescue requires extensive training and specialized equipment.

3. The hazards on the scene of a rescue are dependent on the type of rescue. For example, on the scene of a motor vehicle heavy rescue, broken glass and sharp edges as well as spilled fuel and fluids represent some typical hazards.

4. The most common danger with confined space rescue is the failure of the EMT to identify the hazard. Entering, unprotected, into a confined space the EMT may be exposed to toxic gases as well as low oxygen concentrations in the atmosphere.

5. The first step in a locked entry call is to confirm the address. Provided the address is correct, the EMT should loudly announce her or his presence, pound on doors, and proceed to look for alternative means of entry. In many EMS systems, only law enforcement officers are allowed to force entry.

CASE STUDY   ENTRAPPED PATIENT

Roy thought to himself, "How could so few guys dirty so many dishes?" Once the dishes were done, the duty crew settled down to watch an episode of "Emergency" on syndicated television when the bell rang twice, meaning rescue, and the loudspeaker blared, "Engine Ten, Rescue Nine, and the Rescue Squad respond to a rollover collision with possible entrapment. Time out 19:57."

The engine company rolled up to the scene first, and the crew started to disembark. Smoke and steam were rolling up from the embankment, making it impossible to see the scene at first. Suddenly, as the smoke cleared, Roy spotted the truck. "Over here!" yelled Roy.

As Roy looked at where he was pointing, a queasy feeling flooded over him. At the bottom of the ravine was a tractor-trailer lying on its side. The cab of the truck was twisted and resting on its roof. The roof was partially collapsed. "Well, time to go to work," thought Roy as he grabbed a pry bar in one hand and a step-block in the other.

ADDITIONAL CASE STUDY

It was a dark and stormy night. The road crews had been out salting the roads, but the roads were still slick. A small red sports car took a turn a little too fast and ended up sliding off the road, flipping on its side in the ditch, and eventually coming to rest against a tree.

A passing motorist, seeing headlights where there should not be any, called the highway patrol to report a possible vehicle off the road. As the driver got out of his car, he could faintly here someone yelling, "Help me!"

STOP AND THINK

1. What are some of the hazards present on the scene of a motor vehicle collision?
2. What precautions must an EMT observe?
3. How can an EMT gain quick entry?
4. What can an EMT do to protect the patient while heavy rescue occurs?
5. Are the transportation priorities different after heavy rescue?

ANSWERS TO STOP AND THINK

1. Typical hazards on the scene of a motor vehicle collision include traffic (number-one hazard), spilled fuel and fluids, slippery, uneven surfaces, broken glass, and sharp edges.

2. The EMT should don personal protective equipment to reduce the peril these hazards create. An EMT should wear a helmet or bump-cap, goggles or eyeshield, gloves, and boots, minimally. The EMT should ensure that the vehicle is stabilized, with step-blocks or cribbing, and that the mechanics of the vehicle are rendered inoperative.

3. The quickest entry into a motor vehicle is through an open door. If an open door is not available, the EMT should choose the farthest window from the patient and use a window punch to break the window.

4. While heavy rescue tools are in operation, the EMT should shield the patient with a heavy tarp or wool blanket. If cutting tips are close to the patient, the EMT should shield the patient with a backboard.

5. The transportation priorities are not different after a heavy rescue; however, the delay in transportation often increases the patient's priority.

CASE STUDY   RAPID WATER RESCUE

Last winter's heavy snows and the unrelenting spring rains had swelled the Crystal River to its maximum capacity. The river was cresting at near flood stage, and the river's banks were barely able to hold the river back. This combination of events made the Crystal River especially exciting for white-water enthusiasts, and the river was filled with kayakers and canoeists every weekend.

Because of the inherent danger of the river at this time of year, and the fact that two canoeists had drowned the previous spring, the local fire-rescue was on high alert, and the station was being manned "twenty-four, seven" by a rapid response water team. This team of EMTs had just completed the shore-based rescue course and was part of a larger plan to respond a dive-rescue team and a helicopter-rescue team to the scene of any potential drowning.

The team had just started its morning inspection when the alert was sounded and those fateful words were spoken, "Man in the water." Everybody scrambled to get the equipment assembled as the captain got exact directions to the point the kayaker was last seen in the water.

ADDITIONAL CASE STUDY

Emily took her homemade sailboat down to the river to see if it would sail. Her mother had told her repeatedly not to go near the river that ran behind their house. But Emily was excited so off she went. In the meantime her mother had stopped doing the laundry and paused to look out the window at the river. At that moment she saw Emily slip, fall, and enter the water, her sailboat still clutched in her hand.

Grabbing the portable phone, Emily's mother dashed out the door and was sprinting down the embankment. As she stood helpless on shore, she dialed 9-1-1.

STOP AND THINK

1. What is the difference between swift and flat water?
2. What are the hazards on-scene of a water rescue?
3. What precautions should an EMT take?

ANSWERS TO STOP AND THINK

1. Swift water is moving water whereas flat water appears still. However, flat water can have a current underneath that cannot be observed by the EMT.

2. The greatest hazard of water rescue is when the rescuer becomes a victim. When the rescuer enters the water, he or she potentially becomes the second victim. Other hazards are related to the water and the objects in the water, like low-head dams.

3. No EMT should approach the water without a personal floatation device (PFD). Fire-boots should be replaced with low boots, fire-helmets should be replaced with vented helmets, and the EMT should work with a partner.

CASE STUDY   LOST HIKER

An avid hiker and camper, Mr. Erb had always encouraged his kids to "take to the mountains" and "enjoy the beauty of the great outdoors." Most of his children, on the other hand, were less enthusiastic about hiking then their dad, and they preferred to "camp out" at the local Great Western hotel. The exception was John. Even as a boy, John had a great sense of direction and a great sense of adventure.

So, for his senior year John planned a camping trip to the high Sierras. But this hiking trip was no ordinary hiking trip. John planned to see nature as God intended, and he was going to bushwhack his way from peak to peak, stopping only to replenish his supplies.

With that in mind, his dad parked at the Devil's Fork trailhead and waited for his son to appear. He waited and waited. After 20 hours, he started to think maybe John was in trouble. Calling the local Forest Service office, he explained his concerns. Within hours, the trailhead was swarming with search and rescue (SAR) team members. A command post was set up, and volunteers were being recruited. Local EMTs were being paired with experienced SAR team members and given "fanny-packs" (prepackaged first aid kits).

The first team, dubbed "alpha-alpha," set off down the trail and took up position at the coordinates they were assigned. Andrea, the EMT team member, was asked to walk the trail and look for "clues." As Andrea walked along, she would stop every 50 yards or so and call out "John, John Erb."

ADDITIONAL CASE STUDY

"Another quiet night here at the home," Susan thought to herself as she made her rounds checking on the patients. When she looked into Mr. McKearney's room, she noticed that the bed linen was undisturbed. She turned on the light. Mr. McKearney's dinner was still on the tray where the orderly had left it. Stepping into the hallway, Susan looked down the hallway and saw the open door.

Mr. McKearney had senile dementia and had a habit of walking off without telling anyone. The last time he did this it took the fire department almost 12 hours to find him. Not wanting to take any chances that he would be gone 12 hours again, Susan picked up the telephone and asked the operator to contact the fire department.

STOP AND THINK

1. What are the first actions an EMT should take at a potential search and rescue?
2. What can an EMT do while awaiting professional search and rescue personnel?
3. What medical problems can a lost hiker have?

ANSWERS TO STOP AND THINK

1. The first priority at a potential search and rescue is to establish incident command and confirm the incident.

2. EMS, and other emergency service providers, may establish a command post, a staging area, a rehabilitation area, and a treatment area, and then proceed with a hasty search.

3. Medical problems specific to the out-of-doors include heat or cold illness, animal or insect bites, exposure, and dehydration.

FURTHER STUDY

Anderson, R. (1998). Touchdown: Establishing a helicopter landing zone. *EMS Rescue-Technology*, *1*(2), 64–66.

Sachs, G. Bailey, K., & Hays, C. (1997). Water works: Water rescue. *EMS Rescue-Technology*, *1*(6), 32–36.

Sargent, C. (1999). Close encounters. *Journal of Emergency Medical Services*, *24*(7), 44–49.

Spivak, M. (1998). River rescuers. *EMS Rescue-Technology*, *1*(2), 14–22.

ANSWERS TO TEST YOUR KNOWLEDGE

1. A technical rescue is needed any time special tools or training is needed to safely execute a rescue.

2. All rescues start with establishing incident command, a scene size-up, mobilization and staging of resources, and the technical rescue, and end with the care and transportation of the patient.

3. The appropriate personal protective equipment for flame and flash is full turnout gear. For protection from flying, falling, and sharp objects, the EMT should don protective eyewear, heavy gloves (minimally leather), and a heavy-duty coat. The EMT should wear ear protection for loud noises and use binoculars or a similar device to enhance vision during times of low visibility.

4. Confined spaces include sewer pipes, the hold of a ship, the inside of a tanker, or the inside of a silo.

5. Common hazards that an EMT could encounter in a confined space include low oxygen concentrations, toxic fumes, or explosive gases.

6. The standard of care would have an EMT treat a patient as another EMT, who is similarly trained, would treat the patient under the same or similar circumstances. In the case of rescue, it is widely acknowledged that certain situations, such as confined space or water rescue, require special training and equipment to perform the rescue safely. An EMT who fails to acknowledge this fact, and instead proceeds to try to rescue a patient without this equipment or training would be acting outside of the standard of care.

7. Common hazards on the scene of a motor vehicle collision include spilled fuel and automotive liquids, broken glass and sharp edges, as well as uneven slopes and unstable vehicles.

8. An unstable vehicle represents a hazard to both the patient and the rescuer. If the vehicle shifts unexpectedly, the EMT could become injured or the patient could become injured.

9. When a patient is high-priority, routine immobilization techniques are waived in favor of a rapid extrication. However, if the patient is stable or low-priority, then she or he should be carefully disentangled from the vehicle. If the patient is entrapped, then heavy rescue may be necessary to disentangle the patient from the vehicle.

10. The three most common means of disentanglement are flapping the roof, three-door conversion, and a dash roll-up.

11. Flat water is placid, whereas swift water is moving.

12. A shore-based water rescue for flat water involves establishing command, confirming the incident, donning personal protective equipment such as a personal floatation device, and trying to reach the patient, or throw a rope to the patient, or even row a boat to the patient.

13. A shore-based swift water rescue is similar. After donning personal protective apparel, the EMT

would attempt to locate the patient, then throw a rope-bag, or similar device, to the patient in the water. The EMT would never enter the water himself or herself.

14. After incident command has been established for a search and rescue, it is often customary to send searchers along commonly traveled pathways such as shorelines, roadways, and trails in an effort to discover clues to the patient's whereabouts.

15. The importance of searching for clues is basic. There is only one patient whereas there may be many clues to the patient's whereabouts. Furthermore, clues create a starting point for specially trained search dogs to follow, called a *scent trail.* EMTs walking through the woods can cover or obscure a scent trail.

CHAPTER 45

Advanced Life Support Assist Skills

OBJECTIVES

Upon completion of this chapter, the reader should be able to:

1. Identify the importance of teamwork between basic and advanced emergency providers.
2. Discuss the importance of maintaining a patient's airway using basic techniques.
3. Describe how and when to apply cricoid pressure.
4. List several ways to confirm proper endotracheal tube placement.
5. Describe a method to secure an endotracheal tube orally and nasally.
6. Describe how to ventilate a patient via an oral and a nasal endotracheal tube.
7. Describe how to perform endotracheal suctioning.
8. Describe how to apply different types of cardiac monitoring leads.
9. Describe how to properly prepare a bag of IV solution for administration.
10. Discuss the considerations in maintaining an intravenous line.

GLOSSARY

cricoid pressure   A technique of applying pressure to the cricoid ring to decrease the risk of regurgitation during ventilation and endotracheal intubation.

D5W   An intravenous solution that consists of 5% dextrose in water.

endotracheal intubation   The placement of a plastic tube into the trachea to allow direct ventilation of the lungs.

hyperventilation   A higher than normal ventilatory rate.

lactated ringers   A commonly used intravenous solution.

laryngoscope   A tool that is used to view the lower airway structures during endotracheal intubation.

laryngoscopy   The use of a laryngoscope to view the lower airway structures.

macrodrip   A type of intravenous tubing that is designed to allow large amounts of fluid to flow through it quickly.

microdrip   A type of intravenous tubing that is designed to allow only small amounts of fluid to flow through it at a time.

normal saline   A commonly used intravenous solution that consists of 0.9% sodium chloride.

preoxygenation   Providing high-concentration oxygen to a patient for a period of time before a procedure, such as endotracheal intubation, or suctioning, is performed.

twelve lead ECG   A tracing of the heart's electrical activity from twelve different views.

PREPARATORY

Materials: EMS Equipment: Exam gloves, eye protection, basic airway adjuncts, adult, infant, and child intubation manikins, stethoscopes (1:6), laryngoscope blades (0–4) (1:6), laryngoscope handles (1:6), stylets, endotracheal tubes in various sizes, "C" batteries, spare laryngoscope bulbs, lubricant, suction units, oxygen cylinders, bag-valve mask (1:6), oxygen supply tubing, adult, infant, and child throat models showing anatomy to include trachea and vocal cords, face masks.

Personnel: Primary Instructor: One EMT-Basic instructor with knowledge in basic and advanced airway management techniques. Assistant Instructor: The instructor-to-student ratio should be 1:6 for psychomotor skill practice. Individuals used as assistant instructors should be knowledgeable in basic and advanced airway management techniques.

Recommended Time to Complete: 12 hours (including intubation)

STUDENT OUTLINE

1) Overview
2) Team Concept
    a) Airway
    b) Breathing
    c) Circulation
3) Endotracheal Intubation
    a) Patient Preparation
        i) Hyperventilation
    b) Cricoid Pressure
    c) Assistance with Laryngoscopy
    d) Confirming Placement
    e) Securing Endotracheal Tube
    f) Ventilating via Endotracheal Tube
    g) Endotracheal Suctioning
4) Cardiac Monitoring
    a) Defib Pads
    b) Three Lead
    c) Twelve Lead
    d) Monitor Set-Up
5) Intravenous Therapy
    a) Patient Preparation
    b) IV Solution Selection
    c) Assembly of Fluid and Tubing
    d) Securing an Intravenous Line
    e) Maintaining an Intravenous Line
6) Conclusion

LECTURE OUTLINE

1) Overview
   a) Efficiency
2) Team Concept
   a) Airway
      i) Assist with Intubation
   b) Breathing
      i) Assist with Ventilation via ET
   c) Circulation
      i) Assist with ECG Monitor Setup
      ii) Assist with IV Setup
3) Endotracheal Intubation
   a) Patient Preparation
      i) Psychological
      ii) Good BLS before ALS
         (1) Open, assess, suction, secure
      iii) Hyperventilation
         (1) Pre-Oxygenation
         (2) Nitrogen Washout
   b) Cricoid Pressure
      i) Regurgitation
   c) Assistance with Laryngoscopy
      i) Sellick's Maneuver
   d) Confirming Placement
      i) Look
         (1) Chest Rise
      ii) Listen
         (1) Positive Breath Sounds
             Bilaterally
         (2) Absence of Gastric Sounds
      iii) Feel
         (1) Esophageal Detector Device
             (EDD)
         (2) End-Tidal Carbon Dioxide
             Detector (EndCO$_2$)
   e) Securing Endotracheal Tube
      i) Depth Marking
      ii) Bite Blocks
      iii) Device

         (1) Tape
         (2) Commercial
   f) Ventilating via Endotracheal Tube
      i) Manually Stabilize
      ii) Ventilate to minimal chest rise
   g) Endotracheal Suctioning
      i) Hyperventilate
      ii) Maximum 15 seconds
4) Cardiac Monitoring
   a) Defib Pads
      i) Interchangable AED to Monitor
   b) Three Lead
      i) Leads I, II, III
   c) Twelve Lead
      i) Patient Preparation
         (1) Bare Skin—Shave
      ii) Correct Electrode Placement
   d) Monitor Setup
5) Intravenous Therapy
   a) Patient Preparation
      i) Coats Removal
   b) IV Solution Selection
      i) Normal Saline Standard
   c) Assembly of Fluid and Tubing
      i) Tubing Selection
         (1) Micro-Drip
             (a) Medical Patient
         (2) Macro-Drip
             (a) Trauma Patient
   d) Securing an Intravenous Line
      i) Occlusive Dressing
   e) Maintaining an Intravenous Line
      i) Verification of Placement
         (1) Flashback
         (2) Pain at Site
         (3) Swelling/Infiltration
6) Conclusion
   a) Teamwork

TEACHING STRATEGIES

1. Consider having an ALS provider perform a cardiac arrest simulation (mega-code) and time how long it takes the ALS provider to complete an evolution. Then have the students assist the ALS provider and time how long it takes. Discuss the advantages of multitasking with the students.

2. Consider having the students assist each other with ventilation. Pairing off, first have each student get used to breathing through a mask. Next, add the bag-valve assembly to the mask and have the student get used to breathing through the BVM. Finally, have one student gently assist ventilation of another student by compressing the BVM at the end of inspiration. Ask the students to discuss how they felt during the process.

3. Consider having the students practice running expired IV solutions through IV tubing and placing electrodes on one another. These ALS-assist skills are complex psychomotor skills that are best practiced in the lab before actual experience in the field.

CASE STUDY   ASSISTING WITH BREATHING

The call was for a woman with difficulty breathing. EMS arrived to find Mrs. Anderson leaning over a small plastic bucket that was filled with facial tissues and pink frothy foam. She looked near death, and she could speak only in single words. The EMT, Ira, immediately placed the pulse oximeter on her finger, while Geo, the other EMT, prepared the nonrebreather mask. Then Ira listened to her lungs, and heard loud crackles in all of her lung fields. The initial pulse oximeter reading was 84% on room air.

"Better get the BVM out," declared Ira. "I will contact Medcom and ask them what the ETA is for the paramedic." As Geo assembled the BVM, he started talking calmly to the patient, explaining that he was going to help her with her breathing. Then he placed the mask over her face.

"Breathe easy, Mrs. Anderson. Let me help you," Geo implored as he replaced the mask over her nose and mouth. She was quickly becoming exhausted and had little fight left in her.

ADDITIONAL CASE STUDY

The sound of the collision was horrific and the sight of the mangled cars left little room for doubt that there were seriously injured patients. One patient, apparently ejected through the windshield of the first car, was lying in the middle of the road surrounded by EMTs. Jenny, arriving with the second-due engine, jumped from the engine and was directed to the patient in the middle of the road.

"Get your bag-valve mask out," yelled the captain. "This kid's going to need help with his breathing."

STOP AND THINK

1. What are indications for endotracheal intubation?
2. What can the EMT do to assist in endotracheal intubation?
3. Describe the purpose of cricoid pressure.

ANSWERS TO STOP AND THINK

1. Endotracheal intubation is indicated whenever a patient is incapable of protecting his or her own airway, typically because the patient is unconscious.

2. An EMT can assist an ALS provider with intubation by preparing the intubation equipment, hyperventilating the patient, confirming placement, and assisting with securing the endotracheal tube.

3. Cricoid pressure prevents passive regurgitation, and possible subsequent aspiration, of stomach contents as well as preventing inflation of the stomach.

CASE STUDY   ECG APPLICATION

Dan, the paramedic intern, was busy getting a history on Mr. Briggs, while Mohammed was standing on the sidelines watching. Mr. DeLeon, the paramedic in charge, asked Mohammed if he had ever put a patient on a heart monitor before. Mohammed answered, "No." "OK, kid," said Mr. DeLeon. "If you're going to do it, do it right."

With that introduction, DeLeon launched into a mini-lecture on electrode placement, topographic anatomy, and the importance of placing the electrodes correctly. Mohammed, listening closely, quickly picked up the information and started to apply the electrodes, while Dan started the IV.

ADDITIONAL CASE STUDY

"One, and two, and three," the EMT called out as he completed compressions. The AED was sitting next to the patient and the paramedic, Carri, was getting ready to intubate. "Would you set up my monitor leads while I intubate?" Carri asked the new EMT.

STOP AND THINK

1. Describe how to apply three, four, five, and ten electrodes for ECG monitoring.
2. What should the EMT consider when applying the ECG electrodes?
3. How important is it to place the electrodes in exactly the recommended positions?

ANSWERS TO STOP AND THINK

1. Place the labeled leads on the correct places: one to the right shoulder, one to the left shoulder, and one to the left lower rib margin. A four-lead system has an additional lead placed on the right lower rib margin. Five lead systems permit one more lead to be placed at approximately V^1 or the fourth intercostal space (ICS) at the right sternal border. If a twelve lead ECG is desired, additional leads will have to be placed at the fourth intercostal space (ICS) at the left sternal border, across from V^1. The next electrode (V^4) is placed at the fifth ICS at the midclavicular line (MCL), then the fourth electrode (V^3) is placed midline between the second (V^2) and the third (V^4). The final two electrodes are placed fifth ICS at the anterior axillary line (AAL) and the midaxillary line (MAL), V^{5-6} respectively.

2. Proper preparation prior to placement is imperative. The skin should be degreased with an alcohol prep, abraded with a 2 x 2 or similar material, and then wiped dry of all perspiration. Next, the electrode is placed on the lead, then the electrode is placed on the skin. If the patient is hirsute, it is important to clip the underlying hair to improve adhesion.

3. Misplacement of electrodes can alter the ECG tracing and result in an inaccurate reading.

CASE STUDY PREPPING AN IV

Arriving almost simultaneously with the call for an "unknown, man down in the mall, food court," EMT Sajan and Paramedic Pratt rode the escalator the last several yards to the food court.

Finding the scene was not hard. They simply looked for the crowd of people. In the center of the crowd on the floor was Dean Rome, a diabetic patient who was notorious for having "spells."

"Sajan, after you're done with your initial assessment, could you run a line out for me?" asked Pratt.

ADDITIONAL CASE STUDY

The patient was lying in a heap in the middle of the road. EMTs were already swarmed around her, applying oxygen and a cervical collar. Joy was standing helplessly, looking down at the patient. "Joy! Joy!" shouted the crew chief, "Would you go into the back of the ambulance and set up a couple of bags of saline on a macro-drip tube."

STOP AND THINK

1. Describe how to properly prepare an IV solution for intravenous infusion.
2. What is the concern over keeping the ends of the tubing sterile?
3. How can the EMT prevent bubbles from remaining in the intravenous tubing?

ANSWERS TO STOP AND THINK

1. To properly prepare an IV solution, the EMT would select the correct solution, checking the expiration date, and then squeeze the solution bag to ensure that it is intact as well as observe the solution for particulate matter. Next, the EMT would select the correct administration set, clamp the roller clamp shut, and spike the solution bag with the spike from the administration set. Once the bag is spiked, the drip chamber should be repeatedly squeezed until it is half full, then the roller clamp opened to allow the fluid to run out slowly.

2. Intravenous fluids bypass all the body's defenses from infection and enter the body directly. For this reason it is important that the entire IV administration set be kept sterile.

3. The first step to prevent air from being entrapped in the IV tubing is to half-fill the drip chamber before running the IV out. Next, the EMT should run the fluid through the tubing slowly again, to prevent entrapping air in the IV line. Finally, if air bubbles are in the line and cannot be run out with solution, the EMT can try gently flicking the tubing with a finger and see if the air bubbles will rise.

FURTHER STUDY

Haynes, B. E., & Pritting J. (1999). A rural emergency medical technician with selected advanced skills. *Prehospital Emergency Care, 3*(4), 343–346.
Dougherty, J. E. (1986). The basically advanced provider. *Emergency, 19*(4), 14–16.

ANSWERS TO TEST YOUR KNOWLEDGE

1. Cooperation between basic and advanced EMS providers not only smoothes the way for better patient care but permits multitasking—the accomplishment of several responsibilities simultaneously.

2. If a patient's airway can be maintained using basic airway techniques it may be unnecessary to resort to more dangerous advanced airway techniques. Furthermore, basic airway techniques are the foundation on which advanced airway techniques are based.

3. Cricoid pressure should be applied whenever a patient is being ventilated. To perform cricoid pressure the EMT would apply gentle downward pressure to the cricoid cartilage found just below the larynx (voicebox).

4. The best method of confirming endotracheal intubation is direct visualization of the endotracheal tube entering the trachea. This observation should be followed with indirect methods of confirmation. These methods can be summarized as "look, listen, and feel." The EMT should look to see if he or she can see the chest rise with ventilation. The EMT should look to see if the CO_2 detector is giving a normal reading. The EMT should listen with a stethoscope over the epigastrium as well as both lung fields. The EMT should feel for equal chest rise.

5. Endotracheal tubes can be secured, both orally and nasally, with commercially prepared ET holders (preferred) or with medical tape. Other systems, including use of umbilical tape or a nasal canulla, are acceptable.

6. Ventilation of a patient who is nasally or orally intubated is no different than ventilating any other patient. The EMT should be cautious that she or he does not inadvertently push the endotracheal tube deeper into the patient's trachea or accidentally displace the endotracheal tube into the esophagus.

7. Endotracheal suctioning is a sterile procedure that requires practice. The EMT would first select the suction catheter, and prepare the equipment. Donning sterile gloves the EMT would pick up the suction catheter and introduce it into the endotracheal tube. After the entire length of the catheter is in the endotracheal tube, or the patient coughs, the suction is applied and the catheter is removed. The patient should not be suctioned for more than 10 to 15 seconds. The entire process can be repeated provided the patient is reoxygenated.

8. Place the labeled leads on the correct places—one to the right shoulder, one to the left shoulder, and

one to the left lower rib margin. A four lead system has an additional lead placed on the right lower rib margin. Five lead systems permit one more lead to be placed at approximately V^1 or the fourth intercostal space (ICS) at the right sternal border. If a twelve lead ECG is desired, additional leads will have to be placed at the fourth intercostal space (ICS) at the left sternal border, across from V^1. The next electrode (V^4) is placed at the fifth ICS at the midclavicular line (MCL), then the fourth electrode (V^3) is placed midline between the second (V^2) and the third (V^4). The final two electrodes are placed at the fifth ICS at the anterior axillary line (AAL) and the midaxillary line (MAL), V^{5-6}, respectively.

9. To properly prepare an IV solution for EMT would select the correct solution, checking the expiration date, and then squeeze the solution bag to ensure that it is intact as well as observe the solution for particulate matter. Next, the EMT would select the correct administration set, clamp the roller clamp shut, and spike the solution bag with the spike from the administration set. Once the bag is spiked, the drip chamber should be repeatedly squeezed until it is half full, then the roller clamp opened to allow the fluid to run out slowly.

10. Starting at the patient, maintaining an IV line includes checking the insertion site for swelling, ensuring that the site remains dry, that the drip rate is running at the prescribed rate, and that there is sufficient fluid remaining in the IV solution bag.